Anti-discriminatory Practice in
Mental Health Care for Older People

of related interest

Cultural Perspectives on Mental Wellbeing
Spiritual Interpretations of Symptoms in Medical Practice
Natalie Tobert
Foreword by Michael Cornwall
ISBN 978 1 78592 084 4
eISBN 978 1 78450 345 1

Culture and Madness
A Training Resource, Film and Commentary for Mental Health Professionals
Begum Maitra and Inga-Britt Krause
ISBN 978 1 84905 352 5
eISBN 978 0 85700 701 8

The Equality Act 2010 in Mental Health
A Guide to Implementation and Issues for Practice
Edited by Hári Sewell
ISBN 978 1 84905 284 9
eISBN 978 0 85700 589 2

Racism and Mental Health
Prejudice and Suffering
Edited by Kamaldeep Bhui
ISBN 978 1 84310 076 8
eISBN 978 1 84642 336 9

Anti-discriminatory Practice in Mental Health Care for Older People

Edited by
PAULINE LANE AND RACHEL TRIBE

Jessica Kingsley *Publishers*
London and Philadelphia

Every effort has been made to trace copyright holders and to obtain their permission for the use of copyright material. The author and the publisher apologize for any omissions and would be grateful if notified of any acknowledgements that should be incorporated in future reprints or editions of this book.

First published in 2017
by Jessica Kingsley Publishers
73 Collier Street
London N1 9BE, UK
and
400 Market Street, Suite 400
Philadelphia, PA 19106, USA

www.jkp.com

Library of Congress Cataloging in Publication Data
Title: Anti-discriminatory practice in mental health care for older people / edited by Pauline Lane and Rachel Tribe.
Description: London ; Philadelphia : Jessica Kingsley Publishers, 2017. | Includes bibliographical references and index.
Identifiers: LCCN 2016038898 | ISBN 9781849055611 (alk. paper)
Subjects: | MESH: Mental Health Services | Ageism--prevention & control | Minority Groups | Cultural Competency | Aged | Great Britain
Classification: LCC RC451.4.A5 | NLM WT 31 | DDC 362.1968900846--dc23 LC record available at https://lccn.loc.gov/2016038898

British Library Cataloguing in Publication Data
A CIP catalogue record for this book is available from the British Library

ISBN 978 1 84905 561 1
eISBN 978 0 85700 947 0

Printed and bound in the United States

Contents

Introduction   7
Pauline Lane and Rachel Tribe

Part I: Establishing the Key Principles of Anti-discriminatory Practice in Older People's Mental Health

1. Conceptualising Ageing and Anti-discriminatory Practice   19
    Pauline Lane

2. Humanising the Mental Health Context   48
    Maria Castro Romero

3. Ageing, Ethnicity and Mental Health   69
    Rachel Tribe

4. Common Mental Health Problems   102
    Dr Maureen McIntosh and Dr Afreen Huq

5. The Mental Capacity Act 2005 and Ageing   122
    Ajit Shah

6. Anti-discriminatory Practice: Caring for Carers of Older Adults with Mental Health Dilemmas   147
    Rachel Tribe and Pauline Lane

7. End of Life Issues and Older People's Mental Health   175
    Pauline Lane and Rachel Tribe

Part II: Insights

8. Ageing and Mental Health Issues for People with Learning Disabilities   205
    Musthafar Oladosu and Rena Kydd-Williams

9. Ageing, Sexual Orientation and Mental Health: Lesbian, Gay, Bisexual, Transgender and Intersex Older People   232
    Matt Broadway-Horner

10. Understanding the Lives of Older Gypsies and Travellers and the Impact of Inequality on their Mental Health   258
    Siobhan Spencer and Pauline Lane

11. Social Exclusion and Anti-discriminatory Practice: The Case of Older Homeless People   282
    Peter Cockersell

Part III: Additional Information and Practical Guidance to Support Positive Practice

12. The Rough Guide to Working with Interpreters in Mental Health   315
    Rachel Tribe and Pauline Lane

13. Ageing, Food and Malnutrition   329
    Pauline Lane and Rachel Tribe

    CONTRIBUTORS   344

    ENDNOTES   347

    SUBJECT INDEX   348

    AUTHOR INDEX   353

Introduction

Pauline Lane and Rachel Tribe

Do we not realise that we all grow old? Can we not celebrate the fact that this privilege has been won for us by our collective ingenuity? Do we not realise that the best prospect for our own well-being in old age is to build a world in which equality, independence and active participation of all generations is positively encouraged?

Professor Tom Kirkwood
'The End of Age' Reith Lecture (Kirkwood 2001)

The message is clear. For the first time in history, there will be fewer children in the world than older people, and, as the population ages, this shift will become one of the most significant and powerful forces for social change in the modern world. Consistently low birth rates and increasing life expectancy mean that approximately 700 million people (approximately 10% of the world's population) are already over the age of 60, and it has been estimated that by 2050 Europe will have the world's oldest population (United Nations 2013). In many ways this should be seen as a celebration of human endeavour, as advances in sanitation, medical research, nutrition and education have resulted in millions of people living into old age. Yet, despite these triumphs of progress, many older people do not feel like heroes of human achievement, and they frequently experience age discrimination (Government Office for Science 2015). In other words, simply based on people's membership of a certain social group (i.e. people who have grown old), ageism imposes practices and social attitudes that result in disadvantages and unfair treatment and often exclude older people from their full citizenship rights.

Ageing, however, is only a small part of who we are, and many older people will have experienced a lifetime of discrimination as a result of other personal characteristics, such as living with a disability. If they also come to have a mental health condition in later life, they may find that they are experiencing the adverse effects of multiple forms of intersecting discrimination. The care of older people living with mental health issues raises some of the most significant questions about how society looks at human suffering, and, as Kari Martinsen (1993, cited in E.H. Martinsen 2011) suggests, caring for the most vulnerable raises ethical questions about how we value everyone in our society.

Yet a word of caution is needed, because although this book is about older people who may on occasion be vulnerable, older people living with mental health issues are not simply people in need of protection and care. All older people in society have participated (and continue to participate) in the shaping of all of our lives. Most older people have developed considerable powers of resilience and fortitude having lived through multiple life events. As Professor Tom Kirkwood (a biologist and recognised expert on ageing) suggests in the epigraph to this Introduction, we need to actively celebrate older adults (including their collective histories and ongoing achievements), while at the same time recognising the importance of intergenerational bonds and personal needs. Kirkwood's words acknowledge the importance of working together across generations for the collective good and for the benefit of *all* members of our society. What this holds out for all to see is that reciprocal intergenerational caring (i.e. not just the young caring for the old) matters not only for people who are old today but also for our own futures. So this book, influenced by Kirkwood, is not simply a treatise on how we can care for older people; it seeks to help us to reflect on how we would like to be cared for, when we become old, and if we become vulnerable.

About the book

While this book aims to improve the health and social care of older people from minority and excluded communities by promoting anti-discriminatory practice for professionals working with older adults in mental health, it also seeks to offer a critical understanding of the way in which ageing is lived, experienced and represented and how ageing happens within a 'situated body'. In other words, we age not in a vacuum but in a social context that shapes people's experiences of ageing. In essence, this book examines some of the structural, social and economic forces that shape people's experiences of ageing and mental health, as well as illuminating the concept of 'differentiate ageing', whereby not all older people with or without mental health concerns face the same issues.

The editors and contributors of this book are also keen to stress that older people are not just passive recipients of ideas about themselves; they are also active agents who can represent themselves and change the attitudes of others. Indeed, many older people are starting to redefine what it means to get old. As such, the book aims to support practitioners to develop their reflective skills, and it offers some theoretical understanding and practical advice on how to promote anti-discriminatory practice when working in older people's mental health services. The volume offers an interdisciplinary approach to understanding these complex issues, and it draws on a wide range of expertise.

One of the challenges in writing this edited collection has been that ageing, for many older people, is only one aspect of their identity and it is not always the primary site of their experience of discrimination. For example, in Chapter 8 Musthafar Oladosu and Rena Kydd-Williams suggest that issues concerning ageing and the mental health needs of many older people with learning disabilities are frequently ignored because professionals often focus on a person's primary identity (e.g. the fact that they have a learning disability). Consequently, many practitioners fail to recognise that older people with a learning disability can also experience mental health conditions. In Chapter 9, Matt Broadway-Horner describes how many gay and lesbian older people have felt obliged to hide their sexual identity for most of their lives, and while there is now more acceptance of diverse sexual identities, many older people may still feel that they need to hide this aspect of self. So, we can see that older people will have both visible and invisible aspects of their identity and that ageing may not always be the most significant concern for them. Most older people will be living with multiple identities and may, at times in their lives, experience discrimination on multiple levels. Everyone, no matter their age or situation, can become vulnerable to mental health issues, and many older people living with mental health conditions experience a double, or sometimes triple, burden of discrimination as a result of the intersection of their age and other personal characteristics (such as sexual orientation, ethnicity, etc.) with their mental health. It is therefore impossible to offer a simple 'how to' for promoting anti-discriminatory practice in older people's mental health services. Nonetheless, it is hoped that the diverse perspectives of the contributing authors in this volume will help to illuminate the concept of a differentiated experience of ageing since every person's experience will be unique.

What we hope that you will take away from this book is a deeper understanding of how intersecting inequalities can impact on the lives of older people living with mental health conditions and how you can develop your own anti-discriminatory practice. We also encourage you to work with older people to challenge the organisations that you work in, and to remember that, while you are promoting anti-discriminatory practice for older people today, you are also planning for the future of your own old age.

Structure of the volume

Part I. Establishing the Key Principles of Anti-discriminatory Practice in Older People's Mental Health

The seven chapters within Part I establish the key principles concerning ageing and anti-discriminatory practice in mental health. This part introduces the reader to some of the current theories and conceptual debates in the field.

Chapter 1. Conceptualising Ageing and Anti-discriminatory Practice

In this foundational chapter, Pauline Lane identifies some of the competing theories surrounding ageing, mental health and discrimination, and she discusses care ethics and the intergenerational care contract. She advocates for an understanding of 'intersectionality' as an approach for considering the lives of older people living with mental health issues, and offers some recommendations for developing anti-discriminatory practice.

Chapter 2. Humanising the Mental Health Context

This chapter challenges the reader to think about some of the philosophical debates around our approach to working with older people living with mental health issues. The author, Maria Castro Romero, discusses the impact of 'dehumanising' practices on older people and suggests that humanising requires us to make an ethical commitment. This requires a different approach to practice, with practitioners reflecting on their own humanity as well as that of others.

Chapter 3. Ageing, Ethnicity and Mental Health

In the UK, the proportion of people aged 65 and over within the Black, Asian and Minority Ethnic (BAME) population is increasing. In this chapter Rachel Tribe suggests that some health and social care professionals are failing to give adequate consideration to issues of culture and diversity in their work, and that many fail to consider anti-discriminatory practice to be an essential part of practice within the service they provide. The author also suggests that while much of the research literature within BAME elders' mental health emphasises the vulnerability and the difficulties that older adults face, little attention is given to the resiliency of elders. Yet many BAME elders, including those living with long-term debilitating illness such as dementia, are able to be creative, supportive, expressive and fully engaged with life, and thus continue to make a positive contribution to the world.

Chapter 4. Common Mental Health Problems

In this chapter, Maureen McIntosh and Afreen Huq scope some of the complex issues relating to the labelling of and diagnosis of mental health problems with older adults, as well as some of the challenges in working in therapeutic relationships. The authors suggest that health professionals need to be cognisant of the fact, that working with older adults' can raise personal concerns and emotions for practitioners and conversely, older people may find it difficult to trust practitioners. The authors recommend that one of the ways of promoting anti-discriminatory practice is for practitioners to maintain their curiosity about older people and listen to their needs, working together to find a way forward.

Chapter 5. The Mental Capacity Act 2005 and Ageing

Ajit Shah examines many of the technical aspects of the Mental Capacity Act 2005 (which applies in England and Wales), the implications of ageing, age-related mental disorders and personal characteristics on decision-making capacity and the issues raised for individuals, practitioners and families. The chapter offers examples of good practice, together with strategies to improve the application of the Mental Capacity Act to avoid discrimination.

Chapter 6. Anti-discriminatory Practice: Caring for Carers of Older Adults with Mental Health Dilemmas

This chapter focuses on the vital role of unpaid carers and the ways we can work towards maximising their well-being and that of the person they are caring for. Rachel Tribe and Pauline Lane identify some of the many contextual factors and dilemmas that carers face when looking after a relative or friend living with mental health concerns in old age, and consider how anti-discriminatory practice may need to challenge traditional practices. The chapter stresses the importance of service provision that is relevant and appropriate to the needs of carers and those of the person they care for.

Chapter 7. End of Life Issues and Older People's Mental Health

Pauline Lane and Rachel Tribe examine a range of issues related to dying and suggest how we might maintain anti-discriminatory practice when older people with diminished mental capacity are in the process of dying. The chapter starts by examining how dying has been constructed throughout history, and questions if there can be such a thing as a 'good death'. The authors look at end of life (palliative) care and identify some of the issues that different groups of older people face in trying to access end of life services. The end of the chapter addresses some of the more practical issues concerning advance care plans and issues relating to power of attorney for older people with diminished capacity.

Part II. Insights

Part II contains four chapters and provides an understanding of some of the issues facing older people from specific communities. These 'insight' chapters offer the practitioner an opportunity to reflect on how inequality and discrimination can impact on the lives of people from very different social backgrounds. While each chapter focuses on a specific social group (i.e. older people with learning disabilities; older LGBTi people; older Gypsies; and older homeless people), it is helpful to see these chapters as 'generalised insights' because, as we will see in Chapter 1, the reality is that older people (with or without mental health concerns) have multiple aspects to their identities. It is therefore hoped that these 'insight' chapters will be used as a starting point to reflect on the intersections of older people's identities and how these can impact on individuals. Each chapter provides questions that can be used for private study, as part of a taught session or for group-work discussions.

Chapter 8. Ageing and Mental Health Issues for People with Learning Disabilities

Musthafar Oladosu and Rena Kydd-Williams reflect on the fact that people with learning disabilities and their carers often find it difficult to access mainstream public-sector services. This can result in delays in diagnosis as well as poor health outcomes. When mental health issues in older adults are identified, there is often no clarity as to which service should take the lead in treatment and care, and thus there is a delay in obtaining the appropriate treatment and support. In addition, diagnostic overshadowing (where a behaviour or symptoms may be wrongly dismissed as part of the person's learning disabilities rather than being recognised as a mental health condition) can potentially lead to a lack of access to treatment and, in the worst scenarios, result in premature death.

Chapter 9. Ageing, Sexual Orientation and Mental Health: Lesbian, Gay, Bisexual, Transgender and Intersex Older People

The focus of this chapter is on ageing, sexual orientation and mental health, and Matt Broadway-Horner, as a gay man, looks at some of the issues confronting older lesbian, gay, bisexual, transgender and intersex (LGBTi) people. The majority of older LGBTi people will have felt they needed to hide their sexual identity from the dominant heterosexual society for at least a portion of their lives, and consequently many are still worried about disclosing their sexual identity. This can be especially problematic for older LGBTi people with mental health problems and for their carers.

Chapter 10. Understanding the Lives of Older Gypsies and Travellers and the Impact of Inequality on their Mental Health

In this chapter, Siobhan Spencer and Pauline Lane discuss some of the distinct issues for older Gypsies with mental health issues. They suggest that it is impossible to understand the experience of ageing in Gypsy families without understanding the context of their lives. One of the challenges faced in writing this chapter is that there has been very limited research on Gypsy mental health and even less on older Gypsies. Drawing on Siobhan's first-hand knowledge of Gypsy communities, as well as her experience as an activist and academic, the authors offer some useful insights into how to develop anti-discriminatory practice.

Chapter 11. Social Exclusion and Anti-discriminatory Practice: The Case of Older Homeless People

In this chapter Peter Cockersell, Director of Health and Recovery at St Mungo's (a community housing association that supports rough sleepers and homeless people), offers a personal reflection on older homeless people and identifies that both mental and physical ill health are endemic among older rough sleepers and homeless people. He suggests that institutional discrimination and systemic failure promote the exclusion of rough sleepers and homeless people, and that consequently many older homeless people – and especially those living with mental illness – find that there is little or no care available for them.

Part III. Additional Information and Practical Guidance to Support Positive Practice

In the final part of the book, the editors offer two short chapters with information and practical guidance for practitioners working with older people with mental health concerns.

Chapter 12. The Rough Guide to Working with Interpreters in Mental Health

For many older BAME people facing a language barrier, speaking through an interpreter may be the only way to communicate with practitioners. Being dependent on another person to convey your words and meaning can lead to feelings of immense discomfort, as it requires placing your complete trust in the interpreter to convey your words and feelings accurately. As a professional, working effectively with interpreters in mental health contexts involves a range of skills, and in this chapter Rachel Tribe and Pauline Lane offer an introduction to some of the key issues, as well as providing a range of additional resources. It is recommended that practitioners undertake additional training in this area, as people from different cultures have different ways of presenting their distress (idioms of distress), and therefore it is helpful or practitioners to be receptive to other explanatory health beliefs and to be trained in working with interpreters.

Chapter 13. Ageing, Food and Malnutrition

In the UK more than one in ten older people suffer from malnutrition and its effects, despite the fact that it is largely preventable and treatable and is not a natural consequence of old age. In this chapter the editors look at some of the disturbing facts about malnutrition in older people in the UK and identify some key resources and recommendations for promoting anti-discriminatory practice and healthy eating for older people with mental health concerns.

References

Government Office for Science (2015) *The Barriers to and Enablers of Positive Attitudes to Ageing. Future of an Ageing Population: Evidence Review.* London: Government Office for Science. Available at www.gov.uk/government/uploads/system/uploads/attachment_data/file/454735/gs-15-15-future-ageing-attitudes-barriers-enablers-er06.pdf, accessed on 8 September 2016.

Kirkwood, T. (2001) 'The End of Age.' *The Reith Lectures.* London: BBC Radio 4, 4 April 2001. Transcript available at www.bbc.co.uk/radio4/reith2001/lecture1_print.shtml, accessed on 8 September 2016.

Martinsen, E.H. (2011) 'Care for nurses only? Medicine and the perceiving eye.' *Health Care Analysis* *19*, 1, 15–27.

Martinsen, K. (1993) 'Livsmot og lidelse – den omtenksomme sykepleiers utfordring' [Courage to live and suffering – challenges of the considerate nurse]. In K. Martinsen (ed.) *Den omtenksomme sykepleier* [The considerate nurse]. Oslo: Tano.

United Nations (2013) *World Population Ageing Report.* Report number ST/ESA/SER.A/348. New York: UN Department of Economic and Social Affairs, Population Division.

PART I

Establishing the Key Principles of Anti-discriminatory Practice in Older People's Mental Health

CHAPTER 1

Conceptualising Ageing and Anti-discriminatory Practice

Pauline Lane

As we get older, our rights do not change. As we get older, we are no less human and should not become invisible.

Archbishop Desmond Tutu
(cited in HelpAge International 2015, p.3)

This chapter introduces the reader to some of the key concepts that are discussed throughout the book. It is divided into five sections. Section 1: *Thinking About Ageing* maps out some of the key issues concerning demographic trends, the context of ageing and intersecting inequalities which can impact upon the lives of older people. Section 2: *Approaches to Older People's Mental Health* discusses debates around older people's 'vulnerabilities' and 'capabilities' and briefly outlines those around older people's mental health and well-being. Section 3: *Looking at Ageing Through a Different Lens* suggests that older people have long been 'constructed' through different theoretical perspectives and yet, it is argued, the cultural 'construction' of ageing may tell us more about the worries of a society at a given time than the lived experiences of older people. Section 4: *Thinking About Discrimination* looks at some of the definitions of discrimination and discusses what equity means for our practice. This section also outlines the legal duties of practitioners under the current Equalities legislation. Finally, Section 5: *Thinking About Promoting Anti-discriminatory Practice in Older People's Mental Health* makes some brief recommendations for why we might want to develop anti-discriminatory practice.

Section 1: Thinking About Ageing

Historically, and across the globe, young people have always outnumbered older people. However, life expectancy data suggests that this will be reversed, resulting in dramatic social and economic changes. So, what do we know about global ageing?

The United Nations (2015) has identified the following global trends:

- One in eight people worldwide are already aged 60 years or over, and by 2030 older people are projected to account for one in six people globally. Older people are expected to account for more than 25 per cent of the population in Europe and in North America, 20 per cent in Oceania, 17 per cent in Asia, 17 per cent in Latin America and the Caribbean, but only 6 per cent in Africa.

- The ageing population is increasing fastest in high-income countries. For example, Japan already has the world's most 'aged population', with 33 per cent of Japanese people aged 60 years or over in 2015.

- Women tend to live longer than men by an average of 4.5 years.

- The majority of older people are found to be living in towns rather than in rural areas.

- Most young people living in high-income countries can expect to live until the age of 80 or over, and we therefore need to be planning for an ageing global population.

In the UK and Europe, the increasing population of older people is often explained by a combination of improved healthcare practices and the emergence of a 'population bulge'. This bulge occurred as a result of many families having more children following the end of the Second World War, and is often referred to as the 'baby-boomer generation'.

The International Longevity Centre (2013) has identified the following:

- In England and Wales, 15.7 per cent of the population is aged 65 and above.

- In Scotland, 17.0 per cent of the population is aged 65 and above.

- In Northern Ireland, 14.7 per cent of the population is aged 65 and above.

- Across the UK, the average life expectancy at birth for a child born in 2012 is predicted to be 78.2 years for men and 82.3 years for women.

- Around one-third of babies born in 2012 in the UK are expected to survive to celebrate their 100th birthday.

However, while there is clear evidence of changes in demographic trends based on chronological age, there is some debate as to how we might define 'being old'. Some organisations make distinctions between the 'young old', usually deemed to be 65–74; the 'middle old', 75–84; and people who are called the 'oldest old', who are aged 85 and above (Office for National Statistics 2013). Yet these chronological distinctions do not take into account the individual characteristics and life chances that mean that older people often have very different experiences of 'ageing'. The term 'old' (and other descriptors of ageing, such as 'the elderly', 'senior citizens', 'older adults', 'OAP', 'seniors', etc.) tends to homogenise the experience of millions of people into a primary identity of 'being old'.

Although people's chronological age is a part of their embodied identity (i.e. their physiologically changing body), many of the contributors to this book suggest that ageing is not always the most significant part of a person's identity. Sometimes other personal characteristics (such as disability, ethnicity, sexual orientation, etc.) and/or contextual issues that impact on a person's life (such as homelessness or a change in government policy, for example) can be more significant to people's mental health and well-being than their chronological age.

Thinking about the context of ageing
This subsection looks at the context of older people's lives (i.e. where and how they live) and how this influences quality of life in old age, as well as life expectancy.

The *Global AgeWatch Index* (HelpAge International 2015) assesses the social and economic well-being of older people around the world, and it suggests that older people in most industrialised nations have the best experience of old age. In practical terms, this means that older people living in low- and middle-income countries usually have little or no economic support from the state. Consequently, in most low- and middle-income countries, millions of older people find themselves living in extreme poverty, with limited access to health care or any financial support in old age. In contrast, the majority of older people living in high-income countries have access to both a state pension and healthcare services and therefore may be considered to have provision for a good old age, although a good or happy old age is not defined by economics alone.

Global statistics can often hide the poverty and discrimination that happens *within* countries. For example, in the UK many older people have been hit by cuts in public-sector funding and find that they are no longer eligible for many public services (meals on wheels, for example). This, combined with the rising cost of commodities (including food and utilities), as well as poor returns on life savings, has meant that many older people in the UK are now living in poverty (Centre for Local Economic Strategies 2014; MacInnes *et al.* 2015).

In addition, many older people who contributed to private pensions are now finding that these have been devalued or their terms changed as a result of the global economic crisis (OECD 2013), although some older people from middle- and high-income professions have occupational pensions that are protected from deflation (Institute for Fiscal Studies 2015). Therefore, when considering the context of older people's lives, we should not lose sight of the fact that while there are extreme inequalities between the richest and the poorest older people around the world, there are also extreme inequalities between older people within every nation.

Intersectionality, inequality and ageing

While the *Global AgeWatch Index* (HelpAge International 2015) discusses the context of older people's lives, it does not highlight the contrast between the enduring inequalities some older people (such as those living in the slums of Dhaka, Bangladesh) will face and the intermittent and intersecting inequalities that others, living in the same or different countries, may face at different points in their lives. For many older people, experiences of inequality and discrimination coalesce at certain times in a variety of ways, and these social inequalities can impact on people's mental and physical health. In order to understand the idea of coalescing inequalities, it may be useful to look at the theory of intersectionality that was developed by Kimberlé Crenshaw (1991) in response to some of the debates concerning gender inequality.

Crenshaw pointed out that while feminism traditionally focused on gender inequality, Black feminist theorists had been speaking out for some time about their multiple experiences of oppression and the fact that gender inequality was only one of these experiences. Crenshaw felt that the experiences of Black women were different from White women's because they experienced gender inequality *and* racial inequality, and she felt that feminism did not address these intersecting inequalities. Crenshaw also suggested that these gendered and ethnic inequalities were often amplified by other forms of discrimination (e.g. class, age, disability, etc.) and that these 'intersecting inequalities' varied over a person's lifetime.

Below is an example of how this concept of intersecting inequalities can relate to older people and their mental health.

Case study: Intersecting inequalities in the lives of older Chinese women living in an inner-city area

Some years ago, the editors of this book conducted a study with older Chinese women living in a city in the west of England. Talking through interpreters, a group of older Chinese women described how they had migrated to the UK in the 1950s and had spent most of their working lives in family-run restaurants. The women explained that as a result of traditional gender roles, most of them had worked in the back kitchen (preparing food and washing up) and, consequently, they had little opportunity to interact with the English-speaking community and therefore did not learn to speak English.

Significantly, because they were family-owned businesses, most of the women worked without pay and were not able to save any money or to build up the national insurance contributions required to obtain a full state pension.

Most of the women did have children, and many of their offspring went on to have very successful careers, but this resulted in most of them living far away from their family home.

As the years passed, many of these now elderly Chinese women became widowed and found themselves alone, without financial or emotional support, and unable to speak English.

It was therefore not surprising to hear that many of these elderly Chinese women were struggling with loneliness and that many of them self-identified as feeling depressed (Lane, Tribe and Hui 2010).

However, a local woman set up a Chinese Women's Group for her community to support the health and social care needs of Chinese women and their families in the area. The group offers a range of leisure activities (such as painting and t'ai chi) as well as advocacy, advice and English language lessons. Many of the women we interviewed now find support and friendship in their local community.

A film made by the author and Redmark Films with a Chinese community group in Bristol can be viewed online: https://vimeo.com/19257418.

From this example, we see that the theory of intersectionality can help to make visible the intersection of different forms of oppression and the ways in which they can coalesce at different points in a person's life. The theory of intersectionality helps us to understand that we do not need to locate experiences of oppression within just a single category (such as ageism), and this approach highlights how many people experience multiple forms of oppression.

Thinking about health inequalities in old age

Health inequalities are now starting to be recognised as significant issues for the individual as well as for the funding and delivery of health and social care services (Artazcoz and Rueda 2007). So what do we know about the health of older people? Mortimer and Green (2016) have identified some of the key issues in older people's health in England:

- The majority of the young old are healthy, but as people live longer they are more likely to experience multiple long-term health conditions (co-morbidity). For example, the prevalence of heart disease, hypertension, stroke, diabetes and cancer rises rapidly after the age of 60. However, it is notable that many of these conditions are linked to social determinants of health as well as lifestyle choices, and therefore they are not an inevitable part of ageing.

- The rate of falls also increases with age, although falls are often preventable through effective risk assessments of people's home environments and through fall and walking clinics that aim to improve strength and stability.

- Dementia has a very strong link with ageing, but there is a low risk of the condition in people under the age of 64. Although this risk does increase with age, it only peaks steeply for women (at nearly 30%) and men (20%) when they are 95–99 years old.

- Depression (and other mental health conditions) is frequently not recognised or diagnosed amongst older people, and it has been estimated that 85 per cent of older people living with depression receive no help at all from health services.

Interestingly, despite the demographic changes, there has been comparatively little research looking at health and social care inequalities among older people in the UK. However, a research study by Lee (2009) suggests that inequalities may need to be considered between peers (i.e. groups of older people in the same generation) as well as between generations, and in the context and over the life course of an individual. Indeed, the study by Lee (conducted on behalf of the Equality and Human Rights Commission and Age Concern (now Age UK)) suggests that there is a need to give much more focus to the life-course factors that can produce unequal outcomes in later life. Lee (2009, pp.11–17) draws the following conclusions:

- Poor general health over a person's lifetime is closely associated with being financially poor and socially isolated in later life.

- Older people from lower-income groups are disadvantaged in their use of specific health services; for example, they have lower rates of mammogram uptake, flu vaccinations, eye examinations, dentistry, heart surgery and diabetes care.

- People from less-skilled occupational backgrounds are more likely to be in poor health when they are older, and those who have spent more time unemployed are more likely to have poor health in later life and die at a younger age.

- Gender differences create inequalities throughout life. Although women usually live longer than men, they also spend more years in poor health and are more likely than men to be financially poor when they are older.

- Level of education is one of the strongest and most consistent factors influencing poverty in later life, with a person who has no educational qualifications having a much higher chance of being poor in later life than a person who has educational qualifications.

- People of all ages from ethnic minority groups are more likely to have poor physical and mental health and are also more likely to have lower pension incomes in later life compared with White groups in the UK.

However, issues concerning older people's health often need to be seen in relation to both the context of their lives and their access to services and welfare support. While healthcare provision is a matter for the devolved governments of England, Scotland, Wales and Northern Ireland, it is currently free for all UK citizens. However, social-care services are now means-tested across the UK, and all older people are now means-tested if they need support with personal care needs, or if they need to move into a care home.

Consequently, the number of older people now receiving publically funded social-care support is in steady decline (Mortimer and Green 2016). It has been suggested that the perceived complexity and intrusiveness of means testing may stop some older people who are entitled to state-funded care from applying (Mkandawire 2005). It has also been argued that means testing of welfare benefits not only stigmatises certain groups but also undermines the central objectives of the welfare state, that is, to promote social inclusion and social justice (Van Oorschot 2002), though the counterargument is that targeted welfare benefits and social care can be directed at those with the most need. Mortimer and Green (2016, p.45) also highlight the fact that there is now a 'catastrophic collapse in funding and service provision for older people, and this means that in a time when we are trying to promote older people remaining in their homes and sustaining independence, the very structures to enable this are no longer in place'.

Section 2: Approaches to Older People's Mental Health

In this section we are going to look at some of the trends relating to older people's mental health and explore issues concerning older people's 'vulnerability' and 'capabilities'. This section ends with a brief discussion of the mental health recovery agenda. However, clinical issues concerning older people's mental health are discussed by Ajit Shah in Chapter 5 and are not covered in this chapter. It should also be noted that issues relating to culture, ethnicity and older people's mental health are discussed separately in Chapter 3 by Rachel Tribe.

Before we begin, it is important to acknowledge that, contrary to many of the stereotypes about older people, mental health problems are not an inevitable part of ageing (Moriarty 2005). Indeed, everyone has mental health and emotional needs, and at some points in their life may need professional support with mental health concerns, and so it is helpful to think about mental health as being simply a human, rather than an age-linked, condition. Having said that, older people will more often be exposed to significant life events (such as retirement, the death of a partner or the onset of a long-term health condition), and these factors can mean that some older people are more vulnerable to mental health concerns.

In addition, some older people in marginalised groups – including people from a Black, Asian and Minority Ethnic (BAME) background, lesbian, gay, bisexual and transgender people, people living with a learning disability and people who are homeless – are more vulnerable to mental health concerns due to their experiences of exclusion and discrimination (Mind 2013). These groups are discussed in Chapter 3 and in Part II of this book.

So, what do we know about older people's mental health? NHS England (2015) has identified the following:

- In a 500-bed general hospital, on an average day, 330 beds will be occupied by older people, of whom 220 will have a mental disorder, 100 will each have dementia and depression, and 66 will have delirium.

- For every 1000 people over the age of 65, 250 will have a mental illness, of which 135 will have depression, and of them 115 will have no treatment.

- Of those older people with depression, 85 per cent receive no help from the NHS.

- Older people are a fifth as likely as younger age groups to have access to talking therapies, but are six times as likely to be taking medication for a mental health condition.

- The number of older people being treated in the Improving Access to Psychological Therapies (IAPT) programme rose from 4 per cent in 2008/09 to 6.5 per cent in 2013/14.

- While 50 per cent of younger people with depression are referred to mental health services, only 6 per cent of older people are.

- Around 10 per cent of older people experience loneliness, which can be a contributory factor for depression. Loneliness is reported to have the same negative health effects as smoking 15 cigarettes a day.

The World Health Organization (WHO) (2013a, p.9) suggests that mental health and many common mental health problems are 'shaped to a great extent by the social, economic, and physical environments in which people live', and that social inequalities are associated with an increased risk of many common mental disorders. The social determinant model of mental health accepts that while some older people will experience mental health issues due to organic or physiological causes (such as in the case of dementia), it is often a combination of social conditions and personal attributes that compromises older people's mental health. The case study below offers an example of this interaction.

Case study: Thinking about the social determinants of mental health and social vulnerabilities

Josiah arrived in the UK from Jamaica as a young man with great hopes and expectations for his future life. He married Marjorie when they were both still fairly young and they had hoped to have a big family – but they were not able to have children.

Josiah had always worked hard, but he found it difficult to find employment and there seemed to be few opportunities open to him, especially as he had always struggled with his literacy.

Sometimes, however, Josiah felt that people would not employ him because he was Black, although no one had said this to him directly. During Josiah's working life, he had always been in short-term, insecure or informal employment, and consequently he was never paid enough money to obtain a mortgage or put any money aside for his old age. He had paid his national insurance, though, so he knew he would have a state pension when he retired.

Rent for Josiah and Marjorie's accommodation in London was expensive, and the cost seemed to be rising all the time, but they 'got by' most of the time and were looking forward to their retirement. Having good links with the local Pentecostal church, Marjorie and Josiah envisaged a quiet but active retirement, volunteering within their local community.

However, two years after they had both retired, Marjorie died suddenly. Josiah felt like his world had ended, and he did not feel he could face his friends in the church, as it reminded him of Marjorie. Although friends often called in to see him, Josiah usually felt too low to socialise. He started to struggle to get out of bed in the morning, and he often did not feel it was worth getting washed and dressed or cooking food.

Over the next two years, Josiah became more withdrawn and isolated. With a reduced income and rising rent precipitating his decline into poverty, Josiah was forced to move away from the area he had always lived in.

Luckily, friends at the church had remained committed to visiting him over the years, and when he talked of moving to Liverpool (because the rent was cheaper and it was a place he had liked as a young man), someone from the church helped him to find a room to rent just outside of the city.

The family who offered the room were also Jamaican and they attended a large Pentecostal church in Liverpool. So for the first time in many years, Josiah felt that his life might start to look a bit brighter.

A film made by the author and Redmark Films with a Caribbean community in Luton can be viewed online: https://vimeo.com/channels/redmarkfilms/19266739.

Some authors have discussed the concepts of people's 'vulnerability' and 'capabilities' in relation to mental health. However, the word 'vulnerability' is not used in its common meaning (i.e. of a person at risk and in need of protection), with many now using the term to describe a *process* that arises from the interaction between the characteristics of an individual and the specific context of that individual's life (Delor and Hubert 2000).

Since the early 1970s there has been growing interest in the concept of the 'capabilities' of individuals. This capability discourse originated out of critiques of some aid programmes in low- and middle-income countries that had traditionally blamed the poor for their own poverty (Sen 1993). In response to this negative discourse about the poor, Sen suggested that a discussion about distributional inequalities and how people used resources was needed. He proposed that people's capability is determined by the social and material context of their lives combined with the personal capacities they have developed over their lifetime (meaning their emotional and social skills, as well as material assets such as money, a home, etc.). Unlike the theory of intersectionality (outlined above), which focuses only on the intersecting inequalities in a person's life (also known as the social determinants of health), Sen's capabilities approach shows us that people may respond very differently to the same circumstances due to the interaction between their capabilities and the context of their lives.

Other authors have developed these ideas concerning capabilities further in relation to older people. Schröder-Butterfill and Marianti (2006) identify that older people will often face a number of different negative experiences over their lifetime, and they define these as 'exposure factors'. The authors suggest that while all older people will face a wide range of exposure factors, older people often risk becoming progressively more vulnerable because they can *accumulate* exposure factors as they age. These factors may include the loss of a job and the identity and income it brought, new financial pressures, the death of a loved one, poor housing and physical health problems. Schröder-Butterfill and Marianti also suggest that is not just the *number* of exposure factors that impacts on older people's mental health, but also the *duration* of those factors and their *interaction* within the context of the overall life of the older adult.

However, these authors suggest that while many older people may face similar accumulated exposure factors related to ageing, it is clear that different people will respond to these challenges in different ways. Schröder-Butterfill and Marianti (2006) suggest that older people negotiate different challenges by mobilising different resources at their disposal. They define this as a person's 'capacity' (which is similar to Sen's idea of capability). The authors suggest that the coping capacities of older people fall into three areas – namely:

1. *Individual capacities*: This includes a person's wealth and 'human capital', that is, both the material wealth they have built up over their life (such as pension, savings, property, etc.) and their personal emotional skills and health.

2. *Social network*: This includes an individual's relationships with others (such as a life-partner or children, as well as community links) as these can both provide practical support and help to meet emotional needs. Schröder-Butterfill and Marianti do acknowledge, however, that personal relationships are not always positive and that practitioners need to ask older people about the *quality* of the relationships and networks they have.

3. *Formal social protection*: Schröder-Butterfill and Marianti suggest that formal welfare and social care arrangements can act to 'fill the gap' where individual capabilities and social networks are not able to ameliorate accumulated exposure factors. (However, recent cuts to social-care provision across the UK may mean that this vital aspect of building and maintaining older people's 'capacity' will go into decline.)

In terms of promoting anti-discriminatory practice in older people's mental health, from the discussion above we can see that policymakers and commissioners will need to address many of the social determinants of mental health. However, as practitioners, an understanding of the vulnerability and capacities framework can help us make a very significant difference to the way that we support older people by enabling them to build on their capacities and strengths in order to promote more positive outcomes in later life.

Linked to the idea of capabilities is the idea of mental health recovery. While the word 'recovery' is often used in physical health to imply that someone has been restored to their previous health status, the concept is usually understood in mental health as a way in which people can find a way of living a meaningful life with, or without, the ongoing symptoms of their condition. However, this is not to say that older people with mental health concerns should not seek support. Indeed, talking to a health or social care professional is important, as it enables people to understand what is happening to them and to access support or treatment if required.

The concept of recovery is often seen not as an objective but as part of a philosophy that requires practitioners to understand that, for many people, living with mental health concerns is a part of their life journey. The South London and Maudsley NHS Foundation Trust and South West London and St George's Mental Health NHS Trust (2010) have suggested that recovery involves three interrelated themes:

- *hope*, which is essential to sustaining motivation and supporting the expectation of a fulfilled life

- *agency*, which means that older people remain in control of their own problems and their lives

- *opportunity*, which links recovery with social inclusion and thus people's participation in the community.

Significantly, mental health recovery often involves a shift of control, as service users are understood to be the experts on their own mental health. The purpose of the recovery approach is to enable people experiencing mental health problems to develop resources (personal, social and practical) and skills that will support their quality of life. Consequently, the role of the practitioner within this model is seen as supporting, or facilitating, the service user's own vision of recovery (Roberts and Wolfson 2004). As the recovery approach is about hope and the promotion of person-centred skills and social inclusion, it sits naturally at the heart of the capabilities model, building up older people's coping capacities and social networks, and improving their access to care and support when needed.

Section 3: Looking at Ageing Through a Different Lens

In this section we are going to take a brief look at how older people can be constructed by different theoretical approaches (or 'lenses') — namely, 'disengagement theory', 'active ageing' and 'intergenerational conflict theory' — to see how different social theories of ageing have been influenced by the political landscape of the time. For practitioners, the value of understanding some of the theoretical constructions of older people is to help us think about how older people are portrayed, and why, in the services we provide. However, it could be argued that the interests of different theorists on ageing may actually tell us more about the concerns of a society at a specific time than it does about the reality of older people's lives. We will start by looking at disengagement theory, an early theory of ageing, followed by a brief outline of two more contemporary theories: active ageing theory and intergenerational conflict theory.

Disengagement theory

Disengagement theory emerged in the 1950s and 1960s. The approach suggested that older people needed to withdraw from their social roles in response to their 'natural' biological decline, as this withdrawal would give young people an opportunity to shape society (Cumming and Henry 1961). Disengagement theory used a systems approach to ageing and was concerned with the efficiency of the social and economic systems in society, suggesting that older people had a moral obligation to 'disengage from society for the benefit of the social system' (p.209).

If we look back to the social context of the 1950s, much of Western Europe and the USA was witnessing the emergence of a new 'youth culture'. For the first time in history, many young people had disposable income and they started to be consumers and also creators of new products, leading to the emergence of new markets aimed at young workers and consumers (Abrams 1959). Through into the 1960s, many young people in the UK and the USA were starting to gain collective power, and the development of television and the articulation of youth culture meant that young people were starting to reject the values of the older generation and instead to define the world through their own perspectives (Brake 2013). If we look at the social context of the development of disengagement theory, therefore, we can see that it emerged at a time when young people were gaining social power and traditional post-war values were starting to be rejected, so the emergence of this age-related exclusionary theory was perhaps not so surprising.

Active ageing theory

Active ageing theory, along with intergenerational conflict theory below, is a more contemporary approach but also tells us something about the social values of our time and the ways in which we now view older people. Many modern ageing theorists (see, for example,

Joung and Miller 2007) talk about active ageing in contrast with disengagement theory. While different theorists accentuate different aspects of active ageing, the approach tends to focus on the productive potential of older people (as paid workers or volunteers) and the need to look after the body, living independently and maintaining social activities. It focuses also on the responsibility of individuals to look after their own health and well-being.

Active ageing has been subject to criticism, with writers such as Stenner, McFarquhar and Bowling (2011) suggesting that active ageing is part of an explicitly political strategy to reinvent the very meaning of ageing in a future society and to rethink questions relating to the rights and duties of older citizens. The active ageing discourse may also create different tensions for older people, as it holds out the ideal of a successful and physically vital ageing, where positive mental and physical health are idealised. This ideal of active ageing is also starting to develop into a stereotype and to create a new moral discourse of ageing, where older people are seen to have a duty to stay fit, well and productive (Van Dyk *et al.* 2013). Other authors, such as Higgs and Gilleard (2010), have suggested that active ageing is underpinned by new identity politics, as it implies that the individual should take more responsibility for their own health, and that this is linked to the market and consumerism that encourages older people to make healthy lifestyle choices. Other criticisms have come from Moulaert and Biggs (2013), who suggest that the theory is over-deterministic as it focuses on the contribution of older adults only in the domains of work and work-like activities. These authors suggest that the idea of active ageing creates a narrative that only legitimises very specific ways of growing old and that this excludes the lived experience of many older people, especially those living with a disability or people too poor to make 'lifestyle' choices. It is certainly worth highlighting that the active ageing agenda has gained prominence with governments across Europe and the USA at a time when there is a concern about demographic trends and the global economic crisis, with advanced capitalist societies requiring older citizens to be working longer and remain healthy in order to maintain the economy. However, it is also notable too that 'under the current legal and policy frameworks...little has been done to *enable* older people to remain active and healthy and to live independent lives for longer' (Age Platform Europe 2013, p.2).

Intergenerational conflict theory

The final theory we shall look at is intergenerational conflict theory, which has been growing in prominence in recent years. This discourse concerns the 'burden' of the ageing population and the supposed intergenerational conflict between young people who are working and the retired-old regarding the perceived fairness of the distribution of welfare (Higgs and Gilleard 2010). Some authors, such as Emery (2012), have suggested that a conflict is inevitable between the generations due to limited health and social care resources (with the underlying assumption being that older people use up more of these resources). However, some authors have suggested that focusing on intergenerational conflicts usefully deflects attention away from social inequality at a time when governments are trying to instigate welfare reforms (i.e. financial cuts to public-sector services), and that it may therefore be useful to construct the financial deficit as an intergenerational conflict, rather than addressing the issue of wealth distribution among all citizens (Moore 2006). Another more pragmatic critique of this theory comes from the older people's charity Age UK (2014) who reported that people aged 65 and over were contributing £61 billion to the economy through employment, informal caring and volunteering, and that this amount was six times more than the money that was spent on social care by local authorities in England at that time (Department of Communities and Local Government 2014). Therefore, while the perception is that older citizens are 'using up' welfare resources, the economic evidence suggests that as a social group they contribute more to the economy than they use. In addition, many older people will have spent their working lives contributing to the economy and the building of the welfare state, and so to suggest that they are 'taking it away' from young people may be a misapprehension.

From the brief outlines of the three theories above, it is clear that many theories of ageing are a product of the social concerns of society at a given time. If these debates were merely philosophical discussions, they might not be of any concern to practitioners seeking to promote anti-discriminatory practice. However, theories have informed government policies and they also influence our attitudes towards older people, as well as being influential in how older people feel about themselves. Yet it is notable when looking at different theories of ageing that older people themselves are rarely included as researchers, and nor are they involved in developing new models of ageing (Knight and Ricciardelli 2003). As practitioners trying to develop anti-discriminatory practice, we might therefore like to think about the ways that current narratives construct theories about older people and inform our own attitudes towards them as a social group, and reflect on how contemporary theories are informing the practices of the services that we are working in.

Section 4: Thinking About Discrimination

The fact that people with serious mental illness die an average of 20 years earlier than the rest of the population, the majority from preventable causes, is one of the biggest health scandals of our time, yet it is very rarely talked about.

ReThink Mental Illness (2013)

Discrimination consists of acts, practices or policies that advantage one group over another because of specific characteristics, and this can result in the unequal treatment of others, based on ascribed or claimed characteristics (such as age, ethnicity, gender, class, disability or sexual orientation). All forms of discrimination can have significant consequences for people's mental and physical health, and people who are living with a mental health condition often find that they are discriminated against (Corrigan, Markowitz and Watson 2004).

Pincus (1994) has suggested that discrimination can occur at three levels:

1. *individual discrimination*, referring to the behaviour of an individual that is intended to have a differential and/or harmful effect on others

2. *institutional discrimination*, referring to the policies and practices of the dominant institutions and the behaviour of the people who control them

3. *structural discrimination*, referring to the policies of the dominant institutions and the behaviour of the individuals who *implement* these policies.

What is distinctive about Pincus's definition is that he implies that all of these forms of discrimination are intended and overt and that they aim to have differential or harmful effects. Sometimes this is true; for example, some studies have shown that many lesbian women and gay men are exposed to episodic and day-to-day discrimination, and this can often have an impact on their mental health and well-being (Levine and Leonard 1984; Mays, Cochran and Rhue 1993; Meyer 1995). However, discrimination can sometimes be subtle and unintended, and this can happen when systems, rules and policies have not taken into account the needs of a person who belongs to a group with 'protected characteristics' (see below for details on the Equality Act). Here is a short case study to give an example of indirect discrimination of someone with protected characteristics.

Case study: Gypsies and Travellers trying to access an NHS doctor

Gypsies and Travellers are recognised by law as an ethnic group.

Annie is a Romany Gypsy and she has spent all of her life travelling with her family. Her people have mainly moved around Leicestershire. Annie is 73 years old and often finds it difficult to access an NHS doctor in a local town because the surgeries usually require patients to provide proof of address. But as Annie is nomadic for much of the year, this is not possible.

The receptionist tells Annie that she cannot see the doctor because she has no proof of address, and states that this 'rule' applies to all new patients, regardless of their protected characteristics. But this could be seen as indirect discrimination against Gypsies and Travellers because of their protected characteristic (i.e. race), since this 'rule' has a *worse effect* on this particular ethnic group than others.

A film made by the author and Redmark Films with a Gypsy community about their experiences of trying to access a GP surgery and talk to health professionals can be viewed online: https://vimeo.com/19265453.

When thinking about discrimination, we cannot assume that everyone needs the same thing. Although it seems counter-intuitive, promoting anti-discriminatory practice does not mean treating everyone exactly the same; it means recognising that everyone is unique and that we need to adapt the ways in which we work in order to ensure that everyone is treated fairly and equally, and has access to the same opportunities. We will now discuss ageism as a form of discrimination that is often experienced by older people, but we should also remember that there is often an intersection of different forms of discrimination. For example, an older woman of African origin may meet a combination of sexism, ageism and racism, and this would put her at particular risk of discrimination (Fredman 2001).

Ageism

In most cultures, age-based distinctions are enshrined in law (e.g. the age at which people can vote, drive and get married), and ideas about ageing permeate our language and culture (Wilkinson and Ferraro 2002). Negative and prejudicial attitudes towards people based on their age are common, and the term 'ageism' is used to describe discrimination against individuals as well as discriminatory practices and institutional policies that perpetuate stereotypical ideas about others based on their age (Butler 1969). While young people do experience ageism, what is distinct about young people is that they can leave the status of being 'too young' behind as they grow older, but the status of older people is permanent (Garstka *et al.* 2004). As Nelson (2004) points out, old age is the one social group that most of us will join.

Many of the stereotypes about older people are well known; for example, older people are often defined as vulnerable, frail and impaired (Brewer, Dull and Lui 1981) with little agency. Yet ageism can also include other more gendered stereotypes, such as wealthy older men being constructed as 'elder statesmen', with some older women being constructed as the 'kind grandmother' (Hummert *et al.* 1994; Schmidt and Boland 1986). Theorists such as Sontag (1972) have noted that there are double standards of ageing, and older women are always stereotyped in more brutal ways than older men are. This is because of the cultural obsession in the West with women's looks and beauty.

As shown in the Introduction to this book, the world's population is ageing, and so it seems strange that ageism is still so widespread and that it has been identified as one of the most prevalent forms of discrimination in Europe (Abrams *et al.* 2011). It remains to be seen whether ageism will continue as older people start to become the majority population.

In terms of older people's mental health, ageist assumptions often have implications for older people's well-being, because when there are so many pervasive negative stereotypes about older people in society, it may be difficult for older people not to internalise these (Bennett and Gaines 2010). Some authors have suggested that internalising negative stereotyping can be harmful or detrimental to people's self-image, and this can have an impact on their confidence and abilities (Palmore 1999; Whitbourne and Willis 2006).

Equality and legal obligations for practitioners

This subsection looks briefly at the Equality Act 2010 and the public sector Equality Duty. Although legislation may not seem like the most exciting thing to read, these are really important issues for practitioners, who are simultaneously service providers, employees and perhaps managers and commissioners. Therefore, practitioners have both duties and obligations (as someone providing services), as well as rights (as an employee), and these are all upheld in law. Below is a short introduction to the issues, but it is your legal duty as a professional to stay up to date with any changes in equality legislation and to be aware of any implications for practice.

Equality Act 2010

This Act brought a wide range of past anti-discrimination laws together under a single law to protect individuals from unfair treatment and to promote equality. Everyone in England, Scotland and Wales is protected from unlawful discriminatory behaviour by this Act. (Northern Ireland has different legislation; see section 75 of the Northern Ireland Act 1998.) This is because we all have 'protected characteristics'. These are defined in law as:

- age
- disability
- gender reassignment
- marriage and civil partnership

- pregnancy and maternity

- race

- religion and belief

- sex

- sexual orientation.

Under the 2010 Act, there are four main types of discrimination:

1. *Direct discrimination:* This means that people are treated less favourably because of:

   a. a protected characteristic (listed above) – for example, if a doctor refuses to refer an older person with depression to talking therapies simply because of his or her age

   b. a protected characteristic of someone the person is associated with – for example, an unpaid carer who is looking after someone who is elderly or disabled will be protected by law from direct discrimination or harassment because of these caring responsibilities (because the carer is counted as being 'associated' with someone who is protected because of their age or disability)

   c. a protected characteristic a person is thought to have, regardless of whether this perception by others is actually correct or not – for example, a person facing discrimination because he or she is considered to be gay.

2. *Indirect discrimination:* This kind of discrimination is often more difficult to identify but it occurs when the practices of an organisation or an individual apply to everyone but put certain people at a disadvantage.

3. *Harassment:* This is defined as 'unwanted conduct' and must be related to a protected characteristic or be of a sexual nature, and can be verbal, physical or written. Most importantly, it is based on the victim's perception of the unwanted behaviour, rather than the intent of the person who is the harasser.

4. *Victimisation:* This means treating someone badly because they have undertaken a 'protected act' (or because a person

is believed to have undertaken or to be going to undertake a protected act). A 'protected act' is defined as:

a. making a claim or complaint of discrimination (under the Equality Act)

b. helping someone else to make a claim by giving evidence or information

c. making an allegation that you or someone else has breached the Act

d. doing anything else in connection with the Act.

More information on the Equality Act 2010

The Equality Act is very detailed, and most practitioners will be offered training on it. However, if you want to read more information on the Act, you can take a look at the Equality and Human Rights Commission's website: www.equalityhumanrights.com/en/advice-and-guidance/equality-act-guidance.

Public sector Equality Duty

As a practitioner, it is also important to know about the public sector Equality Duty (PSED), which is part of the Equality Act 2010 and was introduced in 2011. This duty applies to all public authorities in England, Scotland and Wales and obliges them to not simply avoid discrimination but positively promote equality. The PSED also requires all public bodies 'to eliminate unlawful discrimination, advance equality of opportunity and foster good relations between groups' (Age UK 2011, p.6). This duty is intended to ensure that equality informs the delivery of public services and thus to prevent discrimination and advance equality of opportunity in practice. It has two parts: a general duty (which applies across Britain) and specific duties to promote better compliance with the general duty (with different duties in England, Scotland and Wales). Age UK (2011a) suggest that because the Equality Act and the PSED require public authorities to systematically examine the impact of their policies and practices on older people, this will then help them 'to meet the challenges posed by our ageing and increasingly diverse society' (p.6).

As a member of staff employed or contracted in any public-sector organisation, practitioners need to be aware of both and have a duty to work within them.

So, what would anti-discriminatory practice in older people's mental health look like? Of course, the simple answer to this question is to follow the Equality Act 2010 and the PSED as well as any applicable professional or occupational standards, and both the law and professional ethics will guide your practice. However, while these are essential foundations for developing anti-discriminatory practice, in many ways the notion of non-discrimination is much wider, as it requires us to ask deeper questions about others and ourselves. As Maria Castro Romero suggests in Chapter 2, anti-discriminatory practice gets at the very core of who we think we are and how we construct 'others' in relation to ourselves. Anti-discriminatory practice, by its very nature, asks us to think about oppression and our relationships with others. But it is more than simply having an awareness of the way we talk and behave with others. Indeed, as Okitikpi and Ayme (2010) suggest, anti-discrimination has to look at both the internal landscape of the individual practitioner (i.e. attitudes and beliefs) and the external landscape (i.e. social structures, systems, processes, organisational policies, the people we are working with, etc.).

Section 5: Thinking About Promoting Anti-discriminatory Practice in Older People's Mental Health

As a professional working in the public sector with older people who have mental health concerns, promoting equality and non-discrimination should be an integral part of decision-making in everyday practice. Promoting anti-discriminatory practice means that the focus is on meeting the needs of the individual, while at the same time trying to avoid constructing older people as simply victims in need of 'rescuing', and we should not assume that older people are without agency or the capacity to make decisions for themselves.

Practitioners need to be aware of their legal duties under both the Equality Act 2010 (outlined above) and the Mental Health Act 2007 (see Chapter 5 by Ajit Shah in this volume, which concentrates on the Mental Capacity Act 2005). Many professional bodies now offer guidance for their members to ensure that equality and inclusion are at the heart of their practice and that professional guidance is always developed within the framework of national legal and policy mechanisms. However, everyone is unique, and this means that as practitioners we need to have a nuanced approach to our practice that places the individual at the heart of our work.

In thinking about promoting anti-discriminatory practice in older people's mental health, it may be useful to think about health from a human-rights-based perspective. The World Health Organization (2013b) promotes the idea of good health as a 'right' (i.e. a human entitlement) rather than simply a 'need'. The WHO suggests that if we accept that people have a right to good health, including good mental health, then we must also accept that there are core positive human and social values that both promote well-being for the individual but also for the wider society. If these ideas sound a little vague in relation to your own anti-discriminatory practice, you might like to ask yourself what it means for you to be treated well, and why it matters if you are treated differently from your family, friends or others. In other words, why would positive and inclusive social values make a difference to the way that you are treated, and the way you treat others? In order to develop anti-discriminatory practice, we can think about our beliefs, attitudes and actions as well as how the organisations that we work in treat older people.

As practitioners, addressing structural inequalities (i.e. those that are embedded into policies, laws and social systems) can often seem difficult. Below are some suggestions that practitioners might like to use to promote anti-discriminatory practice in their everyday work. As suggested earlier in this chapter, if we take a capabilities approach to promoting and supporting older people's mental health, then we can work towards building on their strengths (as opposed to using a deficit model that focuses on older people's lack of capacity).

- Try to give attention to the lived experience of the individual – older people should have a strong voice in all processes that affect them.

- Try to avoid making assumptions about people on the basis of their age or other characteristics.

- Help older people and their family and friends to navigate the complex health and social care system by referring, signposting and offering information.

- Promote equality in practice-based commissioning, and work to include the views and experiences of older people, especially those from minority and excluded communities. Local data can potentially be useful to find out which groups are benefiting (or being excluded) from public health initiatives, and this should influence commissioning (Hutt and Gilmour 2010).

- Be aware of local services (including voluntary organisations) that older people can be referred to for additional support, company, opportunities to volunteer, etc.

- Maintain high standards in your professional practice through Continuing Professional Development.

- The simple rule when working to promote anti-discriminatory practice with anyone is: *Don't assume – just ask.*

References

Abrams, D., Russell, P.S., Vauclair, C.-M. and Swift, H. (2011) *Ageism in Europe: Findings from the European Social Survey*. London: Age UK. Available at www.ageuk.org.uk/Documents/EN-GB/For-professionals/ageism_across_europe_report_interactive.pdf?dtrk=true, accessed on 17 September 2016.

Abrams, M. (1959) *The Teenage Consumer*. London: London Press Exchange Ltd.

Age Platform Europe (2013) *Older Persons Want Full and Equal Enjoyment of Their Rights*. Brussels: Age Platform Europe. Available at http://social.un.org/ageing-working-group/documents/fourth/AgePlatformEurope.pdf, accessed on 17 September 2016.

Age UK (2014) *Age UK Chief Economist's Report. Spring 2014*. London: Age UK. Available at www.ageuk.org.uk/Documents/EN-GB/For-professionals/Research/Age_UK_chief_economist_report_spring_2014.pdf?dtrk=true, accessed on 17 September 2016.

Artazcoz, L. and Rueda, S. (2007) 'Social inequalities in health among the elderly: A challenge for public health research.' *Journal of Epidemiology and Community Health 61*, 6, 466–467.

Bennett, T. and Gaines, J. (2010) 'Believing what you hear: The impact of aging stereotypes upon the old.' *Educational Gerontology 36*, 5, 435–445.

Brake, M. (2013) *The Sociology of Youth Culture and Youth Subcultures (Routledge Revivals): Sex and Drugs and Rock 'n' Roll?* Abingdon: Routledge.

Brewer, M.B., Dull, V. and Lui, L.L. (1981) 'Perceptions of the elderly: Stereotypes as prototypes.' *Journal of Personality and Social Psychology 41*, 656–670.

Butler, R.N. (1969) 'Age-ism: Another form of bigotry.' *Gerontologist 9*, 243–246.

Centre for Local Economic Strategies (2014) *Austerity Uncovered. Final Report Prepared by the Centre for Local Economic Strategies and Presented to the TUC*. Available at www.cles.org.uk/wp-content/uploads/2015/01/TUC-Final-Report-Dec14.pdf, accessed on 17 September 2016.

Corrigan, P., Markowitz, F. and Watson, A. (2004) 'Structural levels of mental illness stigma and discrimination.' *Schizophrenia Bulletin 30*, 3, 481–491.

Cumming, E. and Henry, W. (1961) *Growing Old: The Process of Disengagement*. New York: Basic Books.

Delor, F. and Hubert, M. (2000) 'Revisiting the concept of "vulnerability".' *Social Science and Medicine* 50, 1557–1570.

Department of Communities and Local Government (2014) *Local Government Financial Statistics No. 242014.* June 2014. Available at www.gov.uk/government/uploads/system/uploads/attachment_data/file/316772/LGFS24_web_edition.pdf, accessed on 17 September 2016.

Emery, T. (2012) 'Intergenerational Conflict: Evidence from Europe.' *Population Ageing* 5, 1, 7–22.

Fredman, S. (2001) *What Do We Mean by Age Equality? A Paper Presented to the IPPR Seminar: 21st November 2001 at the Nuffield Foundation.* Available at www.ippr.org/files/uploadedFiles/projects/Final%20Fredman%20paper.doc, accessed on 17 September 2016.

Garstka, T.A., Schmitt, M.T., Branscombe, N.R. and Hummert, M.L. (2004) 'How young and older adults differ in their responses to perceived age discrimination.' *Psychology and Aging* 19, 2, 326–335.

HelpAge International (2015) *Global AgeWatch Index 2015: Insight Report.* London: HelpAge International. Available at http://reports.helpage.org/global-agewatch-index-2015-insight-report.pdf, accessed on 17 September 2016.

Higgs, P. and Gilleard, C. (2010) 'Generational conflict, consumption and the ageing welfare state in the United Kingdom.' *Ageing and Society* 30, 1439–1451.

Hutt, P. and Gilmour, S. (2010) *Tackling Inequalities in General Practice: An Inquiry into the Quality of General Practice in England.* London: The King's Fund. Available at www.kingsfund.org.uk/sites/files/kf/field/field_document/health-inequalities-general-practice-gp-inquiry-research-paper-mar11.pdf, accessed on 17 September 2016.

International Longevity Centre – UK (2013) *Ageing, Longevity and Demographic Change: A Factpack of Statistics from the International Longevity Centre.* Available at www.ilcuk.org.uk/index.php/publications/publication_details/ageing_longevity_and_demographic_change_a_factpack_of_statistics_from_the_i, accessed on 17 September 2016.

Joung, H. and Miller, N. (2007) 'Examining the effects of fashion activities on life satisfaction of older females: Activity theory revisited.' *Family and Consumer Sciences Research Journal* 35, 4, 338–356.

Knight, T. and Ricciardelli, L. (2003) 'Successful aging: Perceptions of adults aged between 70 and 101 years.' *International Journal of Aging and Human Development* 56, 3, 223–245.

Lane, P., Tribe, R. and Hui, R. (2010) 'Intersectionality and the mental health of elderly Chinese women living in the UK.' *International Journal of Migration, Health and Social Care* 6, 4, 34–41.

Lee, M. (2009) *Just Ageing? Fairness, Equality and the Life Course: Final Report.* London: Equality and Human Rights Commission, Age Concern and Help the Aged. Available at http://justageing.equalityhumanrights.com/wp-content/uploads/2009/06/Just_Ageing_final-report.pdf, accessed on 17 September 2016.

Levine, M.P. and Leonard, R. (1984) 'Discrimination against lesbians in the work force.' *Signs* 9, 700–710.

MacInnes, T., Tinson, A., Hughes, C., Barry Born, T. and Aldridge, H. (2015) *Monitoring Poverty and Social Exclusion.* York: Joseph Rowntree Foundation. Available at www.jrf.org.uk/mpse-2015, accessed on 17 September 2016.

Mays, V.M., Cochran, S.D. and Rhue, S. (1993) 'The impact of perceived discrimination on the intimate relationships of black lesbians.' *Journal of Homosexuality* 25, 4, 1–14.

Meyer, I.H. (1995) 'Minority stress and mental health in gay men.' *Journal of Health and Social Behaviour* 36, 38–56.

Mind (2013) *We Still Need to Talk: A Report on Accessing Talking Therapies.* London: Mind. Available at www.mind.org.uk/media/494424/we-still-need-to-talk_report.pdf, accessed on 17 September 2016.

Mkandawire, T. (2005) *Targeting and Universalism in Poverty Reduction.* United Nations Research Institute for Social Development, Social Policy and Development Programme Paper Number 23. Available at www.unrisd.org/80256B3C005BCCF9/httpNetITFramePDF?ReadForm&parentunid=955FB8A594EEA0B0C12570FF00493EAA&parentdoctype=paper&netitpath=80256B3C005BCCF9/(httpAuxPages)/955FB8A594EEA0B0C12570FF00493EAA/$file/mkandatarget.pdf, accessed on 17 September 2016.

Moore, P. (2006) 'Global knowledge capitalism, self-woven safety nets, and the crisis of employability.' *Global Society* 20, 4, 453–473.

Moriarty, J. (2005) *Update for SCIE Best Practice Guide on Assessing the Mental Health Needs of Older People*. London: Social Care Workforce Research Unit, The International Policy Institute, King's College London. Available at www.scie.org.uk/publications/guides/guide03/files/research.pdf, accessed on 17 September 2016.

Mortimer, J. and Green, M. (2016) *The Health and Care of Older People in England 2015*. London: Age UK. Available at www.ageuk.org.uk/Documents/EN-GB/For-professionals/Research/Briefing-The_Health_and_Care_of_Older_People_in_England-2015-UPDATED_JAN2016.pdf?dtrk=true, accessed on 17 September 2016.

Moulaert, T. and Biggs, S. (2013) 'International and European policy on work and retirement: Reinventing critical perspectives on active ageing and mature subjectivity.' *Human Relations 66*, 1, 23–43.

Nelson, T. (2004) *Ageism: Stereotyping and Prejudice Against Older Persons*. Cambridge, MA: Massachusetts Institute of Technology Press.

OECD (2013) 'Recent Pension Reforms and Their Distributional Impact.' In *Pensions at a Glance 2013: OECD and G20 Indicators*. Paris: OECD Publishing. Available at www.oecd.org/pensions/public-pensions/OECDPensionsAtAGlance2013.pdf, accessed on 17 September 2016.

Office for National Statistics (2013) *What Does the 2011 Census Tell Us about the 'Oldest Old' Living in England & Wales?* London: ONS. Available at http://webarchive.nationalarchives.gov.uk/20160105160709/http://www.ons.gov.uk/ons/dcp171776_342117.pdf, accessed on 6 November 2016.

Okitikpi, T. and Ayme, C. (2010) *Key Concepts in Anti-discriminatory Social Work*. London: Sage.

Palmore, E.B. (1999) *Ageism: Negative and Positive*. 2nd ed. New York: Springer.

Pincus, F.L. (1994) 'From Individual to Structural Discrimination.' In F.L. Pincus and H.J. Ehrlich (eds) *Race and Ethnic Conflict: Contending Views on Prejudice, Discrimination and Ethnoviolence*. Boulder, CO: Westview.

Rethink Mental Illness (2013) *Lethal Discrimination: Why People with Mental Illness Are Dying Needlessly and What Needs to Change*. London: Rethink Mental Illness. Available at www.rethink.org/media/810988/Rethink%20Mental%20Illness%20-%20Lethal%20Discrimination.pdf, accessed on 17 September 2016.

Roberts, G. and Wolfson, P. (2004) 'The rediscovery of recovery: Open to all.' *Advances in Psychiatric Treatment 10*, 37–48.

Schmidt, D.F. and Boland, S.M. (1986) 'Structure of perceptions of older adults: Evidence for multiple stereotypes.' *Psychology and Aging 1*, 255–260.

Schröder-Butterfill, E. and Marianti, R. (2006) 'A framework for understanding old-age vulnerabilities.' *Ageing and Society 26*, 1, 9–35.

Sen, A. (1993) 'Capability and Well-being.' In M.C. Nussbaum and A. Sen (eds) *The Quality of Life*. Oxford: Clarendon Press.

Sontag, S. (1972) *The Double Standard of Aging*. Ontario: Women's Kit.

South London and Maudsley NHS Foundation Trust and South West London and St George's Mental Health NHS Trust (2010) *Recovery is for All: Hope, Agency and Opportunity in Psychiatry. A Position Statement by Consultant Psychiatrists*. London: SLAM/SWLSTG. Available at www.rcpsych.ac.uk/pdf/recovery%20is%20for%20all.pdf, accessed on 17 September 2016.

Stenner, P., McFarquhar, T. and Bowling, A. (2011) 'Older people and "active ageing": Subjective aspects of ageing actively.' *Journal of Health Psychology 16*, 3, 467–477.

United Nations (2015) *World Population Ageing 2015*. New York: United Nations Department of Economic and Social Affairs Population Division. Available at www.un.org/en/development/desa/population/publications/pdf/ageing/WPA2015_Report.pdf, accessed on 17 September 2016.

Van Dyk, S., Lessenich, S., Denninger, T. and Richter, A. (2013) 'The many meanings of "active ageing": Confronting public discourse with older people's stories.' *Recherches sociologiques et anthropologiques 44-1*. Available at https://rsa.revues.org/932#quotation, accessed on 17 September 2016.

Van Oorschot, W. (2002) 'Targeting Welfare: On the Functions and Dysfunctions of Means-Testing in Social Policy.' In P. Townsend and D. Gordon (eds) *World Poverty: New Policies to Defeat an Old Enemy*. Bristol: Policy Press.

Whitbourne, S. and Willis, S. (2006) *The Baby Boomers Grow Up: Contemporary Perspectives on Midlife*. Hove: Psychology Press.

Wilkinson, J.A. and Ferraro, K.F. (2002) 'Thirty Years of Ageism Research.' In T.D. Nelson (ed.) *Ageism, Stereotyping and Prejudice Against Older Persons*. Cambridge, MA: The MIT Press.

World Health Organization (2013a) *Mental Health Action Plan 2013–2020*. Geneva: WHO. Available at http://apps.who.int/iris/bitstream/10665/89966/1/9789241506021_eng.pdf?ua=1, accessed on 17 September 2016.

World Health Organization (2013b) *Investing in Mental Health: Evidence for Action*. Geneva: WHO. Available at http://apps.who.int/iris/bitstream/10665/87232/1/9789241564618_eng.pdf?ua=1, accessed on 17 September 2016.

CHAPTER 2

Humanising the Mental Health Context

Maria Castro Romero

Summary

This chapter will focus on humanisation as a fundamental concept for full citizenship and well-being. It will reflect on critical ideas for humanising care services, policies and social practices with an emphasis on mental health services for older people. However, it is hoped that the philosophical debates and implications for practice discussed in this chapter will be used more widely, especially when considered in relation to working with other populations and contexts.

Introduction

We can understand the humanisation of mental health contexts as the process of transformation through the valuing and respecting of people's full humanity, including the historic, social, economic and political aspects of their lives. Therefore, humanising health care is a central process for the well-being of both professionals working in services as well as the people accessing services. This is particularly important in relation to older people in the UK, since it has been reported that their care 'is failing on dignity' (Commission on Improving Dignity in Care 2012), that they are pervasively marginalised and that age discrimination (ageism) is often implicit and legitimised (Castro Romero 2016). For example, dignity is usually linked to independence (rather than interdependence), beauty is equated with youth, and elders are usually constructed as undesirable (even as sexless), in addition to our society's great fear of ageing and its association with dying/death (Conway 2003).

When thinking about the humanisation of mental health contexts, we might like to reflect on the glorification of scientific knowledge (over other forms of knowledge) that marked modernity, and on how this has contributed to the development of the 'psych' professions. These soon departed from the epistemological meaning of the word *psyche* ('life' as in breath, soul[1]), focusing on the study of mind, as something directly observable (akin to privileged natural sciences), in search for recognition and status. In this context, it is unsurprising that limited attention is paid to humanisation in health services. A literature search yielded only a few relevant references written in English (e.g. Todres, Galvin and Holloway 2009), although there are more in Spanish (e.g. Bermejo 1999), and an impressive body of work in Brazilian Portuguese (among many, Gonçalves Brito and Carvalho 2010; Mattos 2009; Trad and Rocha 2011). In fact, in Brazil there is a National Policy of Humanisation (Política Nacional de Humanização, or PNH; Brazil, Ministério da Saúde 2007) in response to long-term problems in the Sistema Único de Saúde (SUS), the Brazilian equivalent to the UK's National Health Service. However, as seen explicitly in Pasche (2009) and implicitly in Santos Filho, Barros and Gomes (2009), this focus on humanisation goes back to the twentieth century and the legacy of Freire's education for critical consciousness, which is both a humanising and liberating praxis (Castro Romero and Afuape 2016).

Although the focus of this chapter is on services provided for older people, the ideas which are discussed are also central to humanising other services for other populations. It is also important to remember to consider the ideas at all levels: macro (policy, social discourse), meso (organisation and community) and micro (person-to-person interaction). Coherence across levels is necessary for the humanisation of health care as these levels are indivisible; for example, modes of management and attention are mutually influenced and determined, intertwining across all three levels (Pasche 2009). Consequently, the structure of this chapter will follow a reflection on foundational ideas for the challenge of integrating humanisation.

There can be no formula, manual or protocol for the humanising process for, once set, it will lose the ongoing, 'live' nature of all processes and, thus, the capacity to humanise. As author, it is more my intention to raise questions than to provide answers; local solutions will have to be worked out by specific groups of people in each particular context. To facilitate reflection as you read this chapter, and to support you in connecting some abstract notions presented with day-to-day practice, I will utilise three (anonymised) composite stories. These will encompass elements from my own experience and from colleagues across the UK working in NHS Mental Health Services for Older People.

I will begin by briefly contextualising my orientation, then I will discuss generalised dehumanising aspects of current mental health contexts for older people, before I go on to propose key ideas for making humanisation possible in mental health care.

Personal context

For seven years I worked as a clinical psychologist with elders and their families, friends and carers across different Mental Health Services for Older People including: Community Mental Health Team (CMHT), Memory Clinic, Outpatient Psychology, Inpatient and Dementia units and Continuing Care. Being part of these services meant I was also involved in working collaboratively with social services and voluntary organisations (e.g. Alzheimer's Society, and what is now known as Age UK). Since leaving the NHS I have trained and supervised clinical psychologists on their journey to qualifying; much of this work has been in partnership with elders themselves. I have been actively involved in research, presented at conferences and written literature regarding ageing, 'dementia', narrative practice, ethics and liberation psychology. I have discussed my value base and praxis at length elsewhere (e.g. Castro 2015), and for this reason it is sufficient to state here that *siding with* the people who seek our help (or are the focus of a referral) is always my starting point: 'It is only by embodying solidarity alongside elders, by engaging, often struggling, collectively in liberatory praxis that we can humanise (otherwise oppressive) structures and systems' (Castro Romero 2016, p.137).

Institutionalised dehumanisation

We are all human, and yet this does not translate into humanised relationships, practices, structures and discourses. In recent times, consultation papers with seemingly the 'right' intentions have been developed (e.g. the Department of Health's (2012) report *Liberating the NHS: No Decision About Me Without Me*), though sadly these seem to have had little real effect on mental health services and practices. Despite the use of terms such as 'liberating', 'shared decision-making' and 'choice', the structures, underlying assumptions on which services are funded and the way in which professionals are trained have remained unchanged. For example, *High Quality Care for All* (Department of Health 2008) does not once consider 'humanisation', 'citizenship' or 'personhood', and although it does mention 'compassion', 'dignity' and 'respect', particularly regarding the end of life, it does not explain these concepts. It is unclear, too, how they will be achieved, since there is no radical engagement with how we think about high-quality service provision, or with the structures and roles of the different stakeholders within services. The document acknowledges variation in individuals and communities but discursively betrays Western androcentric values,[2] for example around 'independence', and a continued desubjectification[3] (dehumanisation) by calling for 'working together *for patients*' (Department of Health 2008, p.70; my emphasis), rather than 'with people', and asking for change of 'lifestyle' without accounting for the effects of social life and inequalities on health and well-being. Finally, although *High Quality Care for All* proposes that services and professionals be accountable 'to *patients* and communities we serve' (Department of Health 2008, p.61; my emphasis), this is countered by both the dehumanisation of these communities and an individual view of leadership which does not include people and their communities. Care and compassion are only possible when the system sustains them throughout the management, service practices and structures.

Paradoxically, the NHS has focused on the implementation of changes to the point where it seems to be 'ever-changing' and yet maintains the status quo. Partly, this is due to the gap between healthcare workers and guidance policies, where workers become instruments for the delivery of care according to centralised goals and duties, with increased responsibility and decreased autonomy; they are overworked, with excessive care and administrative loads. Consequently, dehumanisation takes place within this 'institutional dictatorship of productivity' (Trad and Rocha 2011, p.1970). What difference would it make to the direction (and realisation) of changes if we explored and built on what inspires and supports staff? Or, indeed, what if we listened to the voices of older people? In not actively engaging elders, allowing time and fully informed decisions, for their participation and autonomy to be exercised, they too are dehumanised, positioned as passive recipients of care and defined by reduced capacity, vulnerability and dependency, which results in diminished citizenship (Hughes and Castro Romero 2015). Further, despite well-meaning efforts, good practice (e.g. person-centred care and personalisation) and caring workers in NHS services for older people, dehumanisation persists as a consequence of political agendas borne out of economic criteria, which not only construct our 'ageing society' and elders as a 'challenge' and burden (Department of Health 2008), but fragment health care into highly specialised and divided services (Bermejo Higuera and Villacieros Durbán 2013).

Service structures

As we grow older, physical health and mental health problems frequently go hand in hand, but there is no true collaborative partnership between these services (e.g. Falls Clinic and CMHT) or even within mental health services. Structures[4] are set according to business models, which emphasise maximising profit and service priorities, such as managing discharge and waiting lists, and measure 'effectiveness' within functionalist and economic frameworks.

Structural discrimination

Health structures force people to fit within their priorities, and in the process they dehumanise both those who access services and those who work in them, not least because of the continued division between the service provider and elders seeking help. Workers are constructed as 'experts', and older people are most often constructed in 'patient' (passive) roles. According to Lindberg *et al.* (2013), many older people find that they 'surrender' their autonomy and freedom to the hands of the 'experts' (even when their study excluded elders who had a diagnosis of dementia, ill health or fatigue). This dehumanising process creates two tasks: making the person into a *patient* (i.e. surrender) and making the patient into a *person* again for successful living in the community. However, the need to become fully a person again is rarely achieved, partially because there is not enough done on the part of services and partially because of wider social conditions. Mental health services seldom discharge older people, even if they return home from hospital; instead, they remain under the care of the CMHT and/or a psychiatrist. What would happen if we worked to maintain personhood in the face of vulnerability or dependence? In some cases, elders are invited into euphemistic 'client' (consumer) roles; this is a market analogy presupposing agency and choice when, in reality, these interventions are limited to treatments approved by the National Institute for Health and Care Excellence (NICE)[5] (see the NHS Choices website).

Although introduced with the intention of providing more equal and improved services for older people and facilitating healthcare delivery for service providers, technicised care (i.e. manualised therapies) and the bureaucratisation of services (e.g. maintenance of both paper files and online systems) have progressively generated structures that are too complex and have become dehumanising (Bermejo Higuera and Villacieros Durbán 2013; Marin, Storniolo and Moravcik 2010). Following protocols or standardised procedures makes the elder an 'object' and the mental health professional a 'factory-line worker'. We all need to be seen and treated as unique individuals with particular contexts and needs; thus, 'treatment' cannot be mechanistic or manualised. The story of Mr Chowdhury and his wife illustrates the rigidity of current policy and politics.

Case study: Mr Chowdhury

Mr Chowdhury, an Asian man in his mid-eighties, has been more and more inactive, and his wife and four daughters had been so concerned that they contacted the GP, who made a referral to mental health services and prompted a hospital admission. After a brief review by the admitting psychiatrist, Mr Chowdhury is started on anti-depressant medication and a referral is made for psychological support. Anna, the psychologist, meets with Mr Chowdhury for an assessment and starts cognitive behavioural therapy, following service practice and nationwide guidelines for 'depression' (NICE 2009), but against her own clinical assessment. Mrs Chowdhury is in the ward every day during visiting hours, waiting for her husband when he is meeting with Anna or other professionals. The nurses feel her presence is not helping Mr Chowdhury to engage in ward activities and is somewhat 'getting in the way' of treatment – hence, they do not engage with her much to discourage her from spending so much time on the ward. After the eight sessions the service offers, despite lack of improvement according to Mr Chowdhury and his family, and minimal improvement shown on routine measuring scales, Anna is ending the work. In their last session, Mr Chowdhury tells her that he and his wife had never separated in the last 40 years of marriage, in fact, not since the birth of their last child. Mr Chowdhury then shares with Anna a family secret he has not told any professional before but wonders if it is related to how he is feeling: he has a son in prison for armed robbery. His son had become involved in drugs; at first he stole things from the family home to fund his addiction, but with time things got worse and they had lost him. Although Mr Chowdhury had been visiting his son every week, he no longer recognises the man facing him as the son he had raised. Family had been the most important thing in his life, but shame had destroyed them and all he has now is his marriage. Anna feels that ending at this time is not appropriate and consults with her supervisor about ways to continue working with Mr Chowdhury and his family, since they have established a good relationship and it has taken Mr Chowdhury eight sessions to trust her with this family secret. Her supervisor, however, decides that Mr Chowdhury needs to be referred for long-term psychodynamic psychotherapy, as their service offers a maximum of eight sessions.

- Think about the opportunities to respect Mr Chowdhury's values and ways of living, and Anna's professional expertise, such as around choice of therapeutic approach, involving Mrs Chowdhury, and referring Mr Chowdhury to another service at this point.

Structural inequality

Presently, elders are objectified through 'gross and multiple inequalities...captured within three interlinked contexts of oppression: historical, political and socio-economic' (Castro Romero 2016, p.129). The Mental Health Foundation (2009) identifies that inequity is reflected in lower quality and service provision for older people[6] in comparison to adults of working age; for example, there are no assertive outreach, crisis or early intervention teams. There is also a financial divide between the remunerated health workforce and older people, who often struggle to live on their retirement pension. Furthermore, pay differentials have always been very high within the NHS; in 2015 the top salary was 15 times greater than the lowest.[7] The Agenda for Change (Department of Health 2004) was introduced to minimise the gap, but it was thwarted from the very beginning by medics[8] and dentists opting out; most senior managers were also exempt from this equality exercise. Not taking into account these posts, there is still great structural inequality: non-medical consultants in the highest pay band get nearly seven times more than support workers at the bottom of the pay banding. Although this is currently under revision, doctors have been receiving an additional supplement of 20–50 per cent when working more than 40 hours a week and outside 7am–7pm Monday to Friday (Health Careers 2015). 'All members of the team are valued' (Department of Health 2008, p.59), yet the same does not apply to nurses or social workers.

Dehumanising practices

The apparent tyranny of technology, and of a mercantile (profit maximisation) approach to how services are run, places an emphasis on costs, risk and risk-management practices instead of the promotion of well-being (e.g. supporting reciprocal and trusting relationships), which would have a positive effect on health and longevity (Diener and Chan 2011). We must continue to ask questions when it comes to sanctioned practices (such as referring older people to a service without their knowledge or consent), for there are many practices in mental health services for older people that are distancing and dehumanising. I will discuss here the most central of these practices: the privileging of diagnostic practices that maintains a hierarchy within mental health teams and in relation to elders, with medical knowledge (and power) as superior to other professions and as holding the 'truth' about older people (Costa, Figeiredo and Schaurich 2009; Trad and Rocha 2011).

Although older people who come into contact with services hold their own life-long knowledges[9] and experiences, these are frequently discounted. I have continually heard the argument made that people who receive diagnoses often find them helpful. This may be true in some way: fears (e.g. of 'going mad') may be allayed; suffering may be legitimised (e.g. by 'high rates of depression'); personal responsibility may be lifted (by virtue of a biomedical explanation of a problem); and support may be made available (since diagnosis is necessary in order to be accepted by services). Nonetheless, diagnoses are problematic (Thomas 2014) as they are, at best, 'thin' descriptions of older people, their predicaments and their particular situations. Providing diagnoses is unlikely to promote elders' healing and personhood. Therefore, when we hear that some older people are relieved to hear that their problems can be explained by having a diagnosis such as 'bipolar disorder', we must inquire into the effects of labelling practices and of the labels:

- Are these practices promoting or maintaining unequal or equal relationships and social status?

- Are they limiting or enriching our understanding of what is going on for elders, and possible solutions?

- Are the labels hindering or facilitating elders' preferred identities or their ability to live by their values and principles?

These diagnostic practices attribute a meaning to elders' experiences that is disconnected from their lives and constructs them as defective and in need of care (more often than not for the rest of their lives), and this further stigmatises and dehumanises them. This is particularly clear around dementia diagnoses, which carry a sense of 'loss of self in life':

Case study: Maureen

Maureen, an Irish woman in her early nineties, is referred to the Memory Clinic for an assessment. She was not happy with the referral, commenting that it is only normal to forget things as one grows old. Nonetheless, Maureen accepts a series of tests for the sake of her family, on whom she has been dependent since becoming wheelchair-bound after a fall and hip-replacement two years earlier. There are no pre-diagnostic discussions or much thinking about the consent process with potential 'patients', since resources are limited and the service is focused on getting the population diagnosed as early as possible, with nursing follow up when service criteria are met. After completing physical (including blood tests and CT, computed tomography, scan), occupational and neuropsychological assessments, Maureen is taken to the clinic to be informed of the outcome of these assessments, although all along she had been telling professionals she was doing these for her family and she wished her family, and not herself, to be informed of the results. Maureen is placed in a wheelchair in the middle of the clinic room, with family and professionals (including medical students) all around her, as there are too many people around the room to make space for the wheelchair. The psychiatrist abruptly gives her a diagnosis of dementia of the Alzheimer's type and then tells her about medication, talking over Maureen, who is quite angrily saying through gritted teeth that she did not 'want to hear anything about the dementia word' and did not understand why it was necessary for her to be told. Some of the professionals in the room feel helpless about the situation because they do not feel empowered to intervene and in any case they do not want to undermine the psychiatrist's authority in front of his students, so they only approach Maureen to show some empathy outside the clinic room, after the psychiatrist concludes the session.

- Think about how the service might be able to fulfil its goal while placing Maureen (not the diagnostic process or her family) at the centre of the referral – what would have been the effects of doing this throughout – and how a non-hierarchical structure would affect the different points of the engagement.

It is fair to assume that people who choose to work in the social, health and care professions do so with a desire to make changes for the better, to at least alleviate, but hopefully also transform, the socio-economic conditions and suffering of fellow humans. To cease being oppressive and dehumanising, the structures that conform mental health services today need to be subordinated to the rights, needs and responsibilities of both the people who access them and the people who work in them. Therefore, as professionals we must become and be treated as actors (rather than instruments) in the care we provide, with elders who access services being protagonists (in leading roles) in their care (Castro Romero 2016; Santos Filho *et al.* 2009). This calls for a bottom-up approach, growing services from the grassroots without them becoming set and stagnant.

A humanising praxis for mental health

Humanisation is a concept with multiple (even contradictory) meanings, which must be left open to allow it to be collectively redefined in the interaction and intersection of healthcare activity, across all relationships, processes, practices and structures (Souza and Mendes 2009). Nonetheless, humanisation is not a fixed state but an active process in continuous movement and flow.[10] Therefore, humanising requires constant awareness and learning in a long-term commitment to joint praxis, because it is only together, in shared experience, that we can advance on the humanising path.

Humanising care is possible only when environmental, clinical, administrative and managerial structures are at the service of human beings, acknowledging, valuing and respecting all aspects of being human (Backes, Koerich and Erdmann 2007). Humanising mental health services for older people necessitates engaging with creative methods to bring individuals into relation, for the co-construction of unique solutions to transform local relationships, conditions and production systems (Brazil, Ministério da Saúde 2007). The Brazilian concept of the National Humanization Policy (2007) articulates methodologies and ethical principles that are inseparable and mutually interdependent, organically and collectively constructed in the intersection of knowledge, power and affectivity in services' everyday practices (Pasche 2009). Since humanising is possible only contextually and relationally, setting concrete rules to be followed would serve to dehumanise. There can be no expert perspective with instructions as to how to carry out the task of humanising, no possible manual for professionals, nor any policy that can enforce it. Instead, I propose some foundational ideas as departure points toward the humanising of services for older people, and I offer a narrative dissection of interrelated aspects for the purpose of examining this process. While I focus on elders and UK contexts, I keep in mind other populations and contexts; I am mindful that we are all part of the same humanity and broader world, despite plurality, differences and even conflicts of lesser or greater magnitude.

Ethical commitment

Bermejo Higuera and Villacieros Durbán (2013) point out that humanisation requires a commitment to the transformation of management, structures, dominant ideologies, training and com-petencies, as well as a focus on preventative care. Further, humanising mental health contexts requires an ethical-political commitment to considering elders in their total humanity, and to the co-construction of contextualised, holistic responses, with the following principles guiding the process.

Integrality

Humanising involves understanding and valuing the full complexity of elders' realities; it 'means bringing back the respect for human life, taking into consideration social, ethical, educational, and psychological circumstances present in every relationship' (Gonçalves Brito and Carvalho 2010, p.222). Mattos (2009) suggests that integrality, with intersubjectivity and dialogue at its centre, must guide all health practices to act as a counter-practice to generalised, reductionist and harming (dehumanising) practices. This calls for multi-professional and multi-level co-ordinated responses via integrated services. Further, the integrity of healthcare staff is also called forth, which means being fully human in our relations with others, opening ourselves to the other person; this was previously referred to as '*true* dialogue', which involves engaging the heart or loving (Castro Romero and Afuape 2016). In recognising and valuing the dialogue between our self and the older person as an 'I and I' encounter, we can go beyond presenting needs and problems in order to mobilise older people's skills and knowledge to confront their predicaments in life together.

Solidarity

This *siding with* demands sensitivity, availability and responsiveness to the other (Gonçalves Brito and Carvalho 2010), challenging ideas about what 'professionalism' means. One such idea is 'boundaries', a reminder of our separateness and disconnection, which dilutes the complexities of relationships in general (around gender, ethnicity, age, etc.) and caring or therapeutic relationships in particular (because of magnified power differentials between caregiver and receiver). Instead, Combs and Freedman (2002) propose a focus on 'ethical relationships', acknowledging both complexities and our interconnectedness. In solidarity, professionals allow themselves to be human, to emotionally connect and be moved in the therapeutic or caring relationship (Backes *et al.* 2007). To become solidary[11] requires us to see elders as equal fellow human beings and to accompany them in becoming more fully human as they actively construct their future and contribute to their communities.

Equality

If the health of nations (i.e. the macro level) is directly correlated to equality (Wilkinson and Pickett 2010), equality will also make for better functioning systems (the meso level) and healthier interpersonal relationships and subjectivities (the micro level). Seeing and treating older people as fully human requires mental healthcare professionals and the elders who seek their help to be equal partners in the process of humanising health care, because

> for elders to have a real position of leadership, not only a willingness to lose one's own professional power but a desire to do so is required, and in doing so we (re)gain the greatest power of all, of humanising ourselves alongside others. (Castro Romero 2016, p.136)

This change in power relations will redefine the spaces and positions in care production, breaking from previous constructions of subjectivities and knowledge and humanising power/knowledge through shared construction of knowledge/power (Foucault 1980). However, to 'take on a new perspective obviously does not mean throwing out all of our knowledge; what it supposes, rather, is that we will relativize that knowledge and critically revise it from the perspective of the popular majorities' (Martín-Baró 1994, p.28) or, in the context of this chapter, that we will critically revise our knowledge from the perspective of older people.

Participation

The natural step that would follow on from the previous principles would be the participation of older people as active subjects in the operational processes and management structures of care production. Indeed, Ceccim and Merhy (2009) have defined participation as 'indissociable from care and management' (p.531) and, in turn, participatory management develops and enhances solidarity in the relationships between professionals and elders (Backes *et al.* 2007). In this way:

> Care becomes a shared outcome between the caregiver and care receiver. This element of personal control is fundamental to the reform of social care systems, particularly for those who are most dependent: people with disabilities, the poor and the marginalized. (Restakis 2010, p.107)

Participation would also mean the involvement and inclusion of networks and social movements as a collective commitment (maintaining the plurality of interests and needs), and would therefore be more able to effect the necessary changes and sustain them (Pasche 2009).

Reciprocity

A true openness to participation not only implies a change in power relations between subjects, but generates the relationships and spaces to manage conflict and differences for long-term sustainability, where the traditional distinction between caregivers and receivers would be blurred. The establishment of bonds in relationships of mutual trust, accountability, respect and appreciation creates the necessary context for workers and elders who access mental health teams or services to become active agents in management and care co-production and co-responsibility, including associated costs (Pasche 2009). While there may be an initial demand in the construction of new subjects and collective spaces for care co-production, concern around increased burden would be minimised by reciprocal relationships – because burden appears in the context of unequal relationships. When we stop seeing ourselves as responsible for others, and see ourselves instead as co-responsible in the relationship we create together (which is then full of potential and teachings for us), we can engage in mutual relationships. There would be a need for support and supervision to maintain a reflexivity that centres elders in working together toward a common ground.

New horizons for mental health contexts

Until we begin to humanise the contexts we have been employing to 'hold' *madness* or mental health problems, we cannot construct alternatives, for these will organically come out of the humanising process. Through this process, which requires iterative reflection on the organisational and social relational contexts (Backes *et al.* 2007), organisational culture is repopulated and transformed. Autonomy and leadership are ethically guided and co-produced in reciprocal relationships (Pasche 2009). An example of how this may look in practice would be establishing an ethics board composed of older people and their relatives (in paid roles), as a counter-practice to business priorities and the privileging of professional knowledge, with a feedback system and a built-in method for checking the implementation of feedback (this has started to be implemented in some NHS mental health services).

Alternative models must 'abandon medical language when talking about emotional distress and disturbing behaviour' (Boyle 2006, p.192) in favour of jointly making sense of these in the contexts of older people's lives and utilising language according to the preference of elders (Castro Romero 2016). Learning from older people about the meaning they give to their past and current stage of life through storytelling allows sense-making, uniqueness and togetherness, and continuity of identity and community (Mota, Reginato and Gallian 2013). However, for storytelling to be a humanising methodology, professionals must invite equal relationships, be influential in asking questions that will open possibilities for healing while maintaining the elder at the centre of the telling (White 2000), and utilise practices that help this process. Such practices involve outsider witnessing (which invites reciprocity through the recognition of the inspiration and learning we derive from joint meaning-making), checking (e.g. of our understanding, that the direction of the story is that preferred by the elder) and transparency (Roberts 2005).

An ethical commitment to humanising can be put into practice in setting the context (e.g. personal and collective dimensions, pre-understandings, who is asking for what) to respond to invitations to engage (as often elders are unaware that they have been referred), before meetings (which will set the tone for any future engagement), for the development of the relationship, and for ongoing critical reflexivity (Fredman, Anderson and Stott 2010). It also creates the space to respect the multiple truths, needs and interests of elders and their family members, which can be conflictual (Denson, Winefield and Beilby 2012). The case study of Helena and her family frames extensively established practices in mental health services for older people.

Case study: Helena

Helena, a Greek woman in her early seventies, is married to Georgios, who is in his late seventies. They have two sons; one lives in Greece with his family (Niko), and another in London, near the parents' home (Andreas). Because of his father's diagnosis of vascular dementia, Andreas is the next of kin. Helena has become very low and forgetful so that taking care of her home and husband has become more and more difficult and she is admitted to a Dementia Unit for assessment whilst her husband is supported at home with a care package. She makes it clear she wants to be at home with her husband and not in the unit, but she is not allowed to go home, so she stops talking or even making eye contact and sits all day staring at the floor. Helena is not under a Mental Health Act Section, nor detained following a Capacity Act assessment, but is kept in the unit for her safety because she has a *likely* diagnosis of Alzheimer's Disease. After a month with no progress despite medication, the team start to plan for a care home placement for her, in consultation with Andreas. He expresses his parents' wish to be together at home supported by Social Services, as he cannot provide the level of attention they need. The doctor explains that due to his mother's diagnosis things will only get worse, so it is a matter of time for his mother to go into care. Andreas informs his mother that she has been allocated a social worker, who is looking for a home for her to move to, and Helena looks at him and cries silently. A nurse observes the interaction and hands it over to the team; Helena's antidepressant medication is increased the next day. When Niko is informed by his brother of the future plans for their mother and her reaction to these, he takes a flight to be present for the forthcoming Care Planning meeting. At the meeting, neither Helena nor Georgios are present; the psychiatrist had considered that it would be too distressing for them because they would not be able to fully understand the discussion. Niko is very vocal in the meeting and states that he wants his mother back home with his father; there is a discussion, however, because it would be Andreas who would be supporting them since Niko lives abroad. Given the insistence of Niko, it is agreed that the occupational therapist (OT) will do an assessment of Activities of Daily Living at the family home, to gather more evidence for the inevitable moving of Helena to a care home. To the surprise of the OT, Helena seems to come to life during the home assessment, showing very good skills in managing kitchen appliances, remembering where things are kept, and looking after her husband and even the OT (offering and making them cups of tea and toast). This is fed back to the team at the following ward-round, although the psychiatrist and social worker still feel it is in Helena's best interest to move her now rather than a few months down the line; they make plans for a homecare package for Helena and Georgios.

- Think about the practices you identify as dehumanising and possible humanising alternatives. What are the turning points in Helena's story and what allowed these to result in Helena and her husband's preferred option?

Older people's citizenship

Older people's ascribed identities often limit their freedom to be full participants, and co-creators, of social life. Insofar as this is the case, they are not allowed full citizenship. Further, older people in the UK do not often shape the currently dominant values and culture, which are more or less explicitly 'anti-age/ing' (e.g. the pursuit of a youthful appearance), but older people are, nonetheless, being shaped by these values. So what does that do to elders' self-concepts? They are constructed as intrinsically 'defective' citizens by virtue of ageist (and Eurocentric) ideals of citizen self-governmentality in which citizens are active and engaged, independent and autonomous (Conway and Crawshaw 2009), roles which many older people will 'fail to perform' at some point or other. Indeed, Conway and Crawshaw (2009) question how possible it is for older people to achieve these cultural ideals when ill health, frailty or dependency may be part of their realities; alternatively, activity and independence may not be their preference even when they are given a choice. For example, the general social valuing of activity over idleness leads to engagement in leisure activities when not at work, but what would 'ageing well' look like from the perspective of older people if they could critically examine this?

Older people are in a paradoxical position in which they are made both responsible for their own health and passive objects of health systems. They are told they have choice, but choice is limited to what is deemed appropriate by experts; they are told they must participate in an active, healthy lifestyle, but they are not afforded the same socio-economic opportunities as younger adults (because of a fixed retirement age) to allow lifestyle options. And in any case, keeping an active lifestyle may not be possible because of physical health problems or it may not be the preferred way of being for some elders, who may feel they have worked hard enough all their life and deserve rest and care. All of these failings in relation to older citizens' self-governmentality are more visible when compounded by mental health problems, with the case of dementia diagnoses erasing citizenship (Brannelly 2011).

Older people's citizenship 'is actually recovered through authenticity, dignity, solidarity, affect and respect for human individuality' (Backes *et al.* 2007, p.35). The respect of elders' rights goes hand in hand with the promotion of their citizenship, which is foundational in all humanising action (Castro Romero 2016).

Thus, through humanisation older people are restored in their right to be active participants in their community, to enjoy close affective relationships and to freely choose their life path. This involves the participation and development of relational systems, with families and broader systems, including the system of care and social-environmental aspects (Bermejo 1999). Further, Pasche (2009) highlights that in order to enhance elder citizenship, the participation of elders in public life must include collective action in public health.

Concluding reflections

Humanisation is a social task; only by humanising all of society can its members be truly humanised and vice versa. This inevitably transforms the world, as humanisation involves fully being in the world, with an awareness of our capacity to be transformative actors, to co-create our realities (Freire 1972). Thus, through humanising praxis (cyclical critical reflection and action) professionals and older people who access mental health services humanise one another and their local services together, departing from their own skills and knowledges. Professional, individual and cultural knowledges become resources for the co-production of health. This will mean that services look very different in diverse parts of the UK, responding to local needs, but also that they will be constantly evolving as the population they serve changes and grows (presenting with different needs). Our constant flexibility to relate to people as individuals and to be inclusive may be more demanding initially as it requires radical change across all levels and structures. However, at the same time, it is more fulfilling and energising to be called to be fully human in healthcare relationships with other human beings, which in turn generates both humanised and humanising practices (Backes *et al.* 2007).

A research focus on humanisation is required (Todres *et al.* 2009), utilising humanising research methodologies. We also need to move beyond limitations in evaluating the prevention of pain or suffering, or the recovery of capacity and well-being, with currently valued outcome measures (Bermejo Higuera and Villacieros Durbán 2013). Given the immeasurability of health promotion and prevention (i.e. measuring what did not happen that would have happened), we need to develop new and integral methodologies based on our knowledge of the effects of dehumanisation; for example, ongoing dialogue and joint reflection.

Pragmatically, I must end the chapter, but there cannot be a conclusion, as humanising is a continuous call for justice, a social praxis towards equity. A better world is possible, but socially valuing elders, and elders equally valuing themselves, is central to the construction of 'a more equal, more just, more peaceful, more joyous and healthy world' (Bermejo Higuera and Villacieros Durbán 2013).

References

Backes, D.S., Koerich, M.S. and Erdmann, A.L. (2007) 'Humanizing care through the valuation of the human being: Resignification of values and principles by health professionals.' *Revista Latino-Americana de Enfermagem 15*, 1, 34–41.

Bermejo, J.C. (1999) *Humanizar los cuidados en la relación con el enfermo de Alzheimer* (Humanising care in the relationship with people with Alzheimers). *Jornadas sobre la ancianidad: El Alzheimer*. Palencia 25 Mayo. Available at http://envejecimiento.csic.es/documentos/documentos/bermejo-humanizar-01.pdf, accessed on 15 December 2014.

Bermejo Higuera, J.C. and Villacieros Durbán, M. (2013) *El compromiso de la humanización en las instituciones sociosanitarias* (The commitment to humanisation in social and health institutions). Available at http://josecarlosbermejo.es/articulos/el-compromiso-de-la-humanizacion-en-las-instituciones-sociosanitarias, accessed on 15 December 2014.

Boyle, M. (2006) 'Developing real alternatives to medical models.' *Ethical Human Psychology and Psychiatry 8*, 191–200.

Brannelly, T. (2011) 'Sustaining citizenship: People with dementia and the phenomenon of social death.' *Nursing Ethics 18*, 5, 662–671.

Brazil, Ministério da Saúde (2007) *Secretaria de Atenção à Saúde. Núcleo Técnico da Política Nacional de Humanização. Humaniza SUS: documento base para gestores e trabalhadores do SUS* (Secretariat of Health Care. Technical Center of the National Humanization Policy. Humanize SUS: base document for managers and workers). 4th ed. Brasília: Editora do Ministério da Saúde.

Castro, M. (2015) 'Teaching Ethics for Professional Practice.' In R. Tribe and J. Morrissey (eds) *Handbook of Professional and Ethical Practice for Psychologists, Counsellors and Psychotherapists*. London and New York: Brunner-Routledge.

Castro Romero, M. (2016) 'Liberatory Praxis Alongside Elders.' In G. Hughes and T. Afuape (eds) *Towards Emotional Well-being Through Liberation Practices: A Dialogical Approach*. London: Routledge.

Castro Romero, M. and Afuape, T. (2016) 'Teaching Liberation Psychology.' In G. Hughes and T. Afuape (eds) *Towards Emotional Well-being Through Liberation Practices: A Dialogical Approach*. London: Routledge.

Ceccim, R.B. and Merhy, E.E. (2009) 'Um agir micropolítico e pedagógico intenso: a humanização entre laços e perspectivas' (An intense micropolitical and pedagogical action: humanization between bonds and perspectives). *Comunicação Saúde Educação 13*, 1, 532–542.

Combs, G. and Freedman, J. (2002) 'Relationships, not boundaries.' *Theoretical Medicine 23*, 203–217.

Commission on Improving Dignity in Care (2012) *Partnership on Dignity in Care*. Available at http://www.nhsconfed.org/~/media/Confederation/Files/Publications/Documents/Delivering_Dignity_final_report150612.pdf, accessed 19 January 2017.

Conway, S. (2003) 'Ageing and imagined community: Some cultural constructions and reconstructions.' *Sociological Research Online 8*, 2. Available at www.socresonline.org.uk/8/2/conway.html, accessed on 17 February 2015.

Conway, S. and Crawshaw, P. (2009) '"Healthy Senior Citizenship" in voluntary and community organisations: A study in governmentality.' *Health Sociology Review 18*, 387–398.

Costa, S.C., Figeiredo, M.R.B. and Schaurich, D. (2009) 'Humanização em Unidade de Terapia Intensiva Adulto (UTI): Compreensões da equipe de enfermagem' (Humanization within an adult intensive care unit (ICU): Understandings among the nursing staff). *Comunicação Saúde Educação 13*, 1, 571–580.

Denson, L.A., Winefield, H.R. and Beilby, J.J. (2012) 'Discharge-planning for long-term care needs: The values and priorities of older people, their younger relatives and health professionals.' *Scandinavian Journal of Caring Sciences 27*, 1, 3–12. doi:10.1111/j.1471-6712.2012.00987.

Department of Health (2004) *Agenda for Change: Final Agreement.* Norwich: DoH.

Department of Health (2008) *High Quality Care for All.* Norwich: DoH.

Department of Health (2012) *Liberating the NHS: No Decision About Me Without Me.* Norwich: DoH.

Diener, E. and Chan, M.Y. (2011) 'Happy people live longer: Subjective well-being contributes to health and longevity.' *Applied Psychology: Health and Well-Being 3*, 1, 1–43. doi:10.1111/j.1758-0854.2010.01045.x

Foucault, M. (1980) *Power/Knowledge: Selected Interviews and Other Writings 1972–1977.* London, Harvester Press.

Fredman, G., Anderson, E. and Stott, J. (2010) *Being with Older People: A Systemic Approach.* London: Karnac Books.

Freire, P. (1972) *Pedagogy of the Oppressed.* Harmondsworth: Penguin.

Gonçalves Brito, N.T. and Carvalho, R. (2010) 'A humanização segundo pacientes oncológicos com longo período de internação' (Humanization according to cancer patients with extended hospitalization periods). *Einstein 8*, 2, 221–227.

Health Careers (2015) *Pay for Doctors.* Available at http://www.healthcareers.nhs.uk/about/careers-medicine/pay-doctors, accessed on 16 April 2015.

Hughes, T. and Castro Romero, M. (2015) 'A processural consent methodology with people diagnosed with dementia.' *Quality in Ageing and Older Adults 16*, 4, 222–234.

Lindberg, E., Hörberg, U., Persson, E. and Ekebergh, M. (2013) '"It made me feel human" – a phenomenological study of older patients' experiences of participating in a team meeting.' *International Journal on Qualitative Studies on Health and Well-being 8*, 20714.

Marin, M.J.S., Storniolo, L.V. and Moravcik, M.Y. (2010) 'Humanization of care from the perspective of the family health strategy teams in a city in the interior of São Paulo, Brazil.' *Revista Latino-Americana de Enfermagem 18*, 4, 7634–7639.

Martín-Baró, I. (1994) *Writings for a Liberation Psychology.* Cambridge, MA: Harvard University Press.

Mattos, R.A. (2009) 'Princípios do Sistema Único de Saúde (SUS) e a humanização das práticas de saúde' (Principles of the Unified Health System (SUS) and the humanization of health practices). *Comunicação Saúde Educação 13*, 1, 771–780.

Mental Health Foundation (2009) *All Things Being Equal: Age Equality in Mental Health Care for Older People in England.* London: Mental Health Foundation.

Mental Health Strategies (2012) *2011/12 National Survey of Investment in Mental Health Services for Older People.* Available at www.gov.uk/government/uploads/system/uploads/attachment_data/file/140099/Finance-Mapping-20112-OPMHS-Nat-Report-03082012.pdf, accessed on 25 November 2014.

Mota, C.S., Reginato, V. and Gallian, D.M.C. (2013) 'A metodologia da história oral de vida como estratégia humanizadora de aproximação entre cuidador/idoso' (Oral life history as a humanistic strategy for the approach between caregivers and the elderly). *Cadernos de Saúde Pública 29*, 8, 1681–1684.

Pasche, D.F. (2009) 'Política Nacional de Humanização como aposta na produção coletiva de mudanças nos modos de gerir e cuidar' (National Humanization Policy as option for collective production of changes in the modes of management and care). *Comunicação Saúde Educação 13*, 1, 701–708.

Restakis, J. (2010) *Humanizing the Economy: Co-operatives in the Age of Capital.* Gabriola Island: New Society Publishers.

Roberts, J. (2005) 'Transparency and self-disclosure in family therapy: Dangers and possibilities.' *Family Process 44*, 45–63.

Santos Filho, S.B., Barros, M.E.B. and Gomes, R.S. (2009) 'A Política Nacional de Humanização como política que se faz no processo de trabalho em saúde.' 'The national humanization policy as a policy produced within the healthcare labor process.' *Comunicação Saúde Educação 13*, 1, 603–613.

Souza, L.A.P. and Mendes, V.L.F. (2009) 'O conceito de humanização na Política Nacional de Humanização (PNH)' (The concept of humanization in the National Humanization Policy (PHN)). *Comunicação Saúde Educação 13*, 1, 681–688.

Thomas, P. (2014) *Psychiatry in Context: Experience, Meaning and Communities.* Ross-on-Wye: PCCS Books.

Todres, L., Galvin, K.T. and Holloway, I. (2009) 'The humanization of healthcare: A value framework for qualitative research.' *International Journal on Qualitative Studies on Health and Well-being 4,* 68–77.

Trad, A.A.B. and Rocha, A.A.R.M. (2011) 'Conditions and work process in the daily of the Family Health Program: Coherency with health humanization principles.' *Ciência & Saúde Coletiva 16,* 3, 1969–1980.

White, M. (2000) *Reflections on Narrative Practice.* Adelaide: Dulwich Centre Publications.

Wilkinson, R.G. and Pickett, K.E. (2010) *The Spirit Level: Why Equality is Better for Everyone.* London: Allen Lane.

CHAPTER 3

Ageing, Ethnicity and Mental Health

Rachel Tribe

Introduction

The number of people in the UK aged over 75 has increased by 89 per cent since 1974, and this age group currently makes up 8 per cent of the population (Office for National Statistics 2015). Approximately 8 per cent of the Black, Asian and Minority Ethnic (BAME) community in the UK are classified as older adults, and this translates to approximately 500,000 older BAME residents in the UK, based on the 2001 census data (PRIAE 2010). This chapter considers issues relating to mental health, ageing and ethnicity. The construction of ageing and mental health and well-being in different cultures will be briefly discussed, while issues of marginalisation and discrimination including indirect discrimination will be reviewed. Finally, issues relating to accessing services and developing appropriate services for BAME older adults with mental health issues will be considered. Some key messages will be presented, which may contribute to anti discriminatory thinking and practice being further developed in this area.

Older adults, culture and identity

Everyone has a personal culture which will be determined by a range of variables including, but not limited to, ethnicity, religion, experiences of life, family background, individual and community values, and meaning-making methods. All individuals are affected by aspects of 'their' personal culture. In addition, the cultural identity an individual develops or selects is multi-layered, often supple and may be influenced throughout life by events and experiences. There has been an unfortunate tendency within psychiatry and psychology in high-income countries to define culture by skin colour, ethnicity or 'difference' from a dominant group (Fernando 2014). This frequently carries racist undertones, involves practices including conscious and unconscious biases, and may replicate or continue discriminatory practices and views (Tribe and Tunariu 2017). There has also been a tendency to essentialise culture, rather than seeing it as dynamic and fluid. The culture of the health or social care practitioner is frequently conveniently forgotten or seen as culturally neutral, which it can never be (Tribe and Tunariu 2017). This is in addition to the mental health or social care context within which the meeting or consultation is situated, where a professional and organisational culture will also be present. The power of the dominant culture was assumed to be the White, Western (Sashidharan 2001; Tribe 2007) and often male perspective within the wider society and mainstream psychiatry and psychology (Patel *et al.* 2000). These cultural perspectives will all intersect in the mental health encounter. Research suggests that culture in the broadest definition may in part define how people construct mental health and illness in terms of causation, help-seeking, 'treatment' options and recovery (Bhugra and Gupta 2011; Bhui 2013).

Health and social care professionals need to guard against stereotyping, 'essentialising' culture or assuming that someone with a particular heritage will make certain choices or hold particular views. Some health and social care professionals fail to adequately consider issues of culture, diversity, ageing and the needs of the whole person in their work (Fernando 2014) and do not consider anti-discriminatory practice to be an essential part of practice within the service they provide. This may mean that BAME older adults with mental health issues do not receive the best and most appropriate service and their needs may not be adequately met. Staff may also lack training and understanding of the significance of culture and mental health or knowledge of how to provide culturally competent or sensitive services (Bhui 2013; Livingston and Sembhi 2003). This may have serious implications for BAME older adults with mental health issues. In addition, people from BAME families often experience problems accessing mental health services (Patel 2003). Therefore, there is a complex set of issues which need to be addressed to ensure that ethnicity, age and mental health are dealt with properly and that anti-discriminatory practice is upheld. This might go some way to ensuring that all members of our community receive the best and most appropriate health and social care services should they require them.

Anti-discriminatory practice would mean that practitioners are well informed, culturally competent and prepared to work with all issues of diversity that arise in their work. In addition, services should be appropriately commissioned and organised to encourage usage by everyone, including BAME older adults with mental health concerns. This chapter focuses on the spectrum running from well-being through to mental ill health, not exclusively on the latter. The definition of BAME communities is very broad, encompassing everyone from newly arrived asylum seekers right through to third- or fourth-generation British nationals with heritage links to other countries.

Case study: Mr Mohammed

The staff at the residential home where Mr Mohammed had recently moved for a short respite stay decided that Mr Mohammed had cognitive impairments and were about to refer him for a specialist assessment. This was because his replies to their standard written questions did not seem to relate to what they were asking him. It was not until his daughter told them that he had not had the opportunity to become fluent in written English that they realised that this was the reason for the breakdown in communication. Had they talked to Mr Mohammed before presenting him with the questions, or considered his life story, this might have become apparent.

The construction of ageing in different cultures

The very process of ageing brings with it many psychological dilemmas and some challenges, including thinking about end of life issues, reviewing life and achievements, and on occasions reflecting on choices made and opportunities taken or not taken. Older adults may experience physical, practical and often related psychological changes. These include retirement, changes in family roles, and often cognitive and physical changes, which may mean that tasks which could be completed in the past now take longer or are more difficult than they had been previously. For many older people these can impact upon their sense of self and well-being and can heighten distress and feelings of uncertainty, worthlessness and loss (World Health Organization 2016). Furthermore, people age at a variety of different rates (known as 'differentiate ageing'), and this can lead to drawing comparisons and experiencing feelings of uncertainty or unfairness (Age UK 2016). Social factors including, but not limited to, changes in circumstances, an increased likelihood of experiencing bereavement, a decrease in economic status, and physical frailty may lead to a loss of independence and decision-making for older adults (Woolfe 1998). Ageing is culturally and socially constructed, and anti-discriminatory practice would require that service users' views and experiences be openly discussed, and that assumptions not be made about how ageing is viewed by an individual, as well as his or her family or carers, but that this concept should be actively explored and considered.

Expectations about age-appropriate behaviour and roles differ greatly. Gawande (2014) compares attitudes and expectations regarding ageing in India and the USA, noting that in India, life goes on much as usual, while in the USA (and many other Western countries) once someone cannot complete the tasks associated with independent living they are seen as being 'at risk' and in need of social care and health interventions. Gawande details how the issue of risk tends to predominate in the USA (and probably other Western societies) and leads to what might be described as the infantalisation of older adults. In addition, the over-medicalisation of the natural ageing process can lead to medical interventions which may not ultimately be in the patient's best interests. Gawande argues that the underlying reasons for this are frequently related to the healthcare staff and service users having unresolved anxieties and fear about death. Perhaps the major message from his work is not to be afraid of having conversations with service users and their families around end of life and death, and the associated anxieties and worries. By avoiding this and hiding behind an expert role, practitioners may inadvertently make these discussions harder to have.

In Uganda, there are several cultural practices that promote the role of older adults and anti-discriminatory practices. For example, among the Baganda group, older people are considered to be custodians of clan and family blessings. They must be contacted or consulted before any decision is taken. This happens at naming ceremonies, at weddings, during funeral rites and at other important events (Mayengo 2016).

Case study: Zubin

Zubin worked in and then ran the family business for all his working life, and he expected always to do so until the day when he felt ready to give up, as his father and grandmother had done before him. He recently had some minor health worries and was advised that he should give up work and rest, as his British GP felt this would be better for his well-being and would minimise any potential health risks. Zubin feels that not to work would be detrimental to his well-being and health, and that if he stops working he might as well 'turn his face to the wall' and stop living. How might you work with Zubin and this dilemma while ensuring that anti-discriminatory practice is upheld?

Ageism within many Western societies can mean that older adults are treated with less respect or are ignored, or that assumptions are made about them and their potential, all of which can lead to a range of difficult emotions for an older person. A change in assumption as to what they are capable of may give rise to feelings and thoughts of surprise, change, reflection, grief, loss, hurt and shock. Ageism and age discrimination are prevalent in many Western societies in a range of contexts and form the backdrop to many older adults' experiences. The Royal College of Psychiatrists (RCP) has stated:

> Age discrimination is now more pronounced in mental health services than in other areas of healthcare…[T]he principles of age-appropriate, non-discriminatory services still appear to be misunderstood by services and commissioners, in particular, the issues of indirect discrimination and age appropriateness. (Anderson 2011, p.2)

This finding was confirmed by work undertaken through the Department of Health both in terms of health (Beecham *et al.* 2008) and also social care (Forder 2008). Older BAME people may therefore find not only that they are dealing with the ageing process but that they are subject to ageism and possibly racism, in addition to potentially experiencing stigma about their mental health status. In addition, the very mental health and social care services that should provide help have been found to discriminate on the basis of age.

Marginalisation, discrimination and social exclusion

Many adults from BAME communities have had to deal with issues of direct individual and institutional racism and discrimination as well as possible marginalisation throughout their lives, and they may therefore have additional health or care needs due to disadvantaged life circumstances (Chakraborty and McKenzie 2002; Fernando 2014). If families have migrated, there may be additional pressures in terms of establishing new lives, and there are often different levels of adaptation and views of belonging across generations (Berry *et al.* 1987). There may be issues relating to where is considered 'home' and possibly issues of displacement, which sometimes become more potent in older age (Walsh and Nare 2016). Older adults from BAME communities are identified by numerous sources as being particularly at risk from social exclusion and poverty (Bowes 2006). The Health Survey for England 2005 found that there was substantial social isolation among older people in England, with 18 per cent of older men and 11 per cent of older women acknowledging a lack of social support from friends or family (Craig and Mindell 2005). Loneliness and feelings of isolation and marginalisation are reported by many older adults (World Health Organization 2016). Age UK Buckinghamshire (2016) states that in the UK in excess of '1 million older people haven't spoken to a friend, neighbour or family member for at least a month'. The charity has launched a campaign to tackle loneliness and now offers a befriending service. However, it is possible that the real numbers are higher, as some people may not feel comfortable admitting this. People from BAME communities (particularly recent migrants or refugees) may not have family members around to support them or have the social capital which some other older adults may have (Carr 2014).

The important role of social support is well documented within mental health and in relation to older adults. A variety of studies have noted the importance of social networks in enhancing mental well-being and even acting as a potential mediating factor in mental distress and ill health, particularly in relation to depression in older adults (Cornwell and Waite 2009; Fiori, Antonicci and Cortina 2006; Litwin 2001). Loneliness and lack of support networks have been found to be detrimental to good mental health. Age Concern and the Mental Health Foundation (2006) identified five key factors which affect the well-being of older adults: discrimination, participation in meaningful activities, relationships and social support, physical health, and poverty. Some BAME older adults may be more at risk of being isolated due to racism, lack of familiarity with services, different cultural constructions and marginalisation. Religious faith can be a considerable source of support and social capital. It may be helpful to encourage people to talk about their faith and beliefs, even if this is something that a practitioner initially feels uncomfortable with. Kaplan and Berkman (2016) noted in the USA that religion and religious community was the largest form of social support for older adults outside their family.

Around two-fifths of people in low-income households come from BAME communities (The Poverty Site 2013). Older people from BAME groups are more likely to be socially excluded than White older adults, and are also more likely to face additional discrimination, especially in relation to income, housing, health, access to services and racial prejudice (Patel 2003). This may mean that older adults from BAME communities are exposed to a range of factors which are not conducive to good mental health and well-being.

These difficulties may be compounded in older age by racism being encountered in conjunction with age discrimination as well as discrimination on mental health grounds, resulting in a 'triple jeopardy' situation for some BAME older adults. The issue of intersectionality where different forms of discrimination interact will be detailed later in this chapter. There may therefore be a number of challenges to a sense of well-being and good mental health for BAME older adults (Cohen and Ahmed 2011).

Discrimination may have influenced the uptake of mental health services by older adults. Goudie (2003) notes that older people are under-represented on the case loads of psychologists and counsellors. In addition, the number of older adults from BAME communities presenting within old-age psychiatry services is reported to be small (Rait and Burns 1997; Shah and Dighe-Deo 1998). Other factors in the low uptake of services may include the resilience of many older adults and the fact that accessing psychological and mental health services is not in many older adults' help-seeking repertoire. Within British society, the concept of discussing feelings with a stranger is a relatively new concept, and the notion of the stiff upper lip was often part of the dominant discourse for older adults. (An international study noted that this cultural phenomenon may actually mean that fewer people seek medical help compared to people in countries with different cultural norms; Forbes *et al.* 2013.) The Improving Access to Psychological Therapies (IAPT) (2009) report on older people states that older adults may 'believe that mental health problems are shameful and should be hidden from everyone, including…health professionals' (p.6). In addition, some of the oldest members of our communities will have lived through war and rationing, and may have been conditioned by a 'coping' discourse whereby showing emotion or requiring help with regard to 'feelings' is a sign of weakness or a 'lack of moral fibre'. Many older adults have shown immense resilience throughout their lives, having lived through difficult times and having experienced and successfully negotiated many difficulties (Centre for Policy on Ageing 2014). Research suggests that resilience does not decline with age and so older adults are just as resilient as younger people (Gooding *et al.* 2012).

Furthermore, mental health services may not be or appear to be appropriate or accessible to older adults for a host of reasons, and this may particularly be the case for older adults from BAME communities. As Shah (2008) writes, 'A multi-faceted approach is needed to ensure that commissioning, design, development and delivery of culturally capable, appropriate and sensitive old age psychiatry actually occurs and improves the equity of service access by BAME older adults' (Shah 2008, p.13).

Therefore, it seems that BAME older adults have a lot of factors and changes to contend with, since most of the factors discussed above will be detrimental to positive well-being and good mental health. The job of practitioners and policymakers is to ensure that we strive to deliver services that are appropriate and accessible for all older adults. These services must promote good mental health; take account of the whole person; foreground the individual and his or her specific individual needs and dignity; aim to maintain independence; and actively uphold anti-discriminatory practice.

Most older adults report living rich and meaningful lives and have good mental health (IAPT 2009; World Health Organization 2016). Despite this, much of the research literature within BAME older adults' mental health emphasises vulnerability and the difficulties that older adults face, giving little attention or prominence to the resiliency of older adults. Many BAME older adults, including many of those living with long-term debilitating illness such as dementia, are able to be engaged with life and to make a positive contribution to society. As practitioners, it is easy to fall back on a 'problems' approach to needs assessment and service delivery, but embracing a holistic approach that takes into account the older adult's personal history and inner resources and that supports anti-discriminatory practice may be a more helpful way forward. For example, reminiscence and life-review therapies are techniques specifically designed for use with older people, helping individuals to achieve a sense of integration through looking back over their lives and integrating memories. Watt and Cappeliez (2000) tested two types of reminiscence therapy which integrate cognitive approaches and found that the interventions led to significant improvements among depressed older adults. In addition, it may be possible to share these personal histories (with the older adult's permission) with local school children, enhancing the children's understanding of the life span, diversity, cultural heritage and personal history and valuing the experiences of older adults.

Case study: Amma

Amma worked for 36 years as a social worker in an inner-city borough, developing a wealth of experience and knowledge. She is now a user of services, but has found that rather than staff asking her about her skills, resources, experience of coping and negotiating multiple challenges, and knowledge, they just treat her as a passive recipient of services with a series of 'problems'. They have not asked her about her working or earlier life and have instead made a range of recommendations for her to follow, most of which she knows are just not realistic. One worker has told her that she knows that Amma's community 'looks after its own well', but in reality Amma is very isolated and has no family living locally. She believes that she is a victim of racism, ageism and stereotyping, but she does not want to make a complaint as she 'knows how stretched workers are'.

Ageing, mental health and indirect discrimination

A report from the Care Services Improvement Partnership (2005) claims that people working with older adults require a different set of skills from those working with younger people. They argue that to treat everyone the same is discriminatory, and to ignore or not consider age is labelled as being age-blind or as the 'chilling effect'. Anderson et al. (2009) argue that the prevalence, nature and aetiology (i.e. the causes or origins of conditions or the predisposing factors) of mental health conditions in older adults may be different. There is some evidence that older adults have frequently been excluded from research (Academy of Medical Sciences 2009; Fortin et al. 2007).

It has been argued that the National Institute for Health and Clinical Excellence (NICE) guidelines may not always account specifically or adequately for issues of age or ethnicity (Mind 2013), which contributes to marginalisation and is a form of indirect discrimination. The needs of BAME older adults with mental health issues may therefore not have been adequately or thoroughly considered and analysed. Many BAME older adults will have been subject to both direct and indirect discrimination (and one example of this is when providing the same service to everyone becomes discriminatory for a particular group, which is discussed further in Chapter 1). Commissioners of services, service providers, researchers, policymakers and individual workers need to actively challenge racism and ageism and prevent indirect discrimination when considering the specific needs of BAME older adults with mental health issues. This will go some way to minimising discrimination, ensuring that services are fit for purpose, good practice is upheld and older BAME people with mental health issues get the services they require.

Within mental health, indirect discrimination might be found in the use of psychometric tests, which have often been developed and normed on younger populations, typically White American college students (Holt Barrett 2005). BAME older adults' scores on these psychometric tests may, as a result, lead to a score which is interpreted as causing concern, even though this would not be the case if the test had been developed and normed for older adults from diverse cultural backgrounds (Rait *et al.* 1997).

Older adults and mental health

There is a variety of statistics relating to the number of people who may be described as having a mental health condition, and this is partly due to the way in which we define mental health being a contested area (Bentall 2010; Boyle 2002; Harper 2013). How mental health is defined is not unproblematic particularly when issues of diversity are concerned. What may be seen as problematic in one culture may be viewed through a different lens or through a different set of explanatory health beliefs in another (see, for example, Patel *et al.* 2000).

So the definitions and measures used, the time period specified and the different populations studied in terms of age and geographical location will all influence any statistics given and should be treated with caution. The World Health Organization (2016) claims the following:

- Over 20 per cent of adults over 60 years of age suffer from a neurological or mental disorder.

- A neurological or mental disorder is the cause of 6.6 per cent of all disability-adjusted life years (DALYs).

- Depression and dementia are the most common disorders.

- Anxiety disorders affect 3.75 per cent of older adults.

- Almost 1 per cent of the world's population of older adults have substance abuse issues.

The IAPT's (2009) *Older People – Positive Practice Guide* states the following:

- Over 25 per cent of older adults (those aged 65 and above) in the UK have depressive symptoms which require intervention.

- Only one third of these older adults talk to their GP about their depressive symptoms.

- Only half of those who talk to their GP receive treatment, which tends to be medication-based. (This is despite guidance from NICE that the full range of treatments, including psychological therapy, should be offered to older adults with depression.)

Case study: Chandra

Chandra is 89 and has multiple health issues. She was struggling with issues related to the end of her life and often talked about them with her family. Her family found this almost impossible to hear and always tried to change the subject or just told her to cheer up. They decided that she should be placed on anti-depressants to 'make her feel better'. Chandra's GP and her family did not consider psychological therapies or the fact that these thoughts and discussions might be an important part of her preparations for leaving this life. In addition, the use of anti-depressants with older adults carries a number of potential risks (Coupland *et al.* 2011).

The UK's Office for National Statistics' report on psychiatric morbidity (The NHS Information Centre 2007) states the following:

- In any year, one in four adults experiences at least one mental disorder.

- People aged over 75 live with common mental disorders at a rate of 12.2 per cent of women and 6.3 per cent of men.

- Any increase in the number of people with mental health issues will come as a result of growth in the population of older people (Wanless, Forder and Fernandez 2006).

Co-morbidities (whereby at least one additional disorder or disease co-occurs with the main condition) in later life may include changes in physical functioning due to frailty or ageing, cognitive disorders, sensory impairments (poor hearing, eyesight or balance) and polypharmacy (taking multiple medications and susceptibility to the adverse effects of medication) (Anderson *et al.* 2009).

BAME older adults and mental health

The statistics on older adults are generally a cause for concern and raise questions about ageing and mental well-being:

- Depression is said to affect 28 per cent of women and 22 per cent of men aged 65 or older (Health and Social Care Information Centre 2007).

- In the UK, 850,000 people are suffering from dementia. Worldwide, the number is 47.5 million (World Health Organization 2016).

- Of those aged 65 or over, 1 in 14 people has dementia, and the prevalence doubles every five years after age 65.

- People with learning disabilities have a higher risk of developing dementia both earlier and at an accelerated rate (Alzheimer's Society 2015).

- Beaumont and Loft (2013), in their report for the Office for National Statistics, found that 20 per cent of people aged 80 or older reported feeling anxious. The percentage of those aged 50 or above who reported feeling anxious was higher than the average for participants of all ages.

- Another relevant and perhaps under-reported finding is that delirium has been found to affect older people who are hospitalised (Inouye 1999). Siddiqi, House and Holmes (2006) also found an increased risk of delirium in older people who were unwell.

- The RCP (2014) estimates that 85 per cent of older adults with depression receive no help from the NHS.

These concerns are magnified when looking at the worrying evidence relating to the mental health of older adults in the BAME community:

- There is a higher rate of depression in South Asian and Caribbean communities in the UK (Nazroo 1997).

- There is a higher incidence of psychosis in people of African-Caribbean ethnicity (Bhugra and Cochrane 2001).

- Within the BAME community in the UK, there are estimated to be approximately 15,000 older adults with dementia, and approximately 6 per cent of them experience the early onset of the condition (Alzheimer's Society 2015; Department of Health 2009).

- General levels of well-being as measured by life satisfaction were found to be lower for Black people. The average score for White people was reported as 7.4 out of 10, while for Black people this was 6.7 out of 10 (Office for National Statistics 2015).

- In 2010, rates of admission to psychiatric hospitals for 'other Black' groups were six times higher than the average (Care Quality Commission 2011).

- Migration is associated with poor health outcomes for marginalised and socially disadvantaged groups (Warfa et al. 2006).

Interestingly, these high prevalence rates of depression and psychosis have not been found in the countries of origin of these groups, as evidenced, for example, by the work of Hickling and Rodgers-Johnson

(1995) in Jamaica. A plethora of reasons for these differential rates have been given, but racism and discrimination in its myriad forms appear to be a strong predisposing factor for mental ill health (Chakraborty and McKenzie 2002; Karlsen and Nazroo 2002; Sharpley *et al.* 2001). The RCP's (2009) position statement on age discrimination in mental health states: 'Sorry isn't good enough... Discrimination against older people must stop: working locally we can do it.' Practitioners and policymakers might like to reflect on the way older adults are segregated into 'Older Adult Services', as there may be times when it would be helpful to think more creatively and outside the usual categorisations. Access to services should be determined by need and not age, and many voluntary projects are very effective in involving all sectors of their community – Camden Chinese Community Centre in London is a good example of this. These projects can have positive effects for older and younger people alike.

BAME older people accessing mental health services

The RCP (2009) launched a position statement on developing age-appropriate, non-discriminatory mental health services, as they were concerned that older adults were not receiving the services they should and that policies had failed to deliver improvements. Older-age psychiatry only became an NHS specialism in 1989, and Odell *et al.* (1997) note that psychological symptoms in BAME older adults may often be missed or ignored by health professionals. BAME older adults are at the greatest risk of non-detection of mental disorders in primary care (Borowsky *et al.* 2000). The reasons for this may include ageism, racism, and different idioms of distress and help-seeking behaviour. Fernando (2014), Mohebati (2012) and Tribe (2014) have all discussed how the methods people use to maintain their psychological equilibrium and find help are in part developed and defined by cultural, societal and health rules and the meanings which they subsequently ascribe to them. A number of authors have also noted that different cultures define different behaviours or feelings as problematic (MacLachlan 2006; Torrey 1972). The explanatory models of health held by those offering help or treatment and those requesting it may differ, and openness, curiosity and consideration are required from both parties if misunderstandings are to be minimised and a meaningful dialogue developed. Power differentials, issues of discrimination and intersectionality, and the subsequent dynamics which can occur in health and social care consultations may require vigilance, consideration, sensitivity and open discussion to ensure that anti-discriminatory practice is upheld and that the best possible service is offered.

Steps need to be taken at every level to ensure that services are appropriate and accessible and are in line with anti-discriminatory practice. The reported barriers to accessing services are said to be many; for example, available services may be viewed as inappropriate, inadequate, inaccessible and culturally insensitive (Fernando 2014; Tribe 2014). If there is no shared language between the service provider and the service user, both parties may be unwilling or unable to enter into a dialogue easily and comfortably. Some older adults and carers find it difficult to access services due to language barriers (CSIP 2005) as some BAME older adults do not speak English fluently or may not have had the opportunity to achieve literacy in their first language (Shah, Chapter 5 of this volume), perhaps due to work patterns and family commitments and/or poor educational opportunities (McCallum 1990). BAME older adults may lose their acquired language (i.e. English) as they age and revert back to, or feel more comfortable conversing in, their mother tongue (Bot and Weltens 1995, 2000; Shah, Chapter 5 of this volume). The use of interpreters or cultural brokers may therefore be required. (For a guide to working with interpreters and cultural brokers, see Chapter 12 of this volume.)

Parity of esteem

Many groups, including the RCP and service users, have argued for parity of esteem in health services, whereby mental health is valued equally with physical health (this is currently not the case), with resources allocated accordingly. There is often an interactive relationship between the physical and mental health conditions, whereby people with physical health issues are at an increased risk of experiencing mental health problems, and vice versa (Mind 2013). It is feasible that BAME older people may have been particularly disadvantaged by this lack of parity because of disadvantaged life circumstances leading to poorer physical health, as well as being affected by the issues discussed earlier in this chapter relating to difficulties in accessing mental health services and questions about the appropriateness of the services provided. The ageing process also can give rise to a number of well-being issues. The principle of mental health having equal priority with physical health is now legally enshrined within the Health and Social Care Act 2012. However, NHS England (2014) notes that the current health system separates physical and mental health in a way that may not provide the best service to service users, and it is working to develop a service based on four principles:

- care that puts patients in control

- care that is fully integrated

- care that is the most clinically effective

- care that provides maximum value.

NHS England (2014) also has a Parity of Esteem programme, which has four priority areas:

- Improving Access to Psychological Therapies (IAPT), which aims to improve access to services for people suffering from depression and anxiety disorders

- improving diagnosis and support for people with dementia

- improving awareness of the Mental Capacity Act 2005 and spotlighting the duties within it

- working with Time to Change to tackle stigma and discrimination.

Statistics on the number of people from BAME communities who have been detained under the Mental Health Act 1983 show that Black people are more likely to present via Accident and Emergency services, to be in crisis and to have the police involved in the process of admission, all of which is cause for concern (Bhui *et al.* 2003; Fernando 2014). Mind (2013, p.14) notes that 'people from some BME groups seem to be treated more neglectfully or coercively in the crisis care system than other people'. They also found that there is variable access to crisis resolution and home treatment (CRHT) teams in relation to the White British group. They note that Bangladeshi, Chinese and Indian people receive low referral rates, while Black Caribbean people have a higher rate of admission to hospital, and

Black men are disproportionally given a diagnosis of schizophrenia. More specifically, Glover and Evison (2009) note that all Black groups use CRHT teams more than White British people do, while Asian, Indian, Pakistani, mixed White and Chinese groups use them less.

The Health and Social Care Information Centre (2013) has shown that once contact with mental health services is established, rates of access to hospital services are higher for all minority groups than for the White British group. Bhui *et al.* (2003) note that the group least likely to be referred to specialist mental health services is that of people of South Asian heritage. As suggested in Chapter 1, intersectionality may offer a useful framework for understanding some of the intersecting inequalities for older BAME people living with mental health concerns. For example, if someone suffers from discrimination on account of their mental health status as well as their older age, the two discriminatory practices intersect and may lead to increased discrimination and difficulties for the individual. Inequalities, stigma, and discriminatory attitudes and practices are often associated with having a mental health diagnosis (Corrigan and Watson 2002; Mental Health Foundation 2015). When racism is also added to the mix, the three forms of discrimination may intersect and lead to negative outcomes. These discriminatory views and associated practices may be even further exacerbated if a person is viewed as 'different' in additional ways that are viewed as negative and to which society ascribes discriminatory practices. For example, this might be with regard to their sexuality, housing status or ethnicity. In addition, older adults tend to have lower incomes than younger adults, often due to a reduction in income after retirement (National Council on Aging 2015), and poverty, too, is associated with poor mental health, with common mental health conditions twice as prevalent among the poor as among the rich (World Health Organization 2000). This intersection of factors may be an additional variable in the equation, leading to anti-discriminatory practice. It is therefore always important to consider how individual factors intersect and interact for each individual and his or her family when considering anti-discriminatory practice with older adults and their carers.

Diagnosing mental illness

How mental illness is diagnosed or labelled is a contentious issue, and it is made more complex by issues of racism and ageism and the overall lack of research on BAME older adults with mental health issues (Shah and MacKenzie 2007). In addition, gender bias or discrimination may be apparent. The *Diagnostic and Statistical Manual of Mental Disorders* (DSM) and the *International Classification of Diseases* (ICD) – the diagnostic tools used by many clinicians to identify and diagnose mental illness – have been criticised for their lack of attention to culture as an organising concept (Fernando 2014; Mezzich *et al.* 1996). We know that all forms of psychological distress are co-produced by a range of factors, including what is loosely defined as 'culture'. Summerfield (2002, p.248) notes:

> DSM and ICD are not, as some imagine, atheoretical and purely descriptive nosologies with universal validity. They are western cultural documents, carrying ontological notions of what constitutes a real disorder, epistemological ideas about what counts as scientific evidence, and methodological ideas as to how research should be conducted.

While the American Psychiatric Association (2013, p.758) states that 'All forms of distress are locally shaped, including the DSM disorders', there are also issues relating to the reification of culture as something that is untouchable and unquestionable (Tribe 2016).

DSM-5 (the latest version of DSM) includes the Cultural Formulation Interview (CFI), which appears to be a move in the right direction, although diagnoses based on the diagnostic manuals may on occasion be reductionist, make assumptions and impose one set of views constructed and produced in one part of the world on to people from other cultures (Bracken 1998; Summerfield 2002). In addition (as touched upon earlier), most psychometric instrumentation has been developed on younger people, with ethnicity often ignored or not considered, and therefore use with older adults from BAME communities must be approached with extreme caution. Moreover, positivistic approaches have often addressed cross-cultural, gender, religious and age-related variations as something that can be categorised and managed, rather than as a central organising concept, examining the amount of variance rather than looking for different underlying constructions and belief systems. It is important that culture and age are adequately accounted for when any mental health diagnosis is made. Culture and age need to be foregrounded rather than seen as add-ons.

Western models of distress have often been positioned as being 'better' and have been imbued with a set of privileged values (see Patel *et al.* 2000 for discussion of this issue). It is important that practitioners are aware of the possible range of idioms of distress and explanatory health beliefs held by different individuals, as discussed below. Otherwise, practitioners may not be able to understand what is being conveyed and may therefore not offer the best help to older adults who require their assistance.

The individuality and personal choices of every service user should be respected. Culture is highly individual and will be influenced by a range of variables including ethnicity, religion, family values, life experiences and life events (Fernando 2014). Certain countries or communities may advocate particular views around what constitutes appropriate sexuality and gender roles or age-appropriate behaviour. These behaviours may be monitored in a range of ways seen as antithetical to international human rights or social justice perspectives. This may lead to a range of emotional dilemmas for BAME older adults, their carers and health and social care professionals. Since ageing may be socially constructed by culture and community, anti-discriminatory practice leads practitioners to try to enable service users to speak freely and openly about their lives and the choices they have made.

Expectations about ageing will vary across countries and cultures. Gibson, Lokae and Truss (2000) argue that age may be viewed as conferring status or social position, power or disempowerment. In addition, there are a multiplicity of views around ageing and end of life issues and beliefs. Banerjee and Chowdhury (2016) have highlighted how cultural psychosocial issues, such as gender discrimination and associated power dynamics, domestic violence and related issues, are not adequately reflected within psychiatric practice. Specifically, they argue that DSM/ICD diagnoses fail to account for the psychosocial dimensions which act as important risk factors for deliberate self-harm and suicide. They suggest that there is a need to think of new dimensions of distress as opposed to those which merely fit with diagnostic criteria. This is an issue which requires further work and consideration.

Stigma and discrimination

The stigma and discrimination often associated with mental illness have been found to be a significant barrier to help-seeking (Corrigan 2004). Ethnicity and age may also play a role, in that older BAME adults do not appear to be seeking help from services (Goudie 2003; RCP 2009). For example, Conner, Copeland and Brown (2010) noted that the impact of social stigma at the macro level (i.e. the negative attitudes held by the public) impacted upon the micro level by affecting the stigmatised individual's subsequent help-seeking behaviour. The study was conducted in the USA with older adults (who were defined as being depressed) through a telephone-based survey. It found that African Americans were more likely to hold more negative attitudes towards seeking mental health treatment than the White participants. The reasons for this may be many, and the findings are not necessarily generalisable. Although society is more comfortable in talking about mental health than previously, discrimination and stigma are still present with regard to mental illness. Stigma concerning mental health is common in many cultures, but levels are higher in some communities than in others (Marwaha 2002; Ng 1997). Some cultures have a preference for private coping strategies, and fear of stigma may also prevent people from seeking help and support outside their family or even *from* their family (Cinnirella and Loewenthal 1999). Evidence of the difficulties associated with having a mental health diagnosis may be partly shown in the findings that people with a mental health diagnosis have poorer physical health (RCP 2015) and tend to earn less (Saraceno and Barbui 1997), although there may also be other factors in play. As Anderson (2011, p.4) notes, 'To deliver non-discriminatory, age-appropriate services on the ground will require mental health services to be much more sophisticated in the way they operate and the way specialties interact.'

Culture, explanatory health beliefs and idioms of distress

The stresses and bodily changes associated with getting older raise a number of new challenges and require physical adaptations, many of which may be involuntary and unwanted by older adults, their families and their friends. These physical changes, while challenging in themselves, can bring about dilemmas and psychological responses. The issue of Cartesian dualism (the mind–body split) is complex, and the exact relationship between the two spheres is complex and still not fully understood. The factors that may mediate this dualism are still being explored (Foster 1991; Kim 2000). Culture, explanatory health beliefs (how someone understands their health, pain, distress or symptoms) (Bhui 2003; Kleinman 1978; Tribe 2014) and idioms of distress (how someone exhibits and describes their distress or pain) may also play a mediating role in how the mind–body relationship is understood and experienced by the individual as well as by health and social care staff and institutions (Hinton and Lewis-Fernandez 2010; Nichter 1981). Emotional distress is not expressed in the same way in all cultures or communities, so BAME older adults may use different idioms of distress or explanatory health models to those in which health professionals have been trained. Health professionals' lack of familiarity with alternative health beliefs and idioms of distress may correspond to BAME older adults' low levels of usage of statutory services (Rait *et al.* 1997; Shah 2008) as discussed elsewhere in this chapter. Therefore, health and social care staff may wish to discuss these explanatory health beliefs and idioms of distress with service users to ensure that they understand the position of the service user and are not inadvertently disregarding or discriminating against a different set of explanatory health beliefs or idioms of distress. This is in line with good anti-discriminatory practice, as not doing so may lead to the needs of service users being ignored and their problems being hidden and possibly getting worse.

Different idioms of distress may include emotional distress being described using the idiom of chronic physical symptoms. Examples of different idioms of distress, health behaviour or what used to be called culturally bound syndromes might include agoraphobia, Type A behaviour and eating disorders in the West, inarun among the Yoruba of Nigeria, quajihaillituq among the Inuit, and tabacazo in Chile (MacLachlan 2006). The meanings that these expressions of distress carry have been labelled as 'cultural explanations of distress' or 'perceived causes' in DSM-5 at the individual and societal level. The authors of DSM-5 write about 'Culturally recognised meaning/s or etiology [meaning the causes] for symptoms, illness or distress' (APA 2013, p.759).

The term 'cultures of distress' refers to the ways in which individuals from particular cultures are likely to express their distress; however, it is important not to stereotype people and make assumptions about their distress, and the best strategy is always to discuss it with the service user. The explanatory health model held by the patient may also determine where he or she seeks help for emotional or physical pain (Helman 2007). The assumption in the West that distress can be explained psychologically or in terms of feelings is not universal but a cultural variant. In some countries, good mental health may be seen as the ability to carry out ascribed tasks or fulfil roles, or it may be attributed to spiritual or other factors (Patel *et al.* 2000). Anti-discriminatory practice requires taking time to discuss how service users understand their distress, what they believe may have caused it and what may help them in dealing with it. Being open and curious – having an open dialogue where practitioners really listen to service users rather than assuming that as professionals they know best – is likely to lead not only to the service user feeling understood but to better outcomes in the longer term.

Appropriate service provision for BAME older adults

Carr (2014), in an empirical review that examined UK-based peer-reviewed articles from 2000 to 2013, argues that statutory care provision for people with 'protected characteristics' under the Equality Act 2010 contains what are labelled 'marginalising dynamics', meaning that services may not be appropriate or accessible to people on account of characteristics including age and ethnicity. Carr argues that people from BAME communities feared that services would be discriminatory and that they were therefore reluctant to engage, with trust being cited as a major and complicated issue. The belief that nothing can be done to assist with a mental health or well-being issue has also been recorded as an issue (Age Concern/Help the Aged Housing Trust 1984; McCallum 1990), and this may contribute to people's reluctance to ask for help and support with mental health concerns. Bowes and Wilkinson (2003) also note that a poor experience of services on a previous occasion is a major factor. Issues of stigma associated with mental health may also play a role (Livingston and Sembhi 2003; Patel *et al.* 2000), and members of BAME communities frequently present to services and receive a mental health diagnosis at a later stage than other groups (Patel *et al.* 2000).

Cultural background may influence the ways in which people seek help as well as their willingness to label issues relating to mental health and well-being. This may prevent BAME older adults and carers from seeking help and support with mental health problems from the health and social care services currently available in the UK (Shah 2008). Services need to be set up in ways which are appropriate to the needs of BAME older adults and which they feel happy and comfortable accessing, but this has not always been the case. (For further discussion of this issue, see IAPT 2009; Tribe, Lane and Hearsum 2009.)

As Drennan and Swartz (1999, p.173) note, 'assumptions of a monolithic culture that can be summarized and commodified for easy psychiatric consumption are inherently problematic and ignore the diversity within any culture or subculture'. Culture is specific to each individual and is influenced by family, upbringing, country of residence or origin, values, life experiences, beliefs, and religious or spiritual values. It is, of course, important to avoid stereotyping and assuming that all people from a particular culture will automatically share a set of beliefs and views. Helman (2007, pp.2–3) describes culture as:

> a set of guidelines (both explicit and implicit) which individuals inherit as members of a particular society, and which tells them how to view the world, how to experience it emotionally, and how to behave in it, in relation to other people, to supernatural forces or gods, and to the natural environment. It also provides them with a way of transmitting these guidelines to the next generation – by the use of symbols, language, art and ritual.

It has been argued that people from BAME communities who have not had to access services previously may find it difficult to understand the services that are available and how to access them (Bhui and Bhugra 2002). There may be a lack of awareness among some members of BAME communities about the role of the GP as a source of information and support for mental health or emotional problems (Jacob *et al.* 1998). Psychological distress may be viewed negatively and may carry notions of stigma or shame (Marwaha 2002; Ng 1997). This may lead to psychological distress being hidden or help not being sought until problems become chronic or difficult for families to deal with (Cinnirella and Loewenthal 1999). The low uptake of health and social care services by older people from BAME communities may lead to their needs being overlooked or underestimated by commissioners

(Fassil and Burnett 2015). This is a cause for concern, as their very absence as service users may mean that future services do not take their needs into consideration when based on previous patterns of usage, establishing a cycle of needs being ignored and no appropriate services being developed.

However, there are a range of self-organised informal networks which have been established in response to this lack of take-up of statutory services. There is a developing research literature which indicates that there is a positive role for self-help and mutual-aid projects which provide BAME (and LGB) older adults with useful support networks. Mutual-aid projects enhance social capital and may play a protective role in maintaining positive well-being and enhancing mental health. Think Local Act Personal (TLAP) (www.thinklocalactpersonal.org.uk), which describes itself as 'a national partnership transforming health and care through personalization and community-based support', has argued for an increase in local not-for-profit provision, while the Community Catalysts organisation (www.communitycatalysts.co.uk) provides practical support and advice to micro-level providers of social care provision.

Key messages for the commissioners of older people's mental health services

The Joint Commissioning Panel for Mental Health's (2013) ten key messages for the commissioners of older people's mental health services are as follows:

1. Given the population changes and the increase in the number of older adults in the UK, commissioners need to ensure that accurate predictions of their local population are conducted as part of their Joint Strategic Needs Assessment to ensure there is adequate capacity in their service provision.

2. Mental health services for older adults should be integrated with social care services (statutory and voluntary) to ensure that people's needs are met and to prioritise independence for older adults.

3. Collaboration between primary care, community and mental health services should take place.

4. The basis of commissioning services should be related to need and not merely to age, to acknowledge that the requirements of older adults may be different.

5. Depression, psychosis and dementia need to be considered, as there is often co-morbidity of dementia, depression and psychosis.

6. Older adults frequently experience physical and mental health problems, and therefore joint and integrated service delivery is recommended.

7. Multidisciplinary teams should be present within mental health services.

8. Community crisis or home treatment services should be available and with longer hours.

9. Psychology services should be available to older adults as they are for younger adults.

10. Liaison services should be available in acute hospitals, as older adults' mental health problems are not always attended to adequately.

Although BAME older adults are not specifically mentioned here, all of the messages are likely to lead to better and more appropriate service provision.

Working to improve access to care services for BAME older adults with mental health problems

Below is an eight-step guide to help build a more inclusive service. This guide was developed in conjunction with five BAME community groups and was supported by the Care Services Improvement Partnership. It has subsequently been developed and updated, and it is reprinted and expanded here with their permission.

Step 1: Deliver on race and age equality in mental health care. This means that there must be commitment from policymakers and those delivering services to the funding, planning, training, service development and delivery of services for all older adults in our communities. Equality demands a 'whole systems' approach, rather than an 'additional extra' approach. If appropriate services are not commissioned for older adults, then no progress can be made.

Step 2: Place person-centred care needs at the heart of service delivery. We need to consult with older adults and carers and ensure that their wishes and needs are central to service delivery. We need to avoid stereotyping, consider culture appropriately and recognise the uniqueness of human experience.

Step 3: Develop services with BAME older adults and carers. Planning mental health services *with* BAME older adults and their carers can help to identify gaps in the current service provision and to design and deliver a more culturally appropriate, effective and responsive service. However, just consulting is not enough – practitioners and policymakers need to move ideas into practice and involve service users and carers in not only planning personal care but also advising on service development, delivery and evaluation (Lane and Tribe 2010).

Step 4: Improve communication. Some older adults and carers find it difficult to access services due to language barriers as some BAME older adults may not speak English fluently (Tribe & Raval, 2003 and a number may also not have had the relevant opportunities to gain literacy in their first language (Shah, 2017).   This may be due to work patterns and family commitments and/or poor educational opportunities (McCallum, 2000). However, many BAME older adults and carers also face other communication challenges, especially if they have never learnt English, have limited English or are experiencing second-language attrition (described above).

Step 5: Don't focus on culture and cultural differences at the expense of systemic inequalities. While it is important to look at BAME older adults and carers' cultural and spiritual needs, this must be undertaken while addressing wider health inequalities. It is widely reported that, as separate groups, people with mental health problems, BAME communities and older people experience social exclusion. It therefore follows, then, that BAME older people with mental health problems are a particularly vulnerable group at risk of social exclusion, which could exacerbate any mental health problems if they go untreated (Department of Health 2005).

Many BAME older adults need practical information when dealing with social inequalities concerning benefits, rights and available services.

Step 6: Practitioners need to work in innovative and appropriate ways with BAME communities. There is a need to recognise the important role played by faith for some BAME community groups in the provision of social, cultural and mental health support for BAME older adults. It is important for practitioners to recognise the value of many community groups in promoting mental health, as well as to acknowledge the expertise held within local BAME communities. Recent policy changes towards direct payments, individualised budgets and the development of social enterprise organisations, as well as the move towards third-sector commissioning, now allow services to work more creatively to provide culturally sensitive solutions to the needs of BAME older adults and carers. It is important for us to recognise that many BAME community groups are under-resourced, and that they will need sustainable funding and community capacity-building if they are to offer service delivery options.

Step 7: Deliver on policy. While there is an avalanche of policy documents promoting equality in health and social care services, it is only through appropriate resource allocation and good service delivery that these objectives can be realised. This will also be achieved through individual workers ensuring that they offer appropriate provision and adhere to anti-discriminatory practice in a range of ways.

Step 8: Develop the workforce. This is essential if practitioners are to keep up to date with changes in mental health and social care policy and practice. Practitioners may need to improve their skills in working across cultures (Patel *et al.* 2000). However, we need to ensure that training is not tokenistic but is part of a wider and systematic approach to service delivery. Often the best teachers are the BAME older adults and carers that we work with.

Questions

1. Nimisha regularly drives and accompanies her mother to health or social care appointments. She notices that despite her mother being the service user, the conversation is frequently directed at Nimisha. If you observed this happening, what would you do at the time or afterwards?

2. You have arranged a second meeting with a service user, Maliq, who speaks very little English, and you do not speak his first language. Your manager tells you that it is too much trouble to get an interpreter, and that you will just have to manage. What action might you take, and on what basis would you do this?

3. You are part of a multi-disciplinary team working with Mrs Mbanga, who is 87. She is finding it difficult to adjust to getting old, as she has multiple health issues and reports feeling distressed and confused about her life and future. You think she would benefit from psychological therapy, but your colleague thinks she should be placed on anti-depressants, as this will be much more straightforward. What might you do in this scenario?

References

Academy of Medical Sciences (2009) *Rejuvenating Ageing Research.* London: Academy of Medical Sciences. Available at www.acmedsci.ac.uk/viewFile/publicationDownloads/ageingwe.pdf, accessed on 19 September 2016.

Age Concern and the Mental Health Foundation (2006) *Promoting Mental Health and Well-being in Later Life: A First Report from the UK Inquiry into Mental Health and Well-being in Later Life.* London: Age Concern and the Mental Health Foundation. Available at www.mentalhealth.org.uk/sites/default/files/promoting_mh_wb_later_life.pdf, accessed on 6 November 2016.

Age Concern/Help the Aged Housing Trust (1984) *Housing for Ethnic Elders.* London: Age Concern.

Age UK Buckinghamshire (2016) *No One Should Have No One.* Available at www.ageuk.org.uk/buckinghamshire/newsandcampaigns1/nooneshouldhavenoone, accessed on 6 November 2016.

Alzheimer's Society (2015) *Factsheet: Learning Disabilities and Dementia.* Available at www.alzheimers.org.uk/site/scripts/download_info.php?fileID=1763, accessed on 10 April 2016.

American Psychiatric Association (2013) *Diagnostic and Statistical Manual of Mental Disorders.* 5th ed. Arlington, VA: American Psychiatric Association.

Anderson, D. (2011) 'Editorial: Age discrimination in mental health services needs to be understood.' *BJPsych Bulletin 35*, 1, 1–4.

Anderson, D., Banerjee, S., Barker, A., Connelly, P., *et al.* (2009) *The Need to Tackle Age Discrimination in Mental Health: A Compendium of Evidence.* London: Royal College of Psychiatrists.

Banerjee, S.D. and Chowdhury, N.A. (2016) 'Globalisation of Pesticide Ingestion in Suicides: An Overview from a Deltaic Region of a Middle-income Nation, India.' In R. White, S. Jain, D. Orr and U. Read (eds) *The Palgrave Handbook for Global Mental Health: Socio-cultural Perspectives.* London: Palgrave Macmillan.

Beaumont, J. and Loft, H. (2013) *Measuring National Well-being: Health.* London: Office for National Statistics.

Beecham, J., Knapp, M., Fernandez, J.-L., Huxley, P., *et al.* (2008) *Age Discrimination in Mental Health Services.* Canterbury: Personal Social Services Research Unit.

Bentall, R. (2010) *Doctoring the Mind: Why Psychiatric Treatments Fail.* London: Penguin.

Berry, J.W., Kim, U., Minde, T. and Mok, D. (1987) 'Comparative studies of acculturative stress.' *International Migration Review 21*, 3, 491–511.

Bhugra, D. and Cochrane, R. (eds) (2001) *Psychiatry in Multicultural Britain*. London: Gaskell.

Bhugra, D. and Gupta, S. (eds) (2011) *Migration and Mental Health*. Cambridge: Cambridge University Press.

Bhui, K. (ed.) (2013) *Elements of Culture and Mental Health: Critical Questions for Clinicians*. London: Royal College of Psychiatrists.

Bhui, K. and Bhugra, D. (2002) 'Mental illness in Black and Asian ethnic minorities: Pathways to care and outcomes.' *Advances in Psychiatric Treatment 8*, 26–33.

Bhui, K., Stansfeld, S., Hull, S., Priebe, S., Mole, F. and Feder, G. (2003) 'Ethnic variations in pathways to and use of specialist mental health services in the UK: Systematic review.' *British Journal of Psychiatry 182*, 105–106.

Borowsky, S.J., Rubenstein, L.V., Meredith, L.S., Camp, P., Jackson-Triche, M. and Wells, K.B. (2000) 'Who is at risk of nondetection of mental health problems in primary care?' *Journal of General Internal Medicine 15*, 381–388.

Bot, K. de and Stoessel, S. (2000) 'In search of yesterday's words: Reactivating a long forgotten language.' *Applied Linguistics 21*, 364–384.

Bot, K. de and Weltens, B. (1995) 'Foreign language attrition.' *Annual Review of Applied Linguistics 15*, 151–164.

Bowes, A. (2006) 'Mainstreaming equality: Implications of the provision of support at home for majority and minority ethnic older people.' *Social Policy and Administration 40*, 7, 739–757.

Bowes, A. and Wilkinson, H. (2003) '"We didn't know it would get that bad": South Asian experiences of dementia and the service response.' *Health and Social Care in the Community 11*, 5, 387–396.

Boyle, M. (2002) *Schizophrenia: A Scientific Delusion?* 2nd ed. London: Routledge.

Bracken, P. (1998) 'Hidden Agendas: Deconstructing Post Traumatic Stress Disorder.' In P. Bracken and C. Petty (eds) *Rethinking the Trauma of War*. London: Free Association Books.

Care Quality Commission (2011) *Count Me In 2010: Results of the 2010 National Census of Inpatients and Patients on Supervised Community Treatment in Mental Health and Learning Disability Services in England and Wales*. Newcastle: Care Quality Commission. Available at www.cqc.org.uk/sites/default/files/documents/count_me_in_2010_final_tagged.pdf, accessed on 20 September 2016.

Care Services Improvement Partnership (CSIP) (2005) *Everybody's Business – Integrating Mental Health Services For Older Adults*. Available at www.changeagentteam.org.uk/index.cfm?pid=34&catalogueContentID=1048.

Carr, S. (2014) *Social Care for Marginalised Communities: Balancing Self-organisation, Micro-provision and Mainstream Support*. Policy Paper 18. Birmingham: Health Services Management Centre, University of Birmingham.

Centre for Policy on Ageing (2014) *Resilience in Older Age*. Available at www.cpa.org.uk/information/reviews/CPA-Rapid-Review-Resilience-and-recovery.pdf, accessed on 6 November 2016.

Chakraborty, A. and McKenzie, K. (2002) 'Does racial discrimination cause mental illness?' *British Journal of Psychiatry 190*, 6, 475–477.

Cinnirella, K. and Loewenthal, K.M. (1999) 'Religious and ethnic group influences on beliefs about mental illness: A qualitative interview study.' *British Journal of Medical Psychology 72*, 4, 505–524.

Cohen, C. and Ahmed, I. (2011) 'Working with Elderly Persons Across Cultures.' In D. Bhugra and K. Bhui (eds) *Textbook of Cultural Psychiatry*. Cambridge: Cambridge University Press.

Conner, K.O., Copeland, V. and Brown, C. (2010) 'Mental health treatment seeking among older adults with depression: The impact of stigma and race.' *The American Journal of Geriatric Psychiatry 18*, 6, 531–543.

Cornwell, E.Y. and Waite, L.J. (2009) 'Social disconnectedness, perceived isolation and health among older adults.' *Journal of Health and Social Behaviour 50*, 1, 31–48.

Corrigan, P. (2004) 'How stigma interferes with mental health care.' *American Psychologist 59*, 7, 614–625.

Corrigan, P. and Watson, A.C. (2002) 'Understanding the impact of stigma on people with mental illness.' *World Psychiatry 1*, 1, 16–20.

Coupland, C., Dhiman, P., Morriss, R., Arthur, A., Barton, G. and Hippisley-Cox, J. (2011) 'Antidepressant use and risk of adverse outcomes in older people.' *British Medical Journal 343*.

Craig, R. and Mindell, J. (2005) *Health Survey for England. Mental Health and Wellbeing: The Health of Older People.* Leeds: NHS Information Centre.

Department of Health (2009) *Living Well with Dementia: A National Dementia Strategy.* London: Department of Health. Available at www.gov.uk/government/uploads/system/uploads/attachment_data/file/168221/dh_094052.pdf, accessed on 20 September 2016.

Drennan, G. and Swartz, L. (1999) 'A concept overburdened: Institutional roles for psychiatric interpreters in post-apartheid South Africa.' *Interpreting 4,* 2, 169–198.

Fassil, Y. and Burnett, A. (2015) *Commissioning Mental Health Services for Vulnerable Adult Migrants: Guidance for Commissioners.* London: Mind. Available at www.mind.org.uk/media/3168649/vulnerable-migrants_2015_mindweb.pdf, accessed on 6 November 2016.

Fernando, S. (2014) *Mental Health Worldwide.* London: Palgrave Macmillan.

Fiori, K.L., Antonicci, T.C. and Cortina, K.S. (2006) 'Social network typologies and mental health among older adults.' *The Journal of Gerontology 61b,* 1.25–32.

Forbes, L.J., Simon, A.E., Warburton, F., Boniface, D. *et al.* (2013) 'Differences in cancer awareness and beliefs between Australia, Canada, Denmark, Norway, Sweden and the UK: Do they contribute to differences in cancer survival?' *British Journal of Cancer 111,* 12, 2382.

Forder, J. (2008) *The Costs of Addressing Age Discrimination in Social Care.* Canterbury: Personal Social Services Research Unit. Available at www.pssru.ac.uk/pdf/dp2538.pdf, accessed on 20 September 2016.

Fortin, M., Soubhi, H., Hudon, C., Baylis, E.A. and Van der Akker, M. (2007) 'Multimorbidity's many challenges.' *British Medical Journal 334,* 1016–1017.

Foster, J. (1991) *The Immaterial Self: Defence of the Cartesian Dualist Conception for the Mind.* London: Routledge.

Gawande, A. (2014) *Being Mortal: Medicine and What Matters in the End.* London: Wellcome.

Gibson, G., Lokae, V. and Truss, K. (2000) 'Older Adults.' In N. Patel (ed.) *Clinical Psychology, 'Race' and Culture.* Leicester: BPS Books.

Glover, G. and Evison, F. (2009) *Use of New Mental Health Services by Ethnic Minorities in England.* Durham: North East Public Health Observatory.

Gooding, P.A., Hurst, A., Johnson, J. and Tarrier, N. (2012) 'Psychological Resilience in young and older adults', *International Journal of Geriatric Psychiatry,* 27, 3, 262–270.

Goudie, F. (2003) 'Psychological Therapy with Older Adults.' In R. Woolfe, W. Dryden and S. Strawbridge (eds) *Handbook of Counselling Psychology.* London: Sage.

Harper, D. (2013) 'On the persistence of psychiatric diagnosis: Moving beyond a zombie classification system.' *Feminism and Psychology 23,* 1, 78–85.

Health and Social Care Information Centre (2013) *Mental Health Bulletin: Annual Report from MHMDS Returns – England, 2011–12, Further Analysis and Organisation-level Data.* Available at http://content.digital.nhs.uk/catalogue/PUB10347, accessed on 6 November 2016.

Helman, C. (2007) *Culture, Health and Illness.* 5th ed. London: Hodder Arnold.

Hickling, F.W. and Rodgers-Johnson, P. (1995) 'The incidence of first contact schizophrenia in Jamaica.' *British Journal of Psychiatry 167,* 193–196.

Hinton, D.E. and Lewis-Fernandez, R. (2010) 'Trauma and idioms of distress.' *Culture, Medicine and Psychiatry 34,* 2, 209–218.

Holt Barrett, K. (2005) 'Guidelines and Suggestions for Conducting Successful Cross-Cultural Evaluations for the Courts.' In K. Holt Barrett and W.H. George (eds) *Race, Culture, Psychology and the Law.* New York: Sage.

Improving Access to Psychological Therapies (IAPT) (2009) *Older People – Positive Practice Guide.* London: Department of Health. Available at www.iapt.nhs.uk/silo/files/older-people-positive-guide.pdf, accessed on 20 September 2016.

Inouye, S.K. (1999) 'Predisposing and precipitating factors for delirium in hospitalised older patients.' *Dementia and Geriatric Cognitive Disorder 19,* 393–400.

Jacob, K.S., Bhugra, D., Lloyd, K.R. and Mann, A.H. (1998) 'Common mental disorders, explanatory models and consultation behaviour among Indian women living in the UK.' *Journal of the Royal Society of Medicine 91,* 66–71.

Kaplan, D.W. and Berkman, B.J. (2016) 'Religion and Spirituality in Older People.' Merck Manuals. Available at www.merckmanuals.com/home/older-people%E2%80%99s-health-issues/social-issues-affecting-older-people/religion-and-spirituality-in-older-people, accessed on 20 September 2016.

Karlsen, S. and Nazroo, J. (2002) 'The relationship between racial discrimination, social class and health among ethnic minority groups.' *American Journal of Public Health 92*, 4, 624–631.

Kim, J. (2000) *Mind in a Physical World.* Cambridge, MA: A Bradford Book, MIT.

Kleinman, A. (1978) 'Concepts and a model for comparison of medical systems as cultural systems.' *Social Science and Medicine 12*, 85–93.

Lane, P. and Tribe, R. (2010) 'Following NICE 2008: A practical guide for health professionals on community engagement with local black and minority ethnic (BME) community groups.' *Diversity, Health and Care 7*, 2, 105–114.

Litwin, H. (2001) 'Social network type and morale in old age.' *The Gerontologist 41*, 516–524.

Livingston, G. and Sembhi, S. (2003) 'Mental health of the ageing immigrant population.' *Advances in Psychiatric Treatment 9*, 31–37.

MacLachlan, M. (2006) *Culture and Health: A Critical Perspective towards Global Health.* Oxford: Wiley.

Marwaha, S. (2002) 'Stigma, racism or choice: Why do depressed ethnic older adults avoid psychiatrists?' *Journal of Affective Disorders 72*, 3, 257–265.

Mayengo, N. (2016) Personal communication.

McCallum, J. (1990) *The Forgotten People: Carers in Three Minority Communities in Southwark.* London: The King's Fund.

Mental Health Foundation (2015) *Fundamental Facts About Mental Health 2015.* London: Mental Health Foundation. Available at www.mentalhealth.org.uk/sites/default/files/fundamental-facts-15.pdf, accessed on 6 November 2016.

Mezzich, J.E., Kleinman, A., Fabrega Jr., H. and Parron, D.L. (eds) (1996) *Culture and Psychiatric Diagnosis.* Washington, DC: American Psychiatric Press.

Mind (2013) *Mental Health Crisis Care: Commissioning Excellence for Black and Minority Ethnic Groups.* Stratford: Mind.

Mohebati, L. (2012) *Time to Change: Challenging Mental Health Related Stigma and Discrimination Experienced by Black and Minority Ethnic Communities.* Available at www.time-to-change.org.uk/sites/default/files/black-minority-ethnic-communities-position-statement.pdf, accessed on 6 November 2016.

National Council on Aging (2015) *Senior Economic Security: Preparing Older Adults and Communities for a New Economic Reality.* Arlington, VA: NCOA. Available at www.ncoa.org/resources/senior-economic-security-preparing-older-adults-and-communities-for-a-new-economic-reality, accessed on 6 November 2016.

Nazroo, J.Y. (1997) *The Health of Britain's Ethnic Minorities: Findings from a National Survey.* London: Policy Studies Institute.

Ng, C.H. (1997) 'The stigma of mental illness in Asian cultures.' *Australian and New Zealand Journal of Psychiatry 31*, 382–390.

NHS England (2014) *A Call to Action: Achieving Parity of Esteem; Transformative Ideas for Commissioners.* Available at www.england.nhs.uk/wp-content/uploads/2014/02/nhs-parity.pdf, accessed on 6 November 2016.

Nichter, M. (1981) 'Idioms of distress: Alternatives in the expression of psychosocial distress: A case study from South India.' *Culture, Medicine and Psychiatry 5*, 4, 379–408.

Odell, S.M., Surtees, P.G., Wainwright, N.W., Commander, M.J. and Sashidharan, S.P. (1997) 'Determinants of general practitioner recognition of psychological problems in a multi-ethnic inner-city health district.' *British Journal of Psychiatry 171*, 6, 537–541.

Office for National Statistics (2015) *Population Estimates for UK, England and Wales, Scotland and Northern Ireland.* Available at www.ons.gov.uk/ons/rel/pop-estimate/population-estimates-for-uk--england-and-wales--scotland-and-northern-ireland/mid-2014/index.html, accessed on 20 September 2016.

Patel, N. (ed.) (2003) *Minority Elderly Care in Europe: Country Profiles.* Leeds: PRIAE.

Patel, N., Bennett, E., Dennis, M., Dosanjh, N. *et al.* (2000) *Clinical Psychology, 'Race' and Culture: A Training Manual.* Leicester: BPS Books.

Policy Research Institute on Ageing and Ethnicity (PRIAE) and the International School for Communities, Rights and Inclusion (ISCRI) at the University of Central Lancashire (2010) *PRIAE–ISCRI: Managing Better Mental Health Care for Black & Minority Ethnic Elders.* Preston: PRIAE and ISCRI, University of Central Lancashire. Available at www.priae.org/assets/4_PRIAE-ISCRI_Managing_Better_Mental_Health_Care_for_BME_Older_People_2010.pdf, accessed on 6 November 2016.

Rait, G. and Burns, A. (1997) 'Appreciating background and culture: The South Asian elderly and mental health.' *International Journal of Geriatric Psychiatry 12*, 10, 973–977.

RCP (2009) *Age Discrimination in Mental Health Services: Making Equality a Reality.* Position Statement PS2/2009. London: RCP. Available at www.rcpsych.ac.uk/pdf/PS02_2009x.pdf, accessed on 20 September 2016.

RCP (2014) *Depression in Older Adults.* Available at www.rcpsych.ac.uk/healthadvice/problemsdisorders/depressioninolderadults.aspx, accessed on 20 September 2016.

RCP (2015) Royal College of Psychiatrists Position Statement PS4 (2010) *No Health Without Public Health.* www.rcpsych.ac.uk/qualityimprovement

Saraceno, B. and Barbui, C. (1997) 'Poverty and mental illness.' *Canadian Journal of Psychiatry 42*, 285–290.

Sashidharan, S.P. (2001) 'Institutional racism in British psychiatry.' *Psychiatric Bulletin 25*, 244–247.

Shah, A. (2008) 'Estimating the absolute number of cases of dementia and depression in the black and minority ethnic elderly population in the UK.' *International Journal of Migration, Health and Social Care 4*, 2, 4–15.

Shah, A. and Dighe-deo, D. (1998) 'Elderly Gujaratis and psychogeriatrics in a London psychogeriatric clinic.' *Bulletin of the International Psychogeriatric Association 14*, 12–13.

Shah, A. and MacKenzie, S. (2007) 'Disorders of Ageing across Cultures.' In D. Bhugra and K. Bhui (eds) *Textbook of Cultural Psychiatry.* Cambridge: Cambridge University Press.

Sharpley, M.S., Hutchinson, G, Murray, R.M. et al. (2001) 'Understanding the excess of psychosis among the African-Caribbean Population in England. Review of current Hypothesis.' *British Journal of Psychiatry,* 178, 47, 60s-80s.

Siddiqi, N., House, A.O. and Holmes, J.D. (2006) 'Occurrence and outcome of delirium in medical in-patients: A systemic literature review.' *Age and Ageing 35*, 4, 350–355.

Summerfield, D. (2002) 'Mental health of refugees and asylum-seekers: Commentary.' *Advances in Psychiatric Treatment 8*, 247–248.

The NHS Information Centre (2007) *Adult Psychiatric Morbidity in England, 2007: Results of a Household Survey.* Available at www.esds.ac.uk/doc/6379/mrdoc/pdf/6379research_report.pdf, accessed on 6 November 2016.

The Poverty Site (2013) *The Poverty Site* (no longer updated). www.poverty.org.uk

Torrey, E.F. (1972) 'What Western psychotherapists can learn from witch doctors.' *American Journal of Orthopsychiatry 42*, 1, 69–72.

Tribe, R. (2007) 'Health pluralism – a more appropriate alternative to Western models of therapy in the context of the conflict and natural disaster in Sri Lanka?' *Journal of Refugee Studies 20*, 1, 21–36.

Tribe, R. (2014) 'Culture, politics and global mental health.' *Disability and the Global South 1*, 2, 251–265.

Tribe, R. (2016) 'Commentary on "Case Studies of Innovative Practice and Policy".' In R. White, U. Read, S. Jain and D. Orr (eds) *Palgrave Handbook of Global Mental Health: Socio-cultural Perspectives.* London: Palgrave Macmillan.

Tribe, R. and Raval, H. (eds) (2003) *Working with Interpreters in Mental Health.* London and New York: Brunner-Routledge.

Tribe, R. and Tunariu, A. (2017) 'Psychological Interventions and Assessments.' In D. Bhugra and K. Bhui (eds) *The Textbook of Cultural Psychiatry.* Cambridge: Cambridge University Press (in press).

Tribe, R., Lane, P. and Hearsum, S. (2009) 'Working towards promoting positive mental health and well-being for older people within BME communities.' *Working with Older People 31*, 1, 35.

Walsh, K. and Nare, L. (2016) *Transnational Migration and Home in Older Age.* Abingdon and New York: Routledge.

Wanless, D., Forder, J. and Fernandez, J.-L. (2006) *Securing Good Care for Older People.* London: The King's Fund.

Warfa, N., Bhui, K., Craig, T., Curtis, S. *et al.* (2006) 'Post-migration geographical mobility, mental health and health service utilisation among Somali refugees in the UK: A qualitative study.' *Health & Place 12*, 4, 503–515.

Watt, L.M. and Cappeliez, P. (2000) 'Integrative and instrumental reminiscence therapies for depression in older adults: Intervention.' *Aging & Mental Health 4*, 2, 166–177.

Woolfe, R. (1998) 'Therapists' attitudes towards working with older people.' *Journal of Social Work Practice 12*, 2, 141–148.

World Health Organization (2000) *The World Health Report 2000. Health Systems: Improving Performance.* Geneva: WHO. Available at www.who.int/whr/2000/en/whr00_en.pdf?ua=1, accessed on 6 November 2016.

World Health Organization (2016) *Mental Health and Older Adults Fact Sheet.* www.who.int/medicaentre/factsheets

Chapter 4

Common Mental Health Problems

Dr Maureen McIntosh and Dr Afreen Huq

Overview

For the first time in recorded history, the population in the UK over age 65, is larger than those under 16 and if this trend extends into the future, we will be faced with major changes in the structure and possible values of our society. This may influence legislation that reflects the rights and values of older adults who will require a new range of services to meet the increasing demand on health services including mental health and social care services. The focus of this chapter is on the challenges of building relationships and working in collaboration with older adults, that are genuinely reciprocal and that will provide the platform for any interventions or services developed and that can be cost effective. We hope to enthuse and inspire clinicians to embrace and explore the challenges and opportunities of working therapeutically with older adults, taking a person centred approach, whilst addressing and countering discrimination and social inequalities, preserving respect and dignity and creating connections between people. We need to be sensitive to ageism and the potential loneliness and invisibility of older adults and make conscious efforts to respond respectfully and warmly.

Anti-discriminatory practice is both an individual, professional and community matter. We need to harness the existing resources and collaborate with service users/experts by experience (EBE) and commissioners to develop effective and safe clinical service provision for older adults which both provides a high quality individualised, appropriate and accessible service and ensures anti discriminatory practice is promoted and upheld.

According to the Office of National Statistics [ONS] (2015), since 1974, the number and proportion of older adults in the UK population (aged 65 and older) has grown by 47 per cent, making up nearly 18 per cent of the total population. The number of people aged 75 and over has increased by 89 per cent over this period and now makes up 8 per cent of the population. There is an awareness globally that communities may not be fully prepared for the continued growth of the older adult population. The current societal discourse reflects the concerns there are regarding the financial cost of health and social care.

According to the Royal College of Psychiatry (2014), depression may affect 1 in 5 older adults in the community and 2 in 5 older adults living in care homes. Siddiqi, House, and Holmes, (2006) have shown that delirium may affect an estimated 14–56 per cent of all hospitalised older adults. Beaumont and Loft (2013) found that anxiety in older adults increased with age, i.e. 14 per cent of 65–69 year olds, 15 per cent of 70–74 year olds, 17 per cent of 75-79 year olds and 20 per cent of 80 years and over, reported experiencing anxiety. Prince (2014) found 1 in 14 older adults aged 65 and over had dementia in 2013.

Mental health difficulties can arise from a combination of factors such as changes in physiology, life experiences, social and cultural shifts. Many older adults will experience common mental health problems such as 'depression, generalised anxiety disorder, social anxiety disorder, post-traumatic stress disorder, panic disorder, obsessive compulsive disorder and body dysmorphic disorder' (NICE 2011, p.5) with co-morbid presentations, this is when more than one physical and or mental health condition [eg: depression, anxiety, arthritis] are happening simultaneously. There are also 'neuro-generative' presentations (e.g. Parkinson's disease) that can impact on the person's psychological well-being (Warren *et al.* 2016,). There is inequity for older adults when trying to access mental health services (Age Concern 2006) and this disparity in health provision (Royal College of Psychiatrists 2013; Department of Health [DH] 2004) demonstrates ageist barriers to meeting the needs of older adults (McIntosh and Sykes 2016).

The needs of older adults are multi-layered and working with this client group is about being able to support them to sustain a good quality of life despite the many challenges they may face. With better resourced older adult services, they can experience tailored support that helps maintain their sense of 'well-being' because they feel valued, respected and understood and the values of anti-discriminatory practice can be upheld. Multi-disciplinary mental health and adult social care teams (MDTs) often struggle to provide adequate services to older adults who present with common mental health problems due to budget reductions created by government driven public sector savings. There are services that adopt ageist practices that do not take account of the person and focus only on age. For example some adult mental health services will routinely transfer cases to older adult community mental health teams, because the individual is 60 or 65 years old without considering whether the transfer is related to problems with ageing. There should be greater resources given to older adult mental health teams so that 'integrated services' can deliver the complex and diverse 'health and social care' needs of older adults (Joint Commissioning Panel for Mental Health 2013, p.4).

Recognising mental health problems and help seeking

The Royal College of Psychiatrists (2009) and the Academy of Medical Royal Colleges have written *No Health without Mental Health* about the importance of recognising that physical health difficulties can be detrimental to a person's psychological health. Many older adults have long term conditions which can mean more medical appointments and a number of medications. It may not always be apparent to those in contact with the older adult that subjective changes in their mood and behaviour happen at a time when overall medical and physical health related matters may increase (Lawrie and Phillips 2016).

Older adults may go to their GP with physical health problems as it may feel less stigmatising talking about medical matters (e.g. somatic problems such as increased pain, sleep difficulties, loss of appetite, poor mobility, having a fall, urinary infection leading to delirium). A family member might notice changes in their behaviour (e.g. withdrawal/isolating themselves, losing interest in pleasurable activities, agitation, tearfulness, lack of confidence, loss of motivation, loss of independence, becoming angry, and being more forgetful) which could have been triggered by a loss or other negative life event.

For the family member, friend or carer the change feels significant and is unlike the older adult's usual way of being and could be an indicator that something could be going on that needs further investigation. Further exploration through a more in depth specialist assessment that examines the older adult's experience (Knight and Pachana 2015; Laidlaw, Kishita and Chellingsworth 2016) may give richer information about what is going on and how the older adult feel.

Referral Pathway

Clinical work with older adults can be across a range of contexts and disciplines including nurses, doctors, social workers, occupational therapists, psychologists, psychotherapists, and residential/nursing home workers, managers of care homes, as well as families and carers. The referral source is usually via the General Practitioners or the Hospital Medical Care Teams and Units.

In general practice, GPs will often refer patients to mental health services for a diagnosis or support from social care workers to provide help to staff and manage the older adult's behavioural and psychological symptoms of distress from a range of mental health conditions such as Dementia, challenging behaviour (BPS and RCP 2007) and Depression, Anxiety Phobia, and other common mental health problem (see NICE 2011). The Department of Health want older adults to receive '…dignified and compassionate care' (DH 2011, p.2). Specialist older adult mental health services usually have a single point of entry referral process to a duty desk where referrals are triaged and then assessed by a member of the MDT. The assessment is discussed during the MDT meeting where recommendations are made to try and meet the needs of the older person. There are referral pathways to other services, for example, clinical health psychology, third sector organisations, social care, Improving access to psychological therapy (IAPT), Physiotherapists, District Nurses, Speech and language therapists, falls service, pain clinic, etc. so that the needs of older adults can be met. However, barriers to receiving help exist when services cannot provide home visits to older adults who cannot attend appointments due to poor mobility caused by becoming frail. Frailty is a broad term that encompasses a number of problems that can impact on older adults, to restrict their mobility and ability to function in their usual way and their mental well-being could subsequently be compromised (Mhaol´ain et al. 2012).

Diagnostic systems, and alternative explanations

The ongoing reforms within the NHS context are dominated by medical diagnostic systems and clinical services are designed and funded on this basis. Following the introduction of the coalition government's Health and Social Care Act (2012), NHS services have faced increased competition for contracts, to explore income generation opportunities, and to meet targets.

The systems for diagnosing mental health problems in older adult services routinely use the Diagnostic and Statistical Manual of Mental Disorders (DSM-V) and International Classification of Diseases [ICD-10]. The Division of Clinical Psychology (DCP, 2013) argue that there ought to be a paradigm shift from a 'disease' model to a 'conceptual system' for all clients with functional presentations. Functional presentations refers to the "limitations" the diagnosis imposes on the individual (e.g. schizophrenia, bipolar disorder, personality disorder, attention deficit hyperactivity disorder, conduct disorders and so on) which interrupts their day to day living (Ustun and Kennedy 2009). Diagnosis provides a flawed basis for evidence-based practice, research, intervention guidelines and the various administrative and nonclinical uses due to its limited reliability and questionable validity. This has been a matter of cross-professional concern for many years (Barker 2011; Bentall 2004; Berger 2013; Boyle 2002; Bracken *et al.* 2012; BPS 2000, 2011; Coppock and Hopton 2000; Johnstone 2008; Moncrieff 2010).

The current classification systems are less controversial for conditions with an identified biological aetiology such as in the fields of neuropsychology, dementias (although not entirely without their controversies) and moderate to severe learning disability. Nevertheless, serious concerns have been raised about the increasing medicalisation of distress and behaviour in both adults and children (BPS 2011; Conrad 2007). The 'functional' diagnoses, for which there is substantial evidence for psychosocial factors in aetiology, and very limited support for a disease model, give rise to a wider range of views and positions and are the primary focus of this statement. This position should not be read as a denial of the role of biology in mediating and enabling all forms of human experience, behaviour and distress (Cromby, Harper and Reavey 2013), as is demonstrated, for example, in emerging epigenetic research (Read and Bentall 2012; Szyf and Bick 2013).

The DCP (2013) posit that a person's experiences can have numerous causes that are intricately connected. Knight and Pachana (2015) suggest that when assessing older adults it is important to know about 'normal ageing', how particular difficulties combine with 'social, psychological and biological' elements in society. We need to acknowledge the growing amount of evidence for psychosocial causal factors that contribute to the experience of distress in older adults, which does not assign an unevidenced role for biology as a primary cause, and that is transparent about the very limited support for the 'disease' model in such conditions. Such an approach would need to be multi-factorial, to contextualise distress and behaviour, and to acknowledge the complexity of the interactions involved, in keeping with the core principles of formulation in clinical psychology (DCP 2011).

Moncrieff (2009) and Whitaker (2010) have suggested that the drug companies use a common narrative with which to explain emotional distress and convert its various manifestations into diagnosable mental illnesses. The Midlands Psychology group (2012) have written about considering distress from a social–materialist perspective, by which they mean that people are social and material beings, our thoughts are continuously shaped by acquired cultural resources and influenced and conditioned by the experiences of the social and material world. Distress arises from the outside inwards as distress is not the consequence of inner flaws or weaknesses. External factors, experiences, difficult life circumstances beyond the person's control can impact on their overall health.

Many psychological therapies attribute distress to some kind of emotional defect (Midlands Psychology group 2012) however acquired, while systemic approaches (Midlands Psychology group 2012) recognise that difficulties do not arise within individuals but in the relationships and interactions between them which are always influenced by social, cultural and material circumstances. Community approaches (Midlands Psychology group 2012) locate distress in the social structures, material circumstances and power relations of everyday life. However, these approaches are limited by the reality of where distress is produced by social and material influences in everyday life. Other writers suggest the effects of trauma, social inequality and life events interact with the experience of poor parenting, friendship, nurturing and caring can all impact on our mental health as we age (Midlands Psychology group 2012). For example being a child evacuee during the Second World War and experiencing prolonged separation from their family.

In summary mental and emotional distress is often influenced by our biology but individuals have different biological and personal capacities and our experiences of mental health can be understood as a continuum with all other experiences and does not fall into discrete categories or diagnoses. Indeed, distress describes an embodied way of being and behaviour and it cannot be separated from context. Medication and therapy can help make a difference to older adults' mental health but not by curing. Effective therapy depends on the successful interaction between both parties' social and material circumstances and the resulting powers and resources that they can mobilise.

Ekdawi and Hansen (2010) describe systemic approaches to working with older adults in the context of difference and discrimination. They advocate supporting preferred identities in older adults, for example, we are more likely to experience 'diminished identity' in contexts where we feel different from others and where this difference is not valued or is seen as negative. For example, using and promoting discourses that inform older adults and improve services, for example, common shared viewpoints such as 'you cannot teach an old dog new tricks', 'it is normal to feel low in old age', etc. need to be noticed as an older adult can accept these expressions of ageism as realities and internalise them. Also dialogues about sexuality and older adults, for example, we need to be mindful of the dominant view of older adults as asexual and heterosexual which can inhibit our curiosity as health and social care professionals about important aspects of their sexual lives.

We need to challenge communication that diminish identities, for example, we need to become aware of our prejudices so that we are able to use these as potential resources where we enable the older adult's preferred version of himself or herself to emerge. The more we are aware of our own prejudices it can enhance our reflective practice so we can work on our assumptions constructively (eg: assuming older adults do not have a sexual life) as well help with effective communication. We may do this by using language that does not denigrate the person and taking care to check with older adult clients what words they prefer to use and what meanings they give to words we use. For example, the term 'old codger' can be experienced as patronising and belittling and not always seen as an affectionate term. We also need to be mindful of addressing difference and discrimination in context in order to learn from others, particularly feedback from experts by experience.

The Medical expert paradigm

Pressures to provide clinical services in a business like way where everyone fits in as led to the service user being disempowered, as the decision making process is in the hands of experts. Al Condeluci (1996) identifies four major themes that are central to the medical/ expert paradigm which is deeply rooted into the fabric of most organised health care systems today. For example, a focus on deficits in the service user, congregative ('...to want people to fit in', p.xxxiii) and segregated services, controlled by experts, attempting to fix or change the service user. For example, the systems we work in have a propensity to want people to fit in, often telling people what their problem is, why this is bad, and then what they need to do to eradicate the problem. Al Condeluci (1996) uses the concept of Interdependence to challenge these four themes and focuses on themes that promote a sense of similarity rather than difference i.e. focus on capacity, promote relationship through inclusion, and advocating action that revolves around the expert by experience and promotes change at the micro and macro level. Biggs (1989) and Knight (2004) both address the patterns of expectations when 'younger therapists' are challenged by the issues that the older adult client may bring; as they may not have expected to have to manage such issues at that point in their own stage of life (Knight 2004).

Dementia, diagnosis and memory services

The economic price of dementia is costed at 26 billion pounds a year (Alzheimer's Society 2014) and 2015 UK figures were predicted to show that 850,000 individuals would be living with dementia (Alzheimer's Society 2014). Dementia is described as a condition that causes changes in brain and impacts on everyday function, for example, 'memory or other thinking skills' like: concentration, communication, language, reasoning and judgement (Alzheimer's Association 2014 p.5). In reality, the scientific basis of the organic narrative of dementia illness is open to serious question (Kitwood 1997; Shenk 2012). For example by the late nineties, the drug companies had launched their cognitive enhancers with large advertising budgets to support the claim that these drugs are effective for memory problems. Bender (2014) examines how the dementia narrative has been used to define the field of cognitive impairment in old age, but argues that the claims are seriously flawed and these have ethical implications for psychologists working with older adults.

There is a growing demand for memory services to diagnose older adults (Alzheimer's Society 2014). The type of service an older adult receives can be patchy where some services may have a dementia care team for instance to provide ongoing support, this is not always the case. In some areas it has increasingly fallen upon Community Mental Health Team (CMHT) secondary care services to provide help into residential settings and within a person's home when the challenging behaviour caused by dementia has created distress for the older adult, or stress for the professional and family caregivers.

Case Study: Sam

Sam, aged 76 is admitted to a Dementia Assessment Ward with a diagnosis (given previously) of advanced dementia. His wife, his main carer, was hospitalised and died from lung cancer a week after his admission. Sam appears disorientated and very sad on the ward. The children in the family have decided that there is no need to inform Sam that his wife has died and do not want him at her funeral. The family members live a considerable distance away and regular visits are not possible. However, the care team strongly disagreed with the family's decision and felt it was not ethical to keep the news of his wife's death from him and that he was deprived of the opportunity to say his last goodbye to his wife at the funeral. The hospital staff offered to provide Sam with transport and a nurse escort to enable his attendance at the funeral. Senior members of the care team spent considerable time liaising with the family and the hospital legal department addressing our duty of care issues.

- What are the multi factorial challenges for the care team?

- How might you work with the team regarding this admission?

All older adults with memory difficulties should be seen quickly and assessed by a memory service. Bender (2014) also raises concerns about the current work culture restricting professionals' ability to act as applied practitioners with reference to the psychologist's limited role in memory clinics.

Mental health needs of older adults

Older adults frequently experience numerous negative life events that may impact upon their everyday life and prevent them from living independently. The needs of older adults are multi-dimensional and there is an impact when adjustments to unexpected negative life events become challenging. These might include, but are not limited to a bereavement or loss, feeling unsafe, social isolation, being housebound, frequent medical appointments, poor mobility, long term conditions (e.g. arthritis, heart conditions, hypertension, diabetes) and/or sensory deficits (e.g. poor eyesight, hearing loss). These might lead to a struggle to maintain good mental health, possible suicidal ideation and social exclusion (Mental Health Foundation 2015). The need to build friendships, support networks, and to maintain psychological and emotional well-being are important. In addition, each older adult's cultural and spiritual needs require active consideration by health and social care professionals if anti-discriminatory practice is to be upheld.

There are a myriad of relational systems the older adult can be located within, depending on their particular circumstances. The interactions within health, social care, family systems, community systems and friendship networks can give rise to complex emotions (McIntosh 2013).

Case Study 2

Iris who is aged 80 with multiple health problems was referred to psychology services for depression. Reading the referral letter you learn that she is angry and frustrated with people treating her like she cannot think for herself, talking down to her, treating her like she is invisible or assuming that she will not understand them.

- What do you think would be an important consideration in how you approach Iris?

- How might you work with such strong emotions in the session?

- What are some ways that you could build trust and engage Iris in the process?

Working Psychologically with frailty

There is an interaction between physical illness and psychological health which may be caused by the life events that older adults face which bring complexity and co morbidity to the therapeutic work, for example 'frailty, losses, dependency, fear of death and survivor guilt' can be experienced as an attack on the older adult's sense of identity (Hyer *et al.* 2004, p.280). Andrew, Fisk and Rockwood (2012) conducted a study about the impact of "frailty" on the older person. They found that the older adult's psychological health is affected because the emotional and physical health changes are frequently experienced as catastrophic (p.1347).

Case Study 3

Shamil is aged 70 and is of Asian origin, with a history of uncontrolled diabetes, and poor mobility due to his arthritis. He is referred to psychology services as the medical team is concerned that he is not compliant with his diabetes medication regime. Due to his frailty he cannot attend your outpatient clinic and you have arranged to visit him at home with an interpreter. On assessment, it is found that he is poorly informed about his condition despite attending regular appointments for diabetes management. He has been given printed information in English which he could not read and they did not share this information with his family. He remembered brief discussions of his condition at the diabetic clinic but he was not able to follow what he was told. He lives with his son and his family and enjoys the meals he is served, and was not keen on imposing changes on them to make him diabetes-friendly meals.

- What are the issues to consider making a home visit and what do you imagine the impact to be on your engagement with Shamil?

- What considerations might you need to make in working with an interpreter?

- How might you consider the family's views and the support they offer Shamil?

In clinical practice, many of the older people with whom we work, have to face challenges of physical, cognitive and social losses and the communication can be dominated by the focus on problems and negative experiences. Listening respectfully to older people's experience of problems, we can work together for a shared understanding of the problems and then move away from problems to focus on strengths, abilities, resources and hopes for the future. Maintaining curiosity about our clients is helpful in exploring possibilities together to find a way forward. Therapeutic outcomes are dependent on the collaborative construction of meaning.

Therapy practices have continued to evolve over time such as systemic therapy, cognitive behaviour therapy, narrative therapy, mindfulness therapy, brief therapy, solution oriented therapy, cognitive analytic therapy, etc. The therapy techniques and tools and understanding the concepts behind their use, one can be creative and adapt therapy to be more appropriate to the needs of older people. Working together in a therapeutic relationship can contribute to the well-being of the client.

The therapy alliance and older adults

There is the potential in therap, that the development of the therapeutic alliance can renew and bring harmony to the older adult's inner world which might be of immense value to them (Newton *et al.* 1986). Fillit and Butler (2009) suggest that the development of a strong therapeutic relationship can help older people who experience frailty to feel heard and understood which can lead to more helpful ways for them to adjust to frailty and the ageing process. Hyer *et al.* (2004) claim that the alliance has a powerful influence when working with the older adults. Therefore, understanding the reciprocal emotional engagement between the therapist and client and its applicability in the therapy environment is important (Sexton *et al.* 1996). The relationship develops from a position of mutual understanding (Safran and Muran 2000) and generates a momentum within the work that has been described as possessing distinctive aspects (Samstag 2002). These facets capture that sense of the individual within the therapy relationship (Duncan 2002) which may be important for the psychology of the older adult; in light of the impact of the life changes that they experience (McIntosh 2013).

There are many considerations that beset the therapist and older adult in clinical practice, which need to be negotiated in order for the alliance to develop. There are times when the same relationship script the older adult may have used with others in their life takes place within therapy and in their everyday life (Knight 2004). The older adult client can associate the therapist with another significant relationship that of a child, grandchild, parent, spouse or a social authority figure (Knight 2004). Whomever the therapist represents for the client there is an opportunity to interpret the transference (Knight 2004). For example, Knight (2004, p.72) suggests that in therapy 'grandchildren' can hold a perfect position within the client's mind or may be; in contrast the 'grandchild' may represent a 'negative transference' where the older adult client may feel on the periphery of the family system and alone. Trying to make sense of how the client perceives what is being triggered within; by talking it through can strengthen the therapeutic bond (Knight 2004) and move therapy forward.

Countertransference is where the conversations within therapy give rise to particular feelings within the therapist. The reality for the therapist and society in general is that the particular life experiences that older adults encompass such as 'illness and disability' and the loss of close relationships might feel quite challenging for some therapists to manage routinely (Knight 2004).

A UK study by Atkins and Lowenthal (2004) also discovered fears and countertransference issues in the therapists who participated in their qualitative research about how they experience delivering therapy to older adults. The authors used a 'heuristic method' to understand the participants' experience (qualified therapists included 6 females and 1 male, aged 45 to 72 working with older adults), using unstructured interviews to explore the therapists' sense of the work (Atkins and Lowenthal 2004). The findings suggested that the therapists' experiences raised a number of personal and professional questions, feelings and thoughts about working with older adults. For example: 'perceptions of old age and ageism; boundaries and settings; changes to practice; culture and experiences; awareness of time; loss; decline and mortality; and parents and children' (Atkins and Lowenthal 2004, p.493).

Atkins and Lowenthal's (2004) findings indicate that the participants thought deeply about the older adult clients and how the challenges they face effect their lives. The participants were also mindful of managing their own 'anxiety and fears' regarding 'ageing and loss' through a reflective process that allowed them to be more cognizant of the intrapersonal issues that arose (Atkins and Lowenthal 2004). The participants' expressed their sense of loss and fears through an awareness of the proximity either to that of the older adults' story or the fear it brought up within them as they drew parallels with their clients (Atkins and Lowenthal 2004). Working with older adults' raised different concerns and emotions that created some anxiety and fear as the participants reflected on themselves or ageing relatives. The participants also contemplated on loss issues that impacted on the older person (Atkins and Lowenthal 2004).

For instance (a quote from a participant): 'When you are older it is a reality and their contemporaries are beginning to die and that can involve perhaps a parent and with these large families a couple of their brothers or sisters and I think that's an awful lot of loss for people in 6 years and "What's that like?" Whatever age, whatever the reasons for death, what that feels like and what it means to them. Loss is in the foreground, present' (Atkins and Lowenthal 2004, p.502).

Additionally, Atkins and Lowenthal (2004) found that the participants' stance of being accepting of the older adults' individual qualities was another way for the participants to adjust to the challenges faced when working with older adults. Moreover, being flexible, adapting the therapy work, being open to experience and letting go of unhelpful frames of reference that serve to confine the older adult within a rigid, negative, ageist, structure was also incorporated by the participants (Atkins and Lowenthal 2004).

Atkins and Lowenthal (2004) produced an interesting study and they claim that the aim of the study was not to create a theoretical framework of therapy with elders; instead they wanted to increase awareness. This is a qualitative study and the results are specific to the participants and demonstrates their subjective experience of working with older adults. Atkins and Lowenthal (2004) acknowledge their own background in the field of psychology and this would have contributed to how much reflexivity played a part in their study. Reflexivity is a vital area within qualitative research and it shows good practice when the researcher can reflect on how they managed the process (Kaskett 2012). Another aspect is the benefit of qualitative studies that highlight how the process of therapy with an older adult is experienced by the therapist using reflective and reflexive skills; moreover, studying the clinical work in this way 'sensitizes' the therapist to the needs of the client (Elliott and James 1989, p.461).

Biggs (1989) and Knight (2004,) both address the patterns of expectations when younger therapists are challenged by the issues that the older adult client may bring; as they may not have expected to have to manage such issues at that point in their own stage of life. Moreover, it can be the case that some therapists may feel conflicted because they are facing similar experiences in their personal lives. For instance there may be a relative that has received a diagnosis of dementia, or who may be depressed and working with a client with those same presentations might create boundary issues If this is the case, it is important that these are discussed in clinical supervision and are kept under review.

Being accepting of older adults' individual qualities was another way for the participants to adjust to the challenges faced when working with older adults. Moreover, being flexible, adapting the therapy work, being open to experience and letting go of unhelpful frames of reference that serve to confine the older adult within a rigid, negative and ageist, structure were found to be useful (Atkins and Lowenthal 2004). Working with older adults the therapist may also begin to learn about how life was for the older person when they were growing up (Knight 2004).

In clinical practice, many of the older adults with whom we work have to face challenges of physical, cognitive and social losses and the communication can be dominated by the focus on problems and negative experiences. By listening respectfully to older people's experiences we can work together for a shared understanding of the problems and then move away from those difficulties to focus on strengths, abilities, resources and hopes for the future. Maintaining curiosity about our clients is helpful in exploring possibilities together to find a way forward. Therapeutic outcomes are dependent on the collaborative construction of meaning. In the current context of the NHS, we can collaborate with practitioners who are committed to a medical model by inviting them to join therapy sessions, meetings, teaching and training sessions and consultations.

Therapy practices have continued to evolve over time such as systemic therapy, cognitive behaviour therapy, narrative therapy, mindfulness therapy, brief therapy, solution oriented therapy, cognitive analytic therapy, etc. The therapy techniques and tools and understanding the concepts behind their use, one can be creative and adapt therapy to be more appropriate to the needs of older people. Working together in a therapeutic relationship can contribute to the well-being of the client and to anti-discriminatory practice.

Learning Lessons

The Francis Report (2013) and the Winterbourne Review (DH 2012), point out malpractice which organisations failed to notice. These reports highlight discrimination and what can go wrong in organisations arising from a compromised capacity to hold compassion and care in mind. It is important for organisations to consider factors such as containment, empowerment, responsible autonomy and internalised accountability to facilitate a culture of compassion, and the dynamics which impact such attributes in individuals and groups.

All three reports demonstrated that within the culture of these organisations there was an emphasis on following procedures without considering the needs of the client and or staff group.

Reflective questions

1. In practice we need to be aware of ethics of complicity, shared decision making, debate around psychiatric medication, informed consent. How would you ensure you are aware of these issues and willing and able/ not able to address these issues?

2. How open, receptive and welcoming are you to older adults individually and within the service where you work?

3. We need to reflect on the language we use to describe people and events and the need to create a consistent blend between the words we use and the actions we show. How would you do this to ensure that you are promoting anti discriminatory practice?

4. Our job is to facilitate and enable people to access services in a manner which makes all involved feel cared for, supported and able to engage on their own terms in line with anti-discriminatory practice, how might you do this?

5. Ethical dilemmas: risk issues, negotiating a shared understanding of risk to promote personal responsibility and boundaries. How and what would you do to address these issues?

Suggested ideas, reading and resources for anti-discriminatory practice

- Listen to older adult service users/experts by experience (EBE)'s feedback and make changes to your clinical practice as appropriate.

- Facilitate reflection with clients, colleagues, teams/services/ organisations and commissioners of services.

- Act upon service user/EBE's views, throughout the process of working together and make any necessary adaptations.

- Uphold your professional code of ethics at all times.

- Undertake self-reflection, attend regular supervision, and engage in dialogue with EBE and community groups for older adults.

- Seek guidance regarding ethical and professional dilemmas before or as they arise.

- Facilitate shared decision making and informed consent.

- The Psychology of Older People: FPOP Bulletin is a useful resource for inspiration and up to date examples of good clinical practice. www.bps.org.uk/publications/member-network-publications/member-publications/fpop-bulletin

- Practitioners should view potential obstacles in a non-definitive way, for example using feedback constructively. Also managing one's expectations: the client, the team and the service in order to maximise clinical service delivery.

- Recognise the importance of group support as an active ingredient to well-being for the service users.

- We recommend 'the discovery that ended Alzheimer's stronghold'. www.youtube.com/watch?v=1ILK8ZQj6Gc

References

Age Concern (2006). *UK Inquiry into Mental Health and Well-Being in Later Life. Coordinated by Age Concern.* www.ageconcern.org.uk

Alzheimer's Society. Dementia 2014 report statistics. Available at *www.alzheimers.org.uk* Accessed 22 October 2016.

Alzheimer's Association (2014) Alzheimer's Disease, Facts and Figures, Alzheimer's and Dementia, Volume 10, 2, 1–80. Accessed 8 December 2016.

Andrew, M. K., Fisk, J. D. and Rockwood, K. (2012). Psychological well-being in relation to frailty: a frailty identity crisis? *International Psychogeriatrics, 24, 8,* 1347–1353.

American Psychiatric Association. (2013). *Diagnostic and statistical manual of mental disorders (5th ed.). Arlington, VA:* American Psychiatric Publishing.

Atkins, D. and Lowenthal, D. (2004). 'The lived experience of psychotherapists working with older clients: An heuristic study.' *British Journal of Guidance and Counselling, 32, 4,* 493–509.

Barker, P. (2011). Psychiatric diagnosis. In P.Barker (Ed.) *Mental health ethics: The human context* (pp.139–148). Abingdon, New York: Routledge

Beaumont, J., and Loft, H. (2013). *Measuring National Well-being: Health.* London: Office for National Statistics.

Bender, M. (2014). The ethics of complicity: Clinical psychologists and the contemporary dementia narrative. Clinical Psychology Forum, 253, 52–56.

Bentall, R.P. (2004). *Madness explained.* London: Penguin.

Berger, M. (2013). *Classification, diagnosis and datasets: Towards an approach for clinical psychology services and electronic records.* Leicester: BPS.

Biggs, S. (1989). Professional Helpers and Resistances to work with Older People. *Ageing and Society, 9, 1,* 43–60.

Boyle, M. (2002). *Schizophrenia: A scientific delusion?* (2nd edn.) Hove, New York: Routledge.

Bracken, P., Thomas, P., Timimi, S., Asen, E., Behr, G., Beuster, C. et al. (2012). Psychiatry beyond the current paradigm. *The British Journal of Psychiatry, 201,* 430–434.

British Psychological Society (2011). *Response to the American Psychiatric Association: DSM-5 development.* Leicester: BPS.

British Psychological Society and Royal College of Psychiatrists. (2007) Dementia: The NICE-Scie guideline on supporting people with dementia and their carers in health and social care. Available on: www.bps.org.uk

Castonguay, L. G., Constantino, M.J. (2006). The Working Alliance: where are we and where should we go? *Psychotherapy: Theory, Research, Practice, Training, 43, 3,* 271–279.

Condeluci, A. (1996). Beyond Difference. Delray Beach, Florida: St. Lucie Press, Inc.

Conrad, P. (2007). *The medicalization of society: On the transformation of human conditions into treatable disorders.* Baltimore, MD: John Hopkins University Press.

Coppock, V. and Hopton, J. (2000). *Critical perspectives on mental health.* London: Routledge.

Cromby, J. and Harper, D. (2013). Paranoia: Contested and contextualised. In S. Coles, S. Keenan and B. Diamond (Eds.), *Madness contested: Power and practice.* Ross-on-Wye: PCCS Books.

DH (Department of Health) (2004). *Patient and Public Involvement in health. The Evidence for policy implementation. London: Department of Health.* www.gov.uk (cited in McIntosh and Sykes, (2016), p.21, op cit).

DH (Department of Health) (2011) *The Operating Framework for the NHS in England 2012/13.* London: Department of Health. Available at: www.gov.uk

DH (Department of Health) (2012). *Transforming Care: A national response to Winterbourne View Hospital. Department of Health Review. Final Report.* London: Author.

Department of Health (2012). *The Health and Social Care Act.* London: The Stationery Office.

DCP (2000). *Recent advances in understanding mental illness and psychotic experiences.* Leicester: British Psychological Society.

DCP (2011). *Good practice guidelines on the use psychological formulation.* Leicester: BPS.

Division of Clinical Psychology (2013). *Classification of behaviour and experience in relation to functional psychiatric diagnosis: Time for a paradigm shift.* The British Psychological Society.

Duncan, B. L. (2002). The legacy of Saul Rosenzweig: The Profundity of the Dodo Bird. *Journal of Psychotherapy Integration, 12,* 32–57.

Ekdawi, I. and Hansen, E. (2010). Working with older people in contexts of difference and discrimination. In Being With Older People: A Systemic Approach, Fredman, G., Anderson, E. and Stott, J. (eds). London: Karnac.

Elliott, R. and James, E. (1989). Varieties of client experience in Psychotherapy: An analysis of the literature. *Clinical Psychology Review, 9*, 443–467.

Fillitt, H. and Butler, R. (2009). The Frailty Identity Crisis. *Journal of American Geriatrics, 57*, 348–352.

Francis, R (Chair) (2013). *Mid Staffordshire NHS Foundation Trust Public Inquiry Report*. London: The Stationery Office.

Garner, J. (2003). Psychotherapies and older adults. *Australian and New Zealand Journal of Psychiatry, 37*, 537–548.

Huq, A. and McIntosh, M. (2015). Professional and ethical issues in working with Older Adults. (cited in Tribe and Morrissey, (2015), p.197-205, op cit). In Chap. 17, Tribe, R. and Morrissey, J. (2015) (Eds) *The Handbook of Professional and Ethical Practice for Psychologists, Psychotherapists and Counsellor* (2nd edn) Hove and New York: Routledge.

Hyer, L., Kramer, D. and Sohnle, S. (2004). CBT with older people: alterations and the value of the therapeutic alliance. *Psychotherapy, Theory, Research Practice, Training, 41, 3*, 276–291.

Johnstone, L. (2008). Psychiatric diagnosis. In T. Turner and B. Tummey (Eds.), *Critical issues in mental health*. Hampshire: Palgrave Macmillan.

Joint Commissioning Panel for Mental Health (2013) Guidance for commissioners of Older People's Mental Health Services. www.jcpmh.info/wp accessed xx

Kasket, E. (2012). The counselling psychologist researcher. *Counselling Psychology Review, 27, 2*, 64–73.

Kitwood, T. (1997). Dementia reconsidered: the person comes first. Open University Press.

Knight, B.G. (2004). *Psychotherapy with Older Adults. (3* red.) London: Sage.

Laidlaw, K., Kishita, N. and Chellingsworth, M. (2016). *A Clinician's Guide to CBT with older people*. University of East Anglia. www.uea.ac.uk/documents/

Lawrie, L. and Phillips, L. H. (2016). A maturing picture of emotion. *The Psychologist, 29*, 12, 908–909.

McIntosh, M. and Sykes, C. (2016). Older Adults' Experience of Psychological Therapy, *Counselling Psychology Review, 31*, 1, 20–30.

McIntosh, M. (2013). 'Older Adults and the Therapeutic Alliance. [Unpublished Manuscript]'. *DPsych research, Chapter 6*: A Critical Review, 200–226.

Mental Health Foundation. (2015). Fundamental facts about mental health. www.mentalhealth.org. uk/publications/fundamental-facts-about-mental-health-2015

Mhaolian, A.M., Wei Fan, C., Ramero-Ortuno, R., Cogan, L., Cunningham, C., Kenny, R. A. and Lawlor, B. (2012). Frailty, depression and anxiety in later life. *International Psychogeriatrics, 24, 8*, 1265–1274.

Midlands Psychology Group (2012). Draft manifesto for a Social Materialist Psychology, Journal of Critical Psychology, *Counselling and Psychotherapy, 12, 2*, 93–107.

Moncrieff, J. (2009). *The myth of the chemical cure: A critique of psychiatric drug treatment*. Basingstoke: Palgrave Macmillan.

Moncrieff, J. (2010). Psychiatric diagnosis as a political device. *Social Theory and Health, 8*, 370–382.

National Institute for Health and Care Excellence (NICE) (2011). Common Mental Health Problems: identification and pathways to care. Available at www.nice.org.uk/guidance/cg123, accessed on 24 January 2017.

Newton, N. A., Brauer, D., Gutmann, D. L., and Grunes, J. (1986). Psychodynamic therapy with the aged: A review. *Clinical Gerontologist: The Journal Of Aging And Mental Health, 5*(3-4), 205-229 (cited in Hyer et al, (2004), p.280, op cit).

Prasko, J., Diveky, T., Grambal, A., Kamaradova, D., Mozny, P., Sigmundova, Z., Slepecky, M. and Vyskocilova, J. (2010). Transference and Countertransference in *Cognitive Behavioral Therapy. Biomedical Papers of the Medical Faculty, 154, 3*, 189–198.

Prince M, *et al.* (2014). *Dementia UK: The Second Edition*. London: Alzheimer's Society.

Read, J. and Bentall, R. (2012). Negative childhood experiences and mental health. *British Journal of Psychiatry, 200*, 89–91.

Royal College of Psychiatrists and Academy of Medical Royal Colleges (2009). 'No Health without Mental Health. The Alert Summary Report. Available at www.rcpsych.ac.uk/pdf/ALERT%20 print%20final.pdf

Royal College of Psychiatrists. (2013). *Whole-person care: from rhetoric to reality Achieving parity between mental and physical health.* Available at www.rcpsych.ac.uk/usefulresources/publications/

Royal College of Psychiatrists (2014). *Depression in OlderAdults.* Available at http://www.rcpsych.ac.uk/healthadvice/problemsdisorders/depressioninolderadults.aspx

Safran, J. D. and Muran, C. J. (2000). *Negotiating the Therapeutic Alliance: A Relational Treatment Guide.* New York: Guildford Press.

Samstag,L, W. (2002). The common versus unique factors hypothesis in psychotherapy research: did we misinterpret Rosenzweig? *Journal of Psychotherapy Integration, 12,* 58-66.

Sexton, H. C., Hembre, K. and Kvarme, G. (1996). The Interaction of the Alliance and Therapy Microprocess: A Sequential Analysis. *Journal of Consulting and Clinical Psychology, 64, 3,* 471–480.

Shenk, D. (2012). *The discovery that ended Alzheimer's stronghold. Retrieved from* www.youtube.com/watch?v=1ILK8ZQj6Gc

Szyf, M. and Bick, J. (2013). DNA methylation: A mechanism for embedding early life experiences in the genome. *Child Development, 84, 1,* 49–57.

Tribe, R. and Morrissey, J. (2015) (Eds) *The Handbook of Professional and Ethical Practice for Psychologists, Psychotherapists and Counsellor* (2nd edn) Hove and New York: Routledge.

Ustun, B. and Kennedy, C (2009). What is "functional impairment"? Disentangling disability from clinical significance. *World Psychiatry 2009, 8,* 82–85.

Warren, E., Eccles, F.J.R., Travers, V. and Simpson, J. (2016). The experiences of being diagnosed with Parkinson's disease, *FPOP Bulletin,* No. 136, 3–8.

World Health Organization. (1992). *The ICD-10 classification of mental and behavioural disorders: clinical descriptions and diagnostic guidelines.* Geneva: World Health Organization.

CHAPTER 5

The Mental Capacity Act 2005 and Ageing

Ajit Shah

Introduction

This chapter examines the implications of ageing, age-related mental disorders and personal characteristics on decision-making capacity and other aspects of the Mental Capacity Act 2005 (MCA) in relation to the relevant literature. Additionally, examples of good practice will be illustrated along with strategies for improved application of the Mental Capacity Act to avoid discrimination.

> You can find a guide to the acronyms used in the MCA here: www.publications.parliament.uk/pa/ld201314/ldselect/ldmentalcap/139/13924.htm.

Background

The MCA is a comprehensive framework for decision-making on behalf of adults aged 16 and over who are unable to make decisions for themselves (i.e. they lack capacity). The Act was developed in 2005 and came into force in England and Wales in 2007. In Scotland, the Adults with Incapacity (Scotland) Act 2000 applies, while in Northern Ireland decisions are made under common law.

The MCA provides a statutory process for those who lack decision-making capacity or who currently have decision-making capacity but would like to plan for the future, when their capacity may decline. There are five principles of the MCA that attempt to ensure anti-discriminatory practice:

- Decision-making capacity is assumed, unless lack of decision-making capacity has been formally established.

- An individual cannot be treated as lacking decision-making capacity unless all practical steps have been undertaken to help the individual to make a decision.

- An individual cannot be assumed to lack decision-making capacity simply because he or she makes or has previously made an 'unwise' decision.

- Any act done or any decision made under the MCA must be in the best interests of the individual who lacks decision-making capacity.

- Before any act is done or any decision is made under the MCA, consideration must be given to whether there is an alternative option that is less restrictive of the individual's rights and freedom.

These points are illustrated in the following scenario.

Case study: George

A 77-year-old man, George, is deaf but is spending most of his savings on buying a series of hearing aids in the hope that they will help him to hear better.

Despite difficulty communicating with him, his support worker assumed that he lacked the capacity to manage his financial affairs. George's doctor was asked to complete a COP3 form supporting an application to place his financial affairs under the Court of Protection.

The doctor was able to communicate with George through writing and subsequently concluded that he did have the capacity to manage his own financial affairs.

Assessment of decision-making capacity

The assessment of decision-making capacity requires a two-stage questioning process.

First, does the individual have an impairment of the mind or brain, or is there some disturbance affecting his or her mentality? This is loosely synonymous with mental disorder. If so, does the impairment or disturbance mean that the individual is unable to make the decision in question, at the time that it needs to be made?

Using the specific four-fold test of capacity under the MCA, an individual is judged to lack decision-making capacity if a person is unable to:

- understand the information relevant to the decision

- retain this information

- use or weigh this information as part of the decision-making process

- communicate his or her decision (whether by talking, using sign language or any other means; specification of these approaches in the MCA intends to reduce any discriminatory practice).

Decision-making capacity should be assessed for each issue of concern individually, as a lack of decision-making capacity for one issue cannot be generalised to other issues. This should also be time-specific, as a person's decision-making capacity can fluctuate and decline. The following scenario offers an example of this.

Case study: Gerard

Gerard, who is 91 years old, has recently been diagnosed with Alzheimer's disease. When his daughter called round to visit, he suddenly became very confused. Worried about his mental state, she took Gerard to hospital.

The doctors found that he was suffering from thyroid problems and dehydration, which may have been the cause of his delirium. The medical team waited to see if his delirium would be resolved through treatment of his physical illness.

The staff did not simply assume that his temporary loss of mental capacity was due to his Alzheimer's disease. In this case, Gerard's mental state improved and he was able to return home and continue with care support provided by his family and private care company.

Making decisions on behalf of someone who lacks decision-making capacity

The MCA stipulates that 'An act done, or decision made, under the Act for or on behalf of a person who lacks capacity must be done, or made, in his best interests'. The Act applies to all decision-makers, including family carers, paid carers, health and social care professionals, donees of lasting power of attorney (formerly enduring power of attorney), court-appointed deputies, and the Court of Protection. It covers all aspects of financial, personal, welfare and healthcare decision-making.

Assessment of 'best interests'

The MCA and the accompanying Mental Capacity Act Code of Practice (Department for Constitutional Affairs 2013) do not formally define best interests but describe a list of factors that must be considered in the determination of an individual's best interests:

- Determination of best interests cannot be based on an individual's age, appearance (including racial appearance or religious dress), condition or behaviour.

- Consideration should be given to all circumstances pertaining to the individual who lacks decision-making capacity.

- Every effort should be made to enable an individual who lacks decision-making capacity to participate in making the decision, including use of appropriate methods of communication (including professional interpreters) and use of other people to facilitate the person to participate in the decision-making process.

- Consideration should be given to the possibility that the decision-making capacity may be regained (e.g. after treatment of a mental illness) and whether the decision-making can be postponed until decision-making capacity is regained.

- Consideration should be given to the past and present wishes, feelings, beliefs and values of an individual who lacks decision-making capacity.

- Consideration should be given to the views of other people who are close to an individual who lacks decision-making capacity, including anyone engaged in caring for the individual, anyone previously nominated by the individual to be consulted with about the decision in question or similar issues, donees of lasting power of attorney, the court-appointed deputies and the Independent Mental Capacity Advocate.

Careful consideration of the above factors may help to avoid discrimination, as demonstrated in the following scenario.

Case study: Florence

Florence, an elderly woman of Jamaican origin, was admitted to a gynaecology ward with uterine cancer, which had spread to her bone, bladder and liver. The urology team wanted to operate on her to relieve the pressure on her bladder and reduce urine retention. She was adamant that she did not wish to have this operation.

The gynaecology team considered this to be an unwise decision and decided that Florence may lack decision-making capacity in relation to the proposed surgery due to her psychiatric history of a delusional disorder. The psychiatric registrar was asked to review the patient, and she also judged her to lack decision-making capacity.

However, the psychiatric registrar spoke also to Florence's sister and her general practitioner. They both confirmed her long-standing view that she did not wish to have any surgery in relation to her cancer, and that she had previously declined surgery at the time of her initial diagnosis. This information was presented to the gynaecology team to include in their deliberations pertaining to her best interests.

Lasting power of attorney

The MCA replaced the former enduring power of attorney (EPA) with the lasting power of attorney (LPA). An LPA is an individual who must be at least 18 years old and must have decision-making capacity him- or herself, who has been given permission to make decisions on behalf of another person. The LPA has the authority to make decisions relating to property and affairs (including financial affairs) as well as personal welfare.

The Court of Protection

The MCA set up a specialist court, the Court of Protection, which has powers to deal with all areas of decision-making covered by the Act. Although the Court of Protection is based in London, most cases are heard by district judges and a senior judge; only the most complicated cases are heard by High Court judges. The Court of Protection can appoint a deputy to make ongoing decisions on behalf of the individual who lacks decision-making capacity. A deputy is usually a close relative or friend of the person who needs help making decisions, although he or she may also be in a paid position (such as accountants or solicitors). If there is no one appropriate for the role, the Court of Protection can appoint a deputy (called a panel deputy).

Advance decisions

The MCA allows people to make advance decisions about specific treatments when they are of sound mind and ensures that these wishes are taken into account in the future if decision-making capacity is lost. As long as they fulfil certain requirements, advance decisions are legally binding, meaning that all healthcare professionals must follow them. When there is a disagreement about an advance decision, professionals must consider all available evidence. If there is still doubt or disagreement, the decision should be referred to the Court of Protection; however, the Court cannot overturn a valid and applicable advance decision.

Equality and the Mental Capacity Act

An Equality Impact Assessment was undertaken for the MCA and its implementation programme, in order to examine the impact on diverse groups of people (Ministry of Justice 2007). The potential impact on people grouped by race, religion or belief, disability, gender, sexual orientation, age and caring responsibilities was assessed through extensive consultation with stakeholders who represented these diverse groups. The overall findings included the following:

- The MCA is anticipated to have an overall positive effect amongst individuals from Black and Minority Ethnic (BME) groups, diverse religious and faith groups, and other disadvantaged groups who lack decision-making capacity.

- The MCA is anticipated to have an overall positive impact for families and carers of BME individuals lacking decision-making capacity.

- All decision-makers must have regard for the statutory principles of the MCA and consider a wide range of factors in the determination of best interests, including wishes, feelings, values and beliefs – all of which may be indicated by cultural and religious background, disability, illness and sensory impairment.

Under the Code of Practice (2013, p.5):

> people taking decisions under the Act must recognise and respect the diverse needs, values and circumstances of each patient, including their race, religion, culture, gender, age, sexual orientation and any disability. They must consider the patient's views, wishes and feelings (whether expressed at the time or in advance), so far as they are reasonably ascertainable, and follow those wishes wherever practicable and consistent with the purpose of the decision. There must be no unlawful discrimination.

However, ageing may lead to disability and change in appearance, and these factors may risk the incorrect application of the MCA (Cairns *et al.* 2005; Mukherjee and Shah 2001; Shah and Dickenson 1999). Individuals who are elderly, have a mental disorder or a disability, and belong to a BME group may also be particularly vulnerable to the incorrect application of the MCA. Selected examples of some common areas of concern in this context are described below.

Communication

The second statutory principle of the MCA, supported by the Code of Practice (Department of Constitutional Affairs 2013), advocates that all practical and appropriate steps to enable an individual to make the relevant decision should be taken before concluding that the individual lacks decision-making capacity. This includes helping the individual to communicate in a manner that reflects his or her personal circumstances. If the individual is deemed to lack decision-making capacity, then every effort should be made to enable that person to contribute evidence towards determining his or her best interest.

Indeed, facilitating individuals to communicate to the best of their capacity should be fundamental across all applications of the MCA.

A formal psychiatric assessment may be needed to establish decision-making capacity, which requires an individual to understand the information relevant to the decision, to retain this information, to use or weigh this information as part of the decision-making process, and to communicate his or her decision. Therefore, it is vital that individuals are provided with information that is appropriate and accessible considering their needs. For example, a doctor who is proposing a specific treatment will need to explain the nature, purpose and the likely effects and side-effects of treatment, the consequences of refusing or accepting the treatment, and the same information for alternative treatments if they are available. Clearly, then, successful application of the MCA is contingent upon good communication between those who apply the MCA and the vulnerable individual (Shah and Heginbotham 2008). This has been well observed in clinical psychiatric practice with patients who are not fluent in English (Bhalia and Blakemore 1981; Shah 1992, 1997a, 1997b, 1999; Shah and MacKenzie 2007), may be hard of hearing (Nnatu 2005) and may have dementia or other mental disorders (Mukherjee and Shah 2001; Shah and Dickenson 1999; Shah et al. 2009a, 2009b, 2009c, 2010a, 2010b).

Some of the issues that have an impact on communication during the application of the MCA may include:

- the fluency of English of both the individual applying the MCA and the individual who may lack decision-making capacity

- the accuracy of interpretation services

- the availability of appropriate vocabulary in the individual's first language

- the degree of cognitive impairment

- the symptoms of mental disorder

- the degree of physical impairment (such as a hearing impairment).

Many BME elders are not fluent in English (Barker 1984; Lindesay *et al.* 1997; Manthorpe and Hettiaratchy 1993; Shah and MacKenzie 2007). Even when BME individuals are fluent in English, some disorders, such as dementia, may lead to loss of fluency in English, and communication in their first language may therefore be more appropriate; this is recognised in Chapter 3 of the Mental Capacity Act Code of Practice (Department for Constitutional Affairs 2013). Ideally, the assessor should conduct the assessment in the individual's first language and preferably have a sound understanding of the individual's culture in order to promote greater accuracy in a culturally appropriate context. However, this approach may not always be possible as bilingual health and social care workers are scarce (Hoxey, Mukherjee and Shah 1999; Phelan and Parkman 1995).

Example of positive practice

A good example of a bilingual worker helping BME people with dementia and their families to deal with financial and related mental capacity issues can be found in Dementia Concern Ealing, a voluntary-sector organisation.

Dementia Concern Ealing provides a Community Legal Service Quality Mark advice and casework service for people with dementia and their carers, including specialist advice and information concerning the MCA. Here, a bilingual staff member of Indian origin supports families from the Indian subcontinent with legal and social issues.

Nonetheless, assessments may be problematic even when the assessor is fluent in the individual's first language if there is an absence of matching vocabulary between English and the languages spoken by BME elders (Shah 1999). For example, the phrase 'decision-making capacity' – a core concept of the MCA – does not have an equivalent translation in several languages spoken by BME elders (such as Gujarati) (Shah and Heginbotham 2008). Vocabulary related to symptoms of illness, diagnosis and treatment may also lack equivalent terms and phrases in some languages. This has been observed in some BME groups in the assessment and management of mental illness (Bhui and Bhugra 2007; Shah 1999; Shah and Heginbotham 2008).

It is also worth noting that some bilingual individuals may withhold information if they are only interviewed in English, as they may not feel comfortable expressing all relevant information in English or may be unable to do so (Bhui and Bhugra 2007). Chapter 3 of the Mental Capacity Act Code of Practice (Department for Constitutional Affairs 2013) suggests that individuals who are applying the MCA should consider the following strategies to facilitate effective communication:

- Ascertain information about the best way to communicate with the individual from others who know him or her well (family members, general practitioner, support workers, etc.). They should also be able to advise on an appropriate time for the assessment; for example, people with dementia may be less alert or experience behavioural disturbances at certain times of day.

- Use simple language with the right volume and tone, break down complex information into smaller points, repeat information as necessary, and pause regularly to ensure the individual has understood everything.

- If appropriate, supplement verbal communication by using pictures, objects or illustrations to demonstrate ideas.

- Invite a trusted person (family member or a friend) or an independent advocate to be present, in case that may facilitate and improve communication. However, it should be noted that the presence of a trusted person can be counterproductive if the trusted person tries to provide answers for the person who is being assessed.

- Use a speech and language therapist or a neuropsychologist to help facilitate communication, particularly if specific language and/or cognitive deficits are identified.

- Use a professional language interpreter, including those for deaf individuals.

- Choose a location for the assessment where the individual feels most comfortable.

All the above strategies should be subject to strict confidentiality. It is important to remember that family members, friends and carers may also have English as a second language and/or may not fully understand some of the technical and legal issues. Therefore, a professional interpreter may still be required in order to communicate with the person being assessed and any trusted person. (For more details on working with an interpreter in mental health services, see Chapter 12 of this volume.)

The use of written material to facilitate communication

Many BME elders cannot read English, and some are also unable to read their mother tongue (Lindesay *et al.* 1997); those with visual impairment and/or dementia may also not be able to read. Any written material given to BME individuals may require either written translation into their first language (if they cannot read English) or audio translation into BME languages (if they cannot read in English or their mother tongue). Similar strategies should be used with people who are visually impaired or cannot read due to dementia.

Interpreters and MCA assessment

As suggested above, professional interpreters should be used at key events including assessments, reviews, case conferences and discussions with carers in clinical psychiatric practice (Centre for Ethnicity and Health *et al.* 2003; Department of Health 2005; Tribe and Thompson 2016). The use of professional interpreters is emphasised because the application of the MCA is a significant legal and personal event (Shah and Heginbotham 2008). The only exception may be if an urgent decision needs to be made in an emergency and a professional interpreter is not readily available (Centre for Ethnicity and Health *et al.* 2003).

The inherent difficulties and limitations in using interpreters in clinical psychiatric practice are well described (Kline *et al.* 1980; Marcos 1979; Shah 1997a, 1997b) and equally apply to the application of the MCA. Any potential difficulties with professional interpreters can be reduced with the guidance developed through clinical practice (Centre for Ethnicity and Health *et al.* 2003; Department of Health 2005; Phelan and Parkman 1995; Tribe and Raval 2003; Tribe and Thompson 2016).

Example of positive practice

For an example of positive practice in communication, this Department of Health video on YouTube depicts interpretation in clinical mental health settings along with strategies to make effective use of interpretation services: www.youtube.com/watch?v=k0wzhakyjck.

Provision of interpretation services

The Mental Capacity Act Code of Practice (Department for Constitutional Affairs 2013) advocates the use of interpretation services in the application of the MCA. Therefore, those determining an individual's best interests and others involved in the application of the MCA have a responsibility for the provision of professional interpretation services for everyone involved in the assessment. This may include employers of paid carers, health and social care professionals, staff of private and local authority nursing and residential homes, Independent Mental Capacity Advocates, court-appointed deputies, staff of the Court of Protection, lawyers, and staff of the Office of the Public Guardian. The Mental Capacity Act Equality Impact Assessment clarifies that interpreters can be made available on request for Court of Protection hearings (Ministry of Justice 2007). The responsibility for the provision of interpretation services for donees of lasting power of attorney is not clarified in the Mental Capacity Act Code of Practice, but it is unlikely that donors (i.e. those who will impart power of attorney) will have appointed donees (those who will hold the power of attorney) that they are unable to communicate with.

Other methods of communication

Chapter 3 of the Mental Capacity Act Code of Practice (Department for Constitutional Affairs 2013) suggests the use of pictures, objects or illustrations as a supplement to verbal communication to demonstrate ideas. In clinical psychiatric practice, audio tapes, DVDs, CDs and diagrammatic representation are all used to complement interpretation services for BME individuals (Lindesay *et al.* 1997). At present, such materials are not widely available in relation to the MCA. However, a summary of the MCA, a leaflet and a series of five booklets have been published in a variety of languages and in audio format for people who may lack decision-making capacity and their families, carers and professionals (Ministry of Justice 2007).

Example of positive practice

The Local Government Association has produced an easy-read guide to explain the Mental Capacity Act for people with learning disabilities. It can be found here: www.local.gov.uk/documents/10180/12137/ntal +Capacity+Act+2005+easy+read+guide/38683f88-4b96-49d6-86ab-89b2404d2e7a.

Cultural and religious factors

The MCA, the Mental Capacity Act Code of Practice and the Mental Capacity Act Equality Impact Assessment all recognise the importance of cultural and religious factors. These factors are considered together because they are closely entwined and are difficult to segregate.

Although detailed information, guidance and case examples on the MCA assessment with regard to cultural and religious factors are lacking, the second statutory principle of the MCA advocates that all practical and appropriate steps to enable an individual to make the relevant decision should be taken before deciding that an individual lacks decision-making capacity. In addition, the Mental Capacity Act Code of Practice clarifies that the MCA assessment should consider the following points:

- A person's 'personal circumstances' should be assessed, including cultural, ethnic and religious factors.

- Communication can be improved by an awareness of the cultural, ethnic and religious factors that shape the individual's thinking, behaviour or communication, and that religious beliefs may influence the individual's approach to medical treatment. (The MCA refers specifically to two religious groups: Jehovah's Witnesses and Christian Scientists.)

- The assessment of decision-making capacity should never be based on age, appearance, assumptions about an individual's condition or any aspect of behaviour. The word 'appearance' covers skin colour (i.e. racial appearance) and the way people dress (including cultural and religious dress).

The Mental Capacity Act Code of Practice reiterates these guidelines for determination of best interests. Careful consideration of the past and present wishes, feelings, beliefs and values of individuals who lack decision-making capacity is required in the determination of their best interests, and these are highly likely to be determined by their cultural, ethnic and religious values.

Chapter 5 of the Mental Capacity Act Code of Practice also states that careful consideration of the views of other people who are close to an individual who lacks decision-making capacity is required (i.e. anyone engaged in caring for the individual, anyone previously nominated by the individual to be consulted on the decision in question or similar issues, the donee of lasting power of attorney, the court-appointed deputy and the Independent Mental Capacity Advocate). Such people are likely to have detailed knowledge of an individual's past and present wishes, feelings, beliefs and values in a culturally appropriate context. Moreover, they may also be able to provide general information about the person's culture and religion, which may be invaluable in the determination of best interests. The importance of these factors was also highlighted in the Mental Capacity Act Equality Impact Assessment. Below are some selected examples of specific cultural and religious issues, which are illustrative but not exhaustive.

Gender

The gender of those who apply the MCA is important in some BME groups (Shah and Heginbotham 2008). For example, due to traditional cultural values, there may be difficulties in establishing rapport, ascertaining accurate information and sharing relevant information if gender-appropriate assessors are not used in the assessment of older people from some cultures. For example, it is often better for female health professionals to assess Indian, Muslim and Gypsy women. Individuals from some BME groups (e.g. Somali and Pakistani) may also prefer to have carers from the same gender, especially for personal care, such as bathing.

Refusal to accept a carer of the opposite gender may trigger an assessment of decision-making capacity, particularly if there are communication difficulties due to having English as a second language. Elderly women from some cultural (e.g. Bangladeshi and Somali) and religious (e.g. Hindu and Muslim) backgrounds may prefer to consult female gynaecologists because of their traditional values. A refusal of a consultation with a male gynaecologist may potentially trigger an assessment of decision-making capacity. The same may apply to elderly Afghan or Arab men with urological problems, who may prefer to be seen by a male urologist.

Case study: Gender

You are a nurse seeing a 72-year-old Iraqi man in a urology clinic. He has a poor command of English and is wearing traditional Iraqi clothes. He is trying desperately to communicate some information to you using frantic gestures and pointing towards different doors in the clinic's waiting room. He has been allocated a young female trainee doctor even though the other three doctors in the clinic are all male.

Questions to consider:

1. How could and should the communication problem be addressed?

2. Is the age and gender of the allocated doctor important when dealing with a urological problem in an elderly Iraqi man?

3. Is this a case of gender discrimination against certain health professionals, or is this an issue of equality for the patient?

Where possible, those who apply the MCA should belong to the same ethnic background as the BME individual or, at least, have a sound understanding of the individual's culture and religion (Shah and Heginbotham 2008). This approach will promote greater accuracy in a culturally appropriate context. However, it may not always be possible, and guidance on how to deal with such situations is provided below.

Personal appearance

Individuals from different cultural and religious backgrounds may wear clothes that have cultural or religious significance (e.g. Sri Lankan women sometimes wear sarees, and Sikh men often wear turbans). They may also carry religious artefacts (e.g. Muslims, Christians and Hindus may all carry religious beads with them). However, the application of the MCA is clear that the process of assessment must not be influenced by clothes or the possession of a religious artefact.[12]

It is also notable that the segregation of men and women is important in many cultures and religions (e.g. in Indian, Pakistani and Gypsy groups as well as for Jains, Muslims and Hindus). In health and social care, this may be required in day centres, day hospitals, inpatient hospital settings and care homes. A BME individual may be reluctant to attend a day centre or day hospital, or to be admitted to hospital or placed in a care home, for fear of enforced mixing with the opposite sex or sharing of sleeping spaces. There is a risk that this may trigger an assessment of decision-making capacity, particularly if there are difficulties with communication because the BME individual lacks fluency in English. The Mental Capacity Act Equality Impact Assessment recommends that the Court of Protection and the Independent Mental Capacity Advocate consider gender-specific accommodation in the determination of best interests.

Religious facilities and services

Those who apply the MCA must give careful consideration to the religious needs of BME individuals in their deliberations around best interests. Religious needs include availability of appropriate prayer facilities, freedom to pray in accordance with religious values, and access to religious leaders and religious rites and ceremonies (Ministry of Justice 2007). Individuals from some religions (such as Jainism and Islam) may be reluctant to consider placement in a care home for fear that their religious needs may not be met. This, again, could trigger an assessment of decision-making capacity, particularly if there are communication difficulties. A strategy that may reassure the BME individual is to enable him or her to visit the relevant home and observe first hand that other residents enjoy access to these religious requirements. Those involved in the application of the MCA must also give careful consideration to the religious and cultural dietary needs of BME individuals in their deliberations.

Refusal of medical treatment on religious grounds

Cultural and religious values may determine the medical treatments that individuals are willing to accept (Shah and Heginbotham 2008). The Mental Capacity Act Code of Practice refers to two religious groups (Jehovah's Witnesses and Christian Scientists) in this context but does not provide further information on how to address the issues. However, those involved in the application of the MCA must always give careful consideration to such religious values in their deliberations. This was evident in a case study of a patient, a Jehovah's Witness, who needed a blood transfusion, which is prohibited by the patient's religion. The patient had dementia and had not made an advance decision to refuse blood transfusion, presenting the medical team with a difficult decision. It was concluded that the MCA and the professional guidelines do not provide clear guidance on this issue (Hegde, Bell and Cole 2006).

Another example of a religious group that may refuse medical treatment is the Jains, who are strict vegetarians. They may decline to take any medication that contains animal products due to their religious beliefs. However, once again there is a risk that a refusal to accept medical treatment due to religious values may trigger an assessment of decision-making capacity, particularly if there are additional communication difficulties. Clearly, such a refusal to accept treatment should never be seen in itself as evidence of lacking decision-making capacity, particularly as it is often possible to find alternative forms of treatment. For example, consultation with the pharmacist may lead to the prescription of a different preparation of the same or similar medication not containing animal products.

Case study: Vegetarian medication

An elderly Jain woman had read in a Gujarati magazine that certain vitamin D preparations contain gelatin, so she decided to stop taking her much-needed vitamin D. A chance discussion with a Gujarati-speaking pharmacist at a social function revealed to her that gelatin-free preparations of this medication are available on prescription.

In some religions, fasting is an important traditional practice. For example, Muslims fast during daylight hours throughout Ramadan, while Jains, Hindus and Christians fast for certain specified religious days. Those who apply the MCA must give careful consideration to this religious practice in their deliberations. For example, during periods of fasting, religious BME individuals may be reluctant to take medication. Once again, this may risk triggering an assessment of decision-making capacity, particularly if there are additional communication difficulties. However, it is often possible for healthcare practices to work with these different religious practices; for example, if the fast is during daylight hours (e.g. during Ramadan for Muslims) it may be possible to take medication at night without significant impact on the medical illness. Also, involvement of a local religious leader, with the individual's agreement, may identify provisions within religious values to cover periods of fasting.

Insight

For an interesting case study on the MCA and religious beliefs, see the discussion of the *Wye Valley NHS Trust v Mr B* [2015] EWCOP 60 case by Alex Ruck Keene (a practising barrister, writer and educator specialising in mental capacity law): www.mentalcapacitylawandpolicy. org.uk/capacity-is-not-an-off-switch.

Last rites

In some religions, when an individual is close to dying, family members wish to perform certain religious rites and ceremonies. This may include prayers, readings from religious texts, quiet chanting, putting a red dot on the forehead of the individual, and each family member giving the individual a spoon of water. Those working in hospitals, hospices and care homes should be aware of these religious values. Such practices should be allowed even if the individual lacks the capacity to make a decision on the issue (and this may be the case if the individual is seriously ill, with a loss or reduction of consciousness) as it is likely to be in their best interests.

Refusal to cooperate with accepted practice in any of the above scenarios should never on its own be considered as evidence of an individual lacking decision-making capacity. Simple clarification from the individual concerned, with the aid of close family or friends and/or a professional interpreter, may resolve the issue. However, if there is further evidence of a lack of decision-making capacity in any of the situations discussed above, then further investigation is required. If a lack of decision-making capacity is determined, then the determination of best interests will also need to take careful account of religious and cultural values.

Delegation of decision-making and ethical dilemmas

In some BME groups, traditional cultural and religious values may mean that some individuals choose to delegate decision-making to other individuals (Shah and Heginbotham 2008). For example, Hindu and Jain elders are expected to disengage themselves from worldly economic, social and domestic responsibility when they reach old age and to adopt a greater spiritual role (Ganguli *et al.* 1999). Therefore, elderly Hindu and Jain men may indicate that any decision should be made by their eldest son. Similarly, women in some BME groups, including a variety of ethnic groups originating from India, may indicate that any decision should be made by their husbands, in accordance with traditional cultural practice. Given that the MCA does not allow other individuals, unless they hold lasting power of attorney (or there is a court-appointed deputy), to consent on behalf of adult subjects, this implied delegation of decision-making raises major ethical difficulties. This has not been recognised or addressed in the MCA other than through the official appointment of an LPA. If individuals from these BME groups can only practise their traditional cultural values through this formal mechanism, then issues of discrimination within the MCA are raised.

Insight

This account is based on an interview the author conducted in Gujarati with an 80-year-old man, Mr X, who only speaks broken English. Mr X is of Indian origin and was born in Kenya, but he has lived in England for the last 40 years. He has continued to practise his religion, Jainism, and was previously unaware of the existence of the MCA.

When discussing the basic components of the MCA, he simply indicated that he does not need the MCA because he will rely totally on his eldest son to help him manage his financial affairs and to deal with issues related to his health. He explained that about two years earlier he had prostate cancer, and he was given the option of receiving traditional treatment by injection or entering a clinical research trial. He relied on his son to take responsibility for making the decision between the two options as he believed that his son was younger and more knowledgeable about medical issues. Similarly, he recently had to decide whether to have his cataracts extracted under a local or general anaesthetic, and again he relied on his eldest son to help him make the decision.

When it was pointed out to him that he could do this more formally by imparting lasting power of attorney to his son (although the health and welfare component could only be used formally if he lost decision-making capacity), he said that traditionally older people from his community have relied on the eldest son to make these important decisions in old age as they retire to a simple spiritual life. As such, he saw no point in formalising this in any way consistent with the MCA. Moreover, he saw the MCA as a difficult process which he may not understand because of his limited command of English. He said that even when he goes to hospital appointments, he usually has to take a member of the family (his eldest son or eldest daughter-in-law) to assist with the interpretation. He felt he would need to see a solicitor for the MCA and that he would need his son or daughter-in-law with him too.

He did not know that under English law nobody can consent for a particular issue on his behalf if he loses decision-making capacity, unless there is a lasting power of attorney in place. He struggled to understand the concept of the MCA and sincerely believed that his eldest son could deal with any issues for him.

Case study: Delegation

A young nurse who works in a hospice is talking to a 78-year-old devout Hindu man with his eldest son. The elderly man has a poor command of English, and his son is interpreting for him. In discussions, the nurse asks him whether or not he has considered resuscitation in the event of cardiac arrest. With the son interpreting, the older man informs the nurse that his son will decide on this issue and that he does not wish to participate further in the discussion. The nurse tries to clarify that his son cannot legally make decisions on his behalf if he loses decision-making power without lasting power of attorney, even if he is aware of his wishes. With his son interpreting, the man replies that the final decision will be made by his son.

Questions to consider:

1. How appropriate is it that the son is interpreting this discussion?

2. Why do you think the elderly Hindu man is disengaged from the process of decision-making?

3. What are some of the ethical issues pertaining to the son being delegated the authority to make the decision?

4. What possible options are available to the nurse?

Working towards understanding cultural and religious values

Several strategies can be used to understand cultural and religious values:

- It may be possible to establish cultural and religious values from BME individuals directly, a person nominated by the BME individual, others who know the individual well (family members, friends, etc.), the donee of a lasting power of attorney, or a court-appointed deputy.

- An advance decision should be developed to include and clarify cultural and religious values and wishes, especially if it influences medical treatment. It may be possible to establish a better understanding of cultural and religious values by consulting family, friends or colleagues of the individual who have better knowledge of the relevant culture and religion; the local community or religious leaders; or representatives of local voluntary-sector organisations that cater for the relevant cultural or religious group.

- Health and social care professionals and lawyers may find it helpful to conduct a web-based literature search to identify case reports of the implications of specific cultural and religious values in the application of the MCA. For example, there is a case study pertaining to the need for blood transfusion in an incapacitated Jehovah's Witness, whose religion prohibits blood transfusion (Hegde *et al.* 2006).

Those who apply the MCA should make an effort to learn about the cultural and religious values of the cultural and religious groups they are most likely to be involved with, perhaps with the aid of some of the above strategies.

Awareness-raising within BME communities with regard to the MCA has also been demonstrated as an effective approach (Shah *et al.* 2010c). The examples of good practice in this chapter could be a good place to start.

The application of these strategies should be complemented by formal diversity training in cultural and religious sensitivity and competence for those who apply the MCA. Models for such training on mental health issues have been described in the government report *Delivering Race Equality in Mental Health Care* (Department of Health 2005) and could be adapted for the purpose of the application of the MCA. The Mental Capacity Act Equality Impact Assessment clearly states that training for judges, court staff and customer contact centre operators should include training on diversity issues (Ministry of Justice 2007). Also, the *Equal Treatment Bench Book* (Judicial College 2013) provided to the judiciary has information and guidance for judges on religious and other beliefs. The standard training of Independent Mental Capacity Advocates covers cultural awareness and sensitivity and includes information on possible issues of concern to people based on their religion and beliefs (Ministry of Justice 2007). The importance of these issues is reiterated in the Mental Capacity Act Code of Practice (Department for Constitutional Affairs 2013).

Conclusion

The above discussion concerning the MCA and equality is by no means comprehensive or exhaustive. However, it provides insight into a wide range of specific issues that those assessing decision-making capacity, determining best interests and responsible for other applications of the MCA are likely to encounter.

Many of these issues are covered theoretically under the statutory principles of the MCA and the general guidance in the Mental Capacity Act Code of Practice. For example, in those judged to lack decision-making capacity on a particular issue, decisions can only be made which are in the best interests of an individual, and determination of their best interests requires consideration of the individual's previous wishes, feelings, beliefs and roles (including culture and religion), and in consultation with other relevant parties. However, many particular issues that may arise in the implementation of the MCA are lost in these general principles, which are open to differing interpretations (Shah and Heginbotham 2008). Those involved in the application of the MCA should be aware of the potential difficulties and take measures to reduce them. Moreover, training materials for the basic application of the MCA have been produced for use in a range of settings (see Stanley *et al.* 2007a, 2007b, 2007c, 2007d, 2007e), which complement much of the guidance provided in this chapter.

There may be occasions when the detailed circumstances of an individual case are complex. On such occasions, careful consideration should be given to the following approaches:

- requesting a second opinion from a colleague

- seeking advice from a lawyer acting on behalf of the decision-maker's employer (e.g. a National Health Service trust or local authority)

- seeking advice from any indemnity organisations the decision-maker may belong to (e.g. the Medical Defence Union or Medical Protection Society)

- seeking advice from professional organisations that the decision-maker may belong to.

References

Barker, J. (1984) *Research Perspectives on Ageing: Black and Asian Old People in Britain.* London: Age Concern Research Unit.

Bhalia, A. and Blakemore, K. (1981) *Elders of the Minority Ethnic Groups.* Birmingham: AFFOR.

Bhui, K. and Bhugra, D. (2007) 'Ethnic Inequalities and Cultural Capability Framework in Mental Healthcare.' In D. Bhugra and K. Bhui (eds) *Textbook of Cultural Psychiatry.* Cambridge: Cambridge University Press.

Cairns, R., Maddock, C., Buchanan, A., David, A.S. *et al.* (2005) 'Prevalence and predictors of mental incapacity in psychiatric inpatients.' *British Journal of Psychiatry 187*, 379–385.

Centre for Ethnicity and Health, University of Central Lancashire, Mental Health Act Commission and NIMHE (2003) *Engaging and Changing: Developing Effective Policy for Care and Treatment of Black and Minority Ethnic Detained Patients.* Accessed at www.kc.nimhe.org.uk/index. cfm?fuseactionItem.viewResources.intItemID=12939, link no longer active.

Department for Constitutional Affairs (2013) *Mental Capacity Act Code of Practice* (revised 2014). Available at www.gov.uk/government/publications/mental-capacity-act-code-of-practice, accessed on 21 September 2016.

Department of Health (2005) *Delivering Race Equality in Mental Health Care: An Action Plan for Reform Inside and Outside Services and the Government's Response to the Independent Inquiry into the Death of David Bennett.* Available at http://webarchive.nationalarchives.gov.uk/20130107105354/http://www.dh.gov.uk/en/publicationsandstatistics/publications/publicationspolicyandguidance/dh_4100773, accessed on 21 September 2016.

Ganguli, M., Dube, S., Johnston, J.M., Pandav, R., Chandra, V. and Dodge, H.H. (1999) 'Depressive symptoms, cognitive impairment and functional impairment in a rural elderly population in India: A Hindi version of the Geriatric Depression Scale (GDS-H).' *International Journal of Geriatric Psychiatry 14*, 807–820.

Hegde, R., Bell, D. and Cole, P. (2006) 'The Jehovah's Witness and dementia: Who or what defines best interests?' *Anaesthesia 61*, 802–806.

Hoxey, K., Mukherjee, S. and Shah, A.K. (1999) 'Psychiatric services for ethnic elders.' *Old Age Psychiatrist 1*, 44–46.

Judicial College (2013) *Equal Treatment Bench Book.* Available at www.judiciary.gov.uk/wp-content/uploads/JCO/Documents/judicial-college/ETBB_all_chapters_final.pdf, accessed on 6 November 2016.

Kline, F., Acosta, F., Austin, W. and Johnson, R. (1980) 'The misunderstood Spanish-speaking patient.' *American Journal of Psychiatry 137*, 12, 1530–1533.

Lindesay, J., Jagger, C., Hibbert, M.J., Peet, S.M. and Moledina, F. (1997) 'Knowledge, uptake and availability of health and social services among Asian Gujarati and white elders.' *Ethnicity and Health 2*, 59–69.

Manthorpe, J. and Hettiaratchy, P. (1993) 'Ethnic minority elders in Britain.' *International Review of Psychiatry 5*, 173–180.

Marcos, L.R. (1979) 'Effects of interpreters on the evaluation of psychopathology in non-English speaking patients.' *American Journal of Psychiatry 136*, 171–174.

Ministry of Justice (2007) *Mental Capacity Act 2005. Equality Impact Assessment.* Available at http://webarchive.nationalarchives.gov.uk/20071204130111/http:/www.justice.gov.uk/docs/mc-equality-impact.pdf, accessed on 21 September 2016.

Mukherjee, S. and Shah, A.K. (2001) 'The prevalence and correlates of capacity to consent to a geriatric psychiatry admission.' *Ageing and Mental Health 5*, 335–339.

Nnatu, I. (2005) 'Assessing cognitive impairment in a prelingually profund deaf person.' *Progress in Neurology and Psychiatry 9*, 34–38.

Phelan, M. and Parkman, S. (1995) 'Work with an interpreter.' *British Medical Journal 311*, 555–557.

Shah, A.K. (1992) 'Difficulties in interviewing elderly people from an Asian ethnic group.' *International Journal of Geriatric Psychiatry 7*, 917.

Shah, A.K. (1997a) 'Interviewing mentally ill ethnic minority elders with interpreters.' *Australian Journal on Ageing 16*, 220–221.

Shah, A.K. (1997b) 'Straight talk: Overcoming language barriers in diagnosis.' *Geriatric Medicine 27*, 45–46.

Shah, A.K. (1999) 'Difficulties experienced by a Gujarati psychiatrist in interviewing elderly Gujaratis in Gujarati.' *International Journal of Geriatric Psychiatry 14*, 1072–1074.

Shah, A.K. and Dickenson, D. (1999) 'The capacity to make decisions in dementia: Some contemporary issues.' *International Journal of Geriatric Psychiatry 14*, 803–806.

Shah, A.K. and Heginbotham, C. (2008) 'The Mental Capacity Act 2005: Some implications for black and minority ethnic elders.' *Age and Ageing 37*, 242–243.

Shah, A.K. and MacKenzie, S. (2007) 'Disorders of Ageing across Cultures'. In D. Bhugra and K. Bhui (eds) *Textbook of Cultural Psychiatry.* Cambridge: Cambridge University Press.

Shah, A.K., Banner, N., Heginbotham, C. and Fulford, B. (2010a) 'The early experience of old age psychiatrists in the application of the Mental Capacity Act 2005: A pilot study.' *International Psychogeriatrics 22*, 147–157.

Shah, A.K., Banner, N., Heginbotham, C. and Fulford, B. (2010b) 'A pilot study of the early implementation of the Mental Capacity Act 2005 in England and Wales: The experience of consultants in old age psychiatry.' *Medicine, Science and the Law 50*, 131–135.

Shah, A.K., Banner, N., Newbiggin, K., Heginbotham, C. and Fulford, B. (2009a) 'The early experience of consultant psychiatrists in the application of the Mental Capacity Act: Issues for black and minority individuals.' *Ethnicity and Inequalities in Health and Social Care 2*, 4–10.

Shah, A.K., Heginbotham, C., Fulford, B. and Banner, N. (2009b) 'The application of the Mental Capacity Act 2005 among geriatric psychiatry patients: A pilot study.' *International Psychogeriatrics 21*, 922–930.

Shah, A.K., Heginbotham, C., Fulford, B., Banner, N., Newbiggin, K. and Kinton, M. (2009c) 'A pilot study of early experience of consultant psychiatrists in the implementation of the Mental Capacity Act 2005: Local policy and training, assessment of capacity and determination of best interests.' *Journal of Mental Health Law 2009*, Winter, 149–164.

Shah, A.K., Heginbotham, C., Fulford, B., Buffin, J. and Newbiggin, K. (2010c) 'The effectiveness of raising awareness event of the Mental Capacity Act among representatives of ethnic minority communities.' *Ethnicity and Inequalities in Health and Social Care 3*, 44–48.

Stanley, N., Lyons, C., Manthorpe, J., Rapaport, J. *et al.* (2007a) *Mental Capacity Act 2005. Core Training Set.* London: Department of Health.

Stanley, N., Lyons, C., Manthorpe, J., Rapaport, J. *et al.* (2007b) *Mental Capacity Act 2005. Community Care and Primary Care Training Set.* London: Department of Health.

Stanley, N., Lyons, C., Manthorpe, J., Rapaport, J. *et al.* (2007c) *Mental Capacity Act 2005. Acute Hospital Training Set.* London: Department of Health.

Stanley, N., Lyons, C., Manthorpe, J., Rapaport, J. *et al.* (2007d) *Mental Capacity Act 2005. Residential Accommodation Training Set.* London: Department of Health.

Stanley, N., Lyons, C., Manthorpe, J., Rapaport, J. *et al.* (2007e) *Mental Capacity Act 2005. Mental Health Training Set.* London: Department of Health.

Tribe, R. and Raval, H. (2003) *Working with Interpreters in Mental Health.* London and New York: Brunner-Routledge.

Tribe, R. and Thompson, K. (2016) *Guidelines for Working with Interpreters in Health Settings.* Leicester: BPS Books.

Chapter 6

Anti-discriminatory Practice: Caring for Carers of Older Adults with Mental Health Dilemmas

Rachel Tribe and Pauline Lane

Many [carers] pay a 'triple penalty': damage to their health; a poorer financial situation; and restrictions in everyday life...[T]heir work and effort saves the public purse £119bn a year – more than the whole budget of the NHS.

Yeandle (2011)

Introduction

This chapter is largely concerned with carers of older adults who have mental health and well-being concerns. Specifically, it focuses on informal and unpaid caring roles, usually carried out by family members or friends of the older adult rather than by paid carers provided through public or private services. However, much of the content of this chapter may also be relevant for paid carers.

A carer has been defined as:

> anyone who cares, unpaid, for a friend or family member who due to illness, disability, a mental health problem or an addiction cannot cope without their support...[T]he variety of tasks that a Carer fulfils can include: practical household tasks, personal care and/or emotional support. The term Carer should not be confused with a care worker, or care assistant, who receives payment. (Carers Trust 2015)

The role of carers in England is recognised in legislation through the Care Act 2014, which details how local authorities are obliged to conduct carer assessments. Every carer is legally entitled to a carer assessment. Although caring relationships are often embedded within existing relationships (such as being a son or a wife), under the Care Act 2014, anyone who seems as though they may benefit from carer support is entitled to an assessment and is eligible for access to support services. The assessment is based on national criteria (there are separate laws about social care in Wales, Scotland and Northern Ireland), and the aim is to ensure that all carers are properly supported and enabled to sustain their caring role. It is hoped that the Care Act 2014 might go some way towards increasing the attention paid to the needs of carers, although it has been reported that difficulties associated with the labelling, accessibility and appropriateness of services may in fact result in carers not seeking help or recognising their own needs and rights to access services. This is particularly likely to happen due to the immense demands placed on many carers (Wirral Carers Strategy 2014–2017). This chapter looks at some of the key issues for carers and makes recommendations for challenging discrimination and building anti-discriminatory practice.

Attitudes towards caring and being a carer are often contradictory, and the apparent ordinariness of caring is deceptive as the role often involves many complex skills. Few people want to be cared for in the sense of being dependent on another person for some or all of their personal needs (Joseph Rowntree Foundation 2008). The 2011 census (Office for National Statistics 2013a) identified that approximately 5.8 million people are providing unpaid care in the UK and that the provision of unpaid care is becoming increasingly common with an ageing population. According to an NHS Information Centre Survey (2010), 40 per cent of carers are caring for their parents or parents-in-law, with an additional 4 per cent caring for their grandparents. Experiences of the transition to becoming a carer will be varied; however, many people do not identify with the term 'carer' and instead see caring as a normal part of their life and family relationships. Some people take up to five years before they begin to think of themselves as 'carers', and some authors (e.g. Smyth, Blaxland and Cass 2011) have suggested abandoning the term altogether as it fails to adequately account for the two-way relationship between the two individuals. A number of studies on carers have focused largely on the negative aspects of the role, with many emphasising what has been labelled the 'burden of care' (Van der Lee, Bakker and Duivenvoorden 2014). While there are undoubtedly considerable pressures associated with being a carer, there can also be many positive aspects and benefits to the role. For example, Ott, Sanders and Kelber (2007) noted that carers described positive effects of their role, which included becoming more caring, compassionate, forgiving, tolerant and helpful, which was viewed by many carers as important for personal growth.

The context of caring

With the global recession, ever increasing restrictions on public spending and an ageing population, unpaid, informal carers have become increasingly important to the economy. The Joseph Rowntree Foundation (2008) has suggested that the emerging rhetoric of 'caring for the carers' was developed to enable them to maintain their caring responsibilities rather than having more people depend on the state economy. However, concerns have been expressed in recent years about the projected need and supply of informal carers for older people. One report has suggested that 'our projection for the older population indicates that there will be a shortage of informal care for some decades, unless the patterns of provision change' (Karlsson et al. 2006, p.202). In part, the projected 'carer deficit' is due to the fact that social patterns are changing. For example, many families live greater distances from each other, families are often smaller so there are fewer people to share the caring role, and it is common for all family members to work full-time outside of the home. These intersecting factors can influence the availability of intergenerational care. Changing social factors combined with the predicted increase in demand for care due to demographic changes suggest that there will be a gap in informal care, with many adult carers being unable to offer informal, unpaid care in the future (Pickard 2008).

Who does the caring?

The probability of needing to provide intergenerational care for an older adult increases with age. Women are more often carers than men, and people who are single are also more likely to provide care (Institute for Research and Innovation in Social Service 2010). For many years, feminists have highlighted the fact that much of the informal care in the home is provided by women, despite there being no reason for this to be the case (Brodolini 2012). The role of caring for an older relative is still often assumed to be the 'natural' role of the females in a family, despite this having been criticised by critical theorists and feminists for over 30 years. This is evident in much research; for example, Finch and Groves (1983) have suggested that the cultural construction of gender roles has meant that women within the family are often given an unequal burden of caring responsibilities. However, as gender roles are becoming increasingly complex, a new reality and theoretical sensitivity is needed to explore the nuances of gender and caring roles. As suggested in the Introduction and Chapter 1, the reality is that many people are caring for older people, and the people offering care live with a range of inequalities, of which gender is often one facet.

How long do people spend a week on their caring role?

Obtaining an accurate estimate of the number of hours that carers spend on their caring role is difficult, as many people see it as an extension of their everyday life, and it has been argued that family members are likely to underestimate the number of hours of their time they give as carers. Nonetheless, Carers UK (2014a) found that 1.4 million people in the UK give over 50 hours of unpaid care per week on average, with almost 4.4 million people providing 1–19 hours of unpaid care per week.

What age are carers?

People can become carers at any age (including in childhood), but almost 1.3 million carers are aged 65 or over (Carers UK 2014a). People in the 50–64 age range are the most likely to have an elderly parent to care for, and this caring role is frequently undertaken in addition to work and other commitments. However, becoming an unpaid carer in your fifties increases your chances of leaving the labour market completely, and this is frequently associated with financial difficulties and restrictions on opportunities for social and leisure activities, which can have a negative impact on health (Office for National Statistics 2013a). Over 2 million people have given up work to care for loved ones for a period of time, and it is estimated that three out of five people will be carers at some point over the course of their lifetime, although this figure includes carers of people who would not be classified as older adults (Carers Trust 2015).

Caring for older adults

Many carers of older adults are adult children, spouses or life partners, and are usually older adults themselves. A quarter of all carers aged 75 and over are providing more than 50 hours of care each week, and many of these older carers find that they face different problems from other carers. This may be due in part to a lack of recognition of their needs, but many carers who look after loved ones with mental health problems also find that they lose contact with friends and family, which can result in isolation (Age UK 2010). The nature of the caring role of a carer of an older person with mental health issues may change over time as the person they care for changes, and this in itself may be a cause of worry for the carer (Shah, Wadoo and Latoo 2010). For example, carers who look after someone with a degenerative mental health condition, such as dementia, know that their caring role may be for the long term and will often involve end of life care. For other carers, their caring role may have lasted a lifetime, such as caring for a partner with a diagnosis of schizophrenia, but the nature of the condition and therefore the nature of the caring may change in older age. For others still, caring may be just a temporary role, such as caring for a family member who is experiencing an episode of depression.

Shah *et al.* (2010) note that being a carer can raise a range of difficult personal issues about duty, family culture, responsibility, adequacy and sometimes guilt, as well as issues relating to role change which can elicit mixed feelings. These can be difficult to manage and may surface in a range of ways. For example, Gosman-Hedström and Dahlin-Ivanoff (2012) looked at the experiences of women who have cared for someone after a stroke and found that many of them reported that they felt the loss of a life companion and their mutual intellectual contact. In addition, many of the carers also reported feeling confined and trapped at home.

Clearly, carers need to maintain their caring role while at the same time trying to minimise the negative effects of caring on their own well-being (Quayhagen and Quayhagen 1998). Research suggests that when carers have a sense of control and have positive feelings towards the person they are caring for, this can have a positive effect in terms of the perceived strain experienced by carers (Horowitz and Shindleman 1983). The paradigm of stress and coping is one that has been used in much of the 'carer' literature (although it is not without its critics). For example, a study of spousal carers for people with Alzheimer's disease showed that carers who felt a lack of control or that they were inadequately prepared and powerless had higher rates of depression (Coppel *et al.* 1985).

Carers from minority and excluded communities

We will now look at some of the most common issues for carers from Black, Asian and Minority Ethnic (BAME) groups, carers living with a learning disability, and lesbian, gay, bisexual, transgender and intersex (LGBTi) carers. This does not mean to imply that these are distinctive communities, but taking a focus on groups may help to identify some of the common issues that carers from these communities face. Many people from minority communities are deemed to have 'protected characteristics' of age, disability, gender reassignment, marriage and civil partnership, race, religion or belief, sex and sexual orientation. The Equality Act 2010 stipulates that discrimination against an individual or community based on any one of these characteristics is unlawful. While many carers with protected characteristics share some common characteristics and experiences, they are not a homogeneous group. 'Carer status' is not recognised as a protected characteristic under the Equality Act 2010 because the protected characteristics are intended to apply to an individual's inherent status or identity and not to what an individual does (Busby 2011).

Research suggests that many carers from marginalised or excluded communities are seemingly 'invisible' to service providers, and therefore practitioners need to develop anti-discriminatory practice to ameliorate this problem. In a review document on social care for marginalised communities, Carr (2014, p.10) notes: 'Across all the groups was a perception or fear of mainstream, traditional care and support as discriminatory which can lead to reluctance to engage.' In other words, many people from marginalised communities do not feel that public-sector services meet their needs. Anti-discriminatory practice needs to actively seek out groups that are not accessing services and develop services that are more appropriate for them, rather than passively assuming that as some groups do not use the services, they do not require them. However, there can be anxieties from health and social care professionals about not interfering or worries about 'getting it wrong' with some minority or excluded communities, and consequently some professionals may not attempt to take significant steps or to engage with carers when issues of diversity are present (Tribe, Lane and Hearsum 2009). The establishment and use of micro-providers and community-based or local initiatives can provide the flexibility, responsiveness and capacity required for groups who have previously suffered from discrimination or who have not seen statutory services as appropriate. In particular, they have been found to be effective in providing support for isolated older people (Walsh and O'Shea 2008).

This type of provision has been labelled 'compensatory self-organisation', and projects can be found for many BAME groups, including South Asian carers, LBGT older adults, Travellers and refugees. Unfortunately, this has sometimes been misunderstood by statutory services, who get the impression that the care needs of these groups are already being met rather than recognising that their own services were not appropriate (Carr 2014), and this can lead to people falling through the cracks. For example, research has shown that BAME carers tend to care in isolation from other resources or carers (Seabrooke and Milne 2009), and this may be particularly true in rural areas where access to community groups tends to be more limited. Mistrust on the part of members of marginalised communities, combined with anxieties on the part of health and social care providers, may inhibit progress towards an improved and more inclusive care system. Anti-discriminatory practice should mean that practitioners are actively establishing links and partnerships with marginalised communities to improve service provision for all members of the community (Lane and Tribe 2010).

Carers from BAME communities

While the experiences of BAME carers and older adults are diverse, the uptake of care services by BAME communities is often identified as minimal. As stated above, research suggests that many BAME carers look to the voluntary sector to find information and support (Gregory 2010). Carers UK (2014a) also suggests that carers from

BAME communities are less likely to be getting support for financial or practical issues relating to caring, although they are more likely to be caring for older or disabled family members. BAME carers are also more likely to report that they are not aware of local services and that these are not appropriate for their needs (Mir and Tovey 2003). There is a stereotypical perspective that BAME people 'look after their own'; however, gender roles and family responsibilities will vary across communities and within families.

It is worth reflecting on the fact that the terms 'carer' and 'caring' are socially and culturally constructed concepts; although caring is a practice conducted throughout all cultures, it may not be constructed in the same way in every culture or family. The role of carer may, for example, be seen as just an extension of ordinary family life and family duties and not defined as an additional role. Culture is a multifaceted and dynamic phenomenon (Fernando 2014; Tribe 2014), and it has been noted that the concept of being a carer does not always translate well into different cultures or languages (National Black Carers and Carers Workers Network 2008). Culture operates at a number of levels and will be affected by a wide range of factors, such as familial and other belief systems, individual experiences and values, and religion. For example, in a study of African/Caribbean and South Asian carers of older relatives, researchers found that many carers saw their role as a continuation of their family role and relationships, despite the disruptions that caring causes to their original relationships (Adamson and Donovan 2005).

Yeandle et al. (2007) surveyed approximately 2000 carers, with just under 10 per cent of their sample being from BAME backgrounds. In comparison with other carers, the researchers found that carers from BAME backgrounds were more likely to report that they struggled to make ends meet, and they were more likely to be caring for someone with a mental health condition. The same study also noted that BAME older adults often have health and social care needs at a younger age than their White counterparts, and consequently BAME carers are also likely to be younger.

While it is worth remembering that cultural issues and family practices may need to be considered when working with carers, it is important not to make assumptions about older adults' or carers' culture based purely on heritage, as the multifaceted nature of any individual's life needs careful consideration. To assist a carer, it is important that practitioners first discuss the concept of being a carer with the carer and explore what this means to them personally. If relevant, this discussion can be opened up to include the wider family. Some older adults and/or carers who do not have English as a first language may benefit from having an interpreter present, but often people do not realise that this is an option. (See Chapter 12 for guidelines on working with interpreters.) Workers also need to be sensitive when offering support to carers with diverse heritage, as they may not share the same cultural, linguistic or spiritual needs as the older adult they care for. Practitioners should never make assumptions with regard to these needs, and it is always better to ask about any issues that are uncertain.

People with learning disabilities as carers

Two-thirds of adults with a learning disability in the UK live with their parents or families. Of these, 40 per cent live with a parent aged over 60, and 33 per cent live with a parent aged over 70 (Emerson and Hatton 2008). The assumption that is often made is that people with a learning disability are being cared for rather than being the carer themselves. However, many people with a learning disability find that as they age, they also become carers for an older relative, partner or friend. It is not known how many people with a learning disability are carers, and most research focuses on caring *for* people with a learning disability and not their role as carers. Many people with a learning disability and their families have developed ways of looking after each other and coping together over many years; this is referred to as 'mutual caring'. The Mental Health Foundation (2015) has noted that people with learning disabilities are often not recognised as carers by professionals and not offered choices about care and support. In addition, most information that is available for carers is not presented in an easy-read or accessible format. This may prevent some carers with learning disabilities from using the resources and also from being able to access services and support.

On occasion, a person with a learning disability and the older family member may worry that if their mutual caring is known to the authorities, they may be separated, and therefore they do not seek help from statutory services. Writing about people with learning disabilities and their ageing family carers, Walker and Walker (1998) noted that anxiety and uncertainty about the future are often experienced by both the carer and the person with a learning disability. They argue that the future needs of this group of carers are predictable due to the ageing process and that statutory services need to work with all family members so that planning for the future can be undertaken in advance. They also suggest that older family carers for people with learning disabilities tend to be the sole carer and often have smaller support networks but wish to support their relative for as long as possible. They often have negative experiences of statutory services, which may make them reluctant to seek help despite feeling undervalued and unsupported. Walker and Walker conclude by arguing that statutory services need to consider how to work with carers with learning disabilities to provide accessible practical support and information, and in particular ensure that they are recognised and accepted as equal partners in the provision of support to their relatives. This would be in line with anti-discriminatory practice. However, it is notable that while there is a growing literature on recognising and meeting the needs of people with a learning disability who are mentally ill, there appears to be very little research on people with a learning disability who are looking after an elderly parent. Furthermore, there is almost a complete absence of research on people living with a learning disability who are caring for an elderly parent who is mentally ill. For practitioners, developing anti-discriminatory practice will involve planning for ageing and ensuring that families of individuals with learning disabilities obtain person-centred support to make plans for both emergencies and the long term.

Carers from lesbian, gay, bisexual, transgender and intersex communities

The needs of carers from lesbian, gay, bisexual, transgender and intersex (LGBTi) communities often go unrecognised by professionals and the public alike. This can be particularly true of LGBTi carers who are also from a BAME background, which may in part be due to the mistaken stereotype that LGBTi people are usually White or that some people from BAME communities may not define themselves as LGBTi even though they are in a same-sex relationship (Fish 2006). Although the LGBTi community is diverse, as many older LGBTi people will have the shared experience of having spent at least part of their life hiding their intimate relationships from others (Heaphy, Yip and Thompson 2003). Same-sex relationships were only decriminalised in 1967 in England and Wales, 1981 in Scotland and 1982 in Northern Ireland. While there is now more public acceptance of LGBTi relationships, for many older adults their sexual orientation may have left them without family support in later life, and many carers may also find that they have limited access to support networks.

Those LGBTi people who are forced to live outside the boundaries of their biological families often work to construct family-like bonds with people they are close to, who may act as a proxy-family (Almack, Seymour and Bellamy 2010). This can be problematic when partners and proxy-family members become carers, as they may not be considered 'family' by statutory and third-sector services. Recent changes to the Carers Act 2014 do allow for non-family carers to have their needs recognised, and this can be a useful tool to help practitioners to meet the needs of LGBTi carers who are looking after elders with mental health problems. However, Almack *et al.* (2010) note that LGBTi carers find only too often that they are 'disenfranchised' from taking part in professional caring discussions and that their role and relationships are ignored. Indeed, there is very little research on LGBTi carers, which tells us something about the normative values of the dominant culture and the lack of recognition of LGBTi carers. With the advent of same-sex marriage and civil partnership, we may witness new forms of kinship becoming absorbed into the wider meaning of family (Shipman and Smart 2007), and it is hoped that LGBTi families will become more accepted as carers.

For practitioners thinking about their own anti-discriminatory practice, it is particularly useful to reflect on their perceptions and biases in the construction of family and carers. An anti-discriminatory approach should be person-centred to ensure that the specific needs of LGBTi carers and older adults are recognised and met and that this group is adequately represented in consultations and the planning of services.

Potential health issues for carers

Looking after an older adult with mental and/or physical disabilities can become difficult and place a strain on the health and well-being of carers themselves. While on a personal level caring is an important and valuable role, many carers who provide high levels of care for relatives and friends on an unpaid basis are more than twice as likely to suffer from poor health compared to people without caring responsibilities (Carers UK 2014a). Carers can sometimes neglect their own health and well-being to the extent that they are forced to give up their caring role (Henwood 1998). A report by Wilson *et al.* (2015) noted that approximately 50 per cent of carers with health problems reported that their condition began after they started being a carer, while Carers UK (2015) noted that approximately 70 per cent of carers who dedicated over 50 hours per week to their caring role had a long-standing health condition. Understandably, many carers have reported that it is extremely difficult to find time for their own medical care due to their caring responsibilities (Carers Week 2012). Caring can have an impact on the carer's mental health, and in the last National Census (Office for National Statistics 2013b) 92 per cent of carers stated that their role had a detrimental effect on their mental health, often causing depression and stress-related illnesses.

A report by the Audit Commission in 2004 found that most primary care staff including GPs were not referring carers for support – or even identifying them as carers – and most GPs did not offer carers home or telephone appointments despite being aware of their caring responsibilities. Many carers require not just health support but also information, training or assistance to provide them with the knowledge and skills to undertake their role safely. For example, they may need training in the use of hoists, advice on incontinence care or guidance on how to support an older adult who is agitated. They may also need help to identify pathways to practical as well as emotional support. It is important not to assume that all carers need specialist services or cannot access mainstream support; it is possible that the services in place already meet their needs, but work may be needed to improve pathways to this support. Where the need for specialist services arises, practitioners may need to be creative and innovative in meeting the carer's needs; for example, it is possible that local voluntary or specialist agencies may be able to offer more appropriate services. Part of anti-discriminatory practice may be to ensure that the carers you come across in your work know about the relevant help and support available and how to access this.

As discussed, health issues for carers may be considerable, and this can put them under additional pressure. Therefore, the implications relate to how to develop anti-discriminatory practice which helps to mitigate against the many pressures carers face in ways that enhance their own well-being and health. Anti-discriminatory practice means that all service providers should be monitoring the well-being and physical health of all carers as a matter of course and providing appropriate respite and additional support. The Care Act 2014 provides a framework for this, but real change will only be realised through the actions of service providers and individual practitioners working with carers.

Addressing social exclusion and isolation

The role of social support and good networks in promoting positive mental health and resilience and reducing stress has been noted for some time and by a number of researchers (Cohen and Willis 1985). Carers UK (2014b) found that social isolation and exclusion are serious problems for many carers and that it can be difficult to maintain relationships while being a carer. Research reviewed by Kessler, Price and Wortman (1985) also highlighted the important role of social support in stress buffering, a concept that is supported by the findings of Boen, Steffen Dalgard and Bjertness (2012) in a study specifically related to older adults. As such, good anti-discriminatory practice would concern itself with addressing the social isolation of carers and older adults with mental health problems. As carers can easily become isolated and socially excluded, it is important that they have the opportunity and space for active contact with the outside world, and time for themselves.

There are a range of networks and events that carers can join, as well as internet discussion forums that offer online support. In addition, there are Facebook pages, Twitter feeds and other forms of social media, which are a good way of getting fast responses to specific queries, connecting with other people in a similar position or just asking for information or advice. It is important to acknowledge that carers in rural locations are often geographically isolated and may not have access to a local group, so online options can be particularly helpful; however, they may not compensate for actual human contact. Another source of support can be self-help groups (also known as mutual-aid groups); based on reciprocal peer support, these offer a valuable type of resource in the community that is not replicable in professional–

client relationships. It has been proposed that self-help groups offer an additional, but not alternative, 'space' that enables members to transcend their identity as a 'carer' (Caring for Carers 2004).

Working carers and associative discrimination

Some carers do manage to maintain their paid employment alongside their caring role. This is often a struggle, however, and some carers feel that they experience discrimination at work because of their caring role. This is a complex area of law, because although the Equality Act 2010 protects those with 'protected characteristics' from discrimination, which may include the person being cared for, this does not extend to carers even though they may find that they experience associative discrimination. Associative discrimination occurs when someone is discriminated against because of their relationship, or perceived relationship, with another person who is subject to discrimination. For example, carers may suffer discrimination on account of their relationship with the older person that they care for due to that person's age and/or mental health status. Associative discrimination is outlawed in the Equality Act (as well as in European law and in the legislative detail of many countries), and the Act also prohibits 'associative' disability discrimination.

Clearly, the law itself does not prevent discrimination from happening, but it does give people a recourse for action, and potential sanctions include legal proceedings against the offenders. However, in law employers do *not* have a duty to make reasonable adjustments where an individual, typically a carer, has an association with a disabled person. Outside of the Equality Act 2010, workers have the right to request flexible working, which covers all employees (full-time and part-time), but carers need to be aware that an employer can refuse flexible working for business reasons – the right is to *request* flexible working, not to be given flexible working. An employer could still face a claim of associative disability discrimination in relation to direct discrimination and harassment against a carer, and there have been a number of associative disability discrimination cases brought by carers against their employers, including cases against private companies and a government department.

The financial impact of caring

It is well documented that unpaid carers save the economies of many countries vast amounts of money: Carers UK and the University of Leeds (2011) have claimed that the care provided by unpaid carers in the UK is worth an estimated £119 billion each year. However, Age UK (2012) claim there is also a cost of £5.3 billion each year to the British economy through lost earnings and tax revenues and the additional benefit payments claimed by people undertaking caring responsibilities. Certainly, caring roles can impact negatively upon the financial circumstances of an individual, causing a range of difficulties for the carer, and this can also have an impact on people who are being cared for (Carers UK 2013, 2014a, 2014c). In a study conducted by Carers UK (2014c), 53 per cent of carers stated that financial concerns were adversely affecting their health and that many carers themselves have a disability or illness. They also noted that carers are more likely to be in debt and have higher levels of debt. The contribution carers make to society should not be underestimated, particularly as it is a role that is often taken on suddenly and without preparation, leaving carers to struggle with the vital responsibilities that they have assumed (Carers UK 2015).

Given the nature of the work, carers often miss out on job opportunities as many carers are unable to accept full-time employment, while over half of those carers who are not working say that they would like to be in paid employment (Carers Trust 2015). This finding of missed job opportunities was echoed in further research, which also found that many carers experienced a loss of skills and confidence about returning to work, which has hampered their opportunities for work (Carers UK 2015). For many, the role of caring is a full-time job, and Carers UK (2014) reported that 40 per cent of carers had not had a complete day off for over a year and had not been able to take a holiday within the last five years.

Financial worries have been shown to be linked to poor mental well-being and health (Mind 2015). Research suggests that many carers of people with mental disorders have elevated rates of mental ill health themselves compared to the general population as a direct consequence of their caring role, although the mental health symptoms exhibited by carers tend to be in the moderate range (Shah *et al.* 2010). Clearly, anti-discriminatory practice needs to be concerned with ensuring that services, support and benefit entitlement are all widely available, not only to the person requiring care but also to the carers themselves. Discriminatory attitudes and subsequent practices may be compounded when the carer is looking after someone who is an older person, as ageism can also play a role.

Support for carers

Older people's mental health services are concerned with the care and treatment of people, some of whom will have complex histories of health inequalities which may interact with and be affected by the biological process of ageing. The impact of older people's mental health needs is wide-ranging, and this can have an impact not only on older people themselves but also on their families, friends and carers. In order to support older people with mental health conditions in their homes, it is important for commissioners, service providers and practitioners not only to meet the needs of the client, but also to be aware of the needs of their carers – especially as many of them may be older adults themselves. Maintaining the mental health and well-being of carers is also important in enabling older people to remain in the community for as long as possible, should this be what they want (Joint Commissioning Panel for Mental Health 2013). A carer's needs assessment (as well as a separate community care assessment for the person who is being cared for) should be the start of the process. The local council should provide this under the Care Act 2014, and the assessor should discuss and develop an agreed care plan with the carer. As a result of the assessment, some people will be eligible for funding support from the council. Others will not, but this process can be useful to help carers to recognise their own financial and health needs and to develop strategies for self-care.[13] Sharing the care responsibility through respite care can help carers cope better and offer them time to look after themselves. This may involve day care, home care and respite residential care. Much of the support available for carers comes from the voluntary or third sector rather than statutory services.

However, many conventional respite care services do not accept people with mental health issues, and older people and carers from some communities (e.g. LGBTi or BAME groups) may not feel that the services are appropriate for their needs. For example, older adults and carers from BAME communities may have a number of cultural, linguistic and spiritual issues that need to be taken into consideration when planning respite care. However, most of these issues can be addressed if respite care is planned with the involvement of the older adult and the carer. As stated earlier, specific attention should also be given to the particular needs of carers with learning disabilities, as in many cases people with learning disabilities start to care for their ageing parents while still needing some care themselves. It can be difficult to ensure that everyone has the care and support they require, especially as many older parents will not recognise that their caring role has changed, and many people with learning disabilities will not be able to seek advice or support. It is also important to be sensitive to carers from other minority groups, for example LGBTi carers, who may be concerned that statutory or voluntary sector services may not be accepting or friendly. Therefore, good practice that is anti-discriminatory needs to address these issues and ensure that services are meeting the needs of individual carers as well as the people who are cared for.

Carers, personalisation and direct payments

As discussed in earlier chapters, the personalisation agenda has been significant over the past few years. Personalisation is a process of thinking about services from the perspective of the service user and is aimed at ensuring better outcomes that focus on the service user's needs. This process involves seeing service users and their carers not so much as passive consumers of services but as active participants who are empowered to make decisions about their own care. For many older service users and carers, this can be problematic as they are familiar with the professional expert model where decisions about care are made for them; the expert by experience approach can be difficult to adapt to. In this new model, carers often find that they are located in a dual position of being both someone who offers care and at times someone in need of care and support themselves. Carers may find that they need to take on new roles – for example, acting as an advocate when they are supporting someone with impaired cognitive ability, communicating the needs and wishes of the person they are caring for.

Many carers also find themselves responsible for the management of the personal budget of the person they are caring for. There is often confusion about the terminology used in the personalisation agenda and allocated budgets, so here is a quick overview:

- *Self-directed support* gives service users choice and control over how their needs are met, and personal budgets and direct payments are part of self-directed support. Previously, money was automatically paid to statutory services to provide the relevant support to people in need of services, thus giving service users little choice about service provision. Self-directed services should improve choice for service users, but the caveats noted above are important concerns with regard to carers.

- *A personal budget* is the amount of money that a local authority has calculated is needed to meet a person's social care needs, after a needs-based assessment and financial assessment have been conducted. (England, Scotland, Wales and Northern Ireland all have different systems of support.) Some people are deemed to have adequate financial resources and do not qualify for state support; they will need to meet the cost of their own care needs. However, recent policy indicates that a 'care cap' will be put in place in 2020, which means that people will not be expected to fund more than £72,000 of their own care. Some carers can also receive a personal budget themselves following a carer's assessment by their local authority.

- *Direct payments* are one way of receiving this personal budget, and it allows people to arrange their own social care support. This personal budget is awarded in money (not credits) so that people can buy their own support directly and easily. The person will be informed about how much money has been allocated to them.

Despite this personalisation agenda and allocated budgets, many carers find themselves 'brokering' the relationship between many different agencies; for them, self-directed support may feel like an additional burden. For example, it has been suggested that while carers do play an important role in working with professionals to develop assessment and care planning for the personal budgets for the people they care for, the professionals tend to see carers primarily as a resource rather than as co-clients and individuals with personal needs themselves (Glendinning, Mitchell and Brooks 2015). Little research has been conducted so far on the impact of personal budgets on carers despite the essential role of carers in helping the person they are caring for to claim and use the budget.

The underlying philosophy of direct payments is that they improve choice and control for service users who usually have complete control over the budget, though it is possible for the council or another organisation to manage the money if required, with the person still directing how it is spent. Direct payments may enable more choice over services, which allows service users to identify options that are better tailored to their particular requirements. It also means that a person can pay a member of their family or friend to provide the care, if that is their preference. BAME older adults including Gypsies and Travellers are likely to benefit from direct-payment arrangements as they offer them the opportunity to choose more culturally appropriate services. In some areas, self-directed personal budgets have been used in innovative ways, such as to create a collective budget between two or more people by pooling personal budgets together. For example, the West Lothian Council in collaboration with the Minority Ethnic Carers of Older People Project (MECOPP) have adopted a service brokerage model which supports Asian women to pool their direct payments to purchase tailored support.

The value of partnership working

Carers are often the people who best know the people they are caring for, and they can provide valuable insight and information about the care needed by that person. They will therefore be crucial in the planning and delivery of care offered to older people with well-being or mental health needs. 'Carers are the experts about their relative's illness: they live with it day in and day out, whereas [we as] healthcare professionals can go home at the end of a shift' (BBC Caring for Carers 2006). If, as practitioners, we develop a collaborative ongoing working relationship with carers, mental health services for older adults as a whole can only improve. It is of course vital that the older adult is consulted, although this may on occasions usefully be done in collaboration with the carer if the older adult believes this will be helpful. The importance of listening to and involving service users/experts by experience and carers in planning service provision is increasingly being recognised (Wallcraft et al. 2011). In reality, however, these policies and intentions for collaboration and partnership are not always translated into practice on the ground and are inconsistently implemented.

There are currently a lot of regional and national variations in practice across mental health services, despite a number of recommendations and resolutions, including the Madrid Declaration on Ethical Standards for Psychiatric Practice (World Psychiatric Association 2011). The World Psychiatric Association Task Force on Best Practice in Working with Service Users and Carers within Mental Health (Wallcraft *et al.* 2011) made a number of recommendations, including the need to develop a comprehensive and integrated approach to advocacy for service users and carers within mental health and to ensure that this is located within a context that works to enhance the related human rights issues at both national and international levels. In the past, consultations concerning service change or development have tended to be led by health professionals, but groups or communities (including service users/experts by experience and carers) can also call consultations to ensure that they are listened to and taken into account. Local Healthwatch[14] initiatives can often help with this as they act as a recognised independent body to liaise with local service providers. Real consultations and partnership working might be one way of ensuring that the needs of older carers and service users are understood, and this has the potential to challenge current practice and ensure that some aspects of anti-discriminatory practice are upheld, as well as ensuring services are appropriate and accessible.

Promoting anti-discriminatory practice: Some key ideas

Ensuring the views of service users and carers are heard and listened to at all levels is essential to developing anti-discriminatory practice. Other things to be considered include the following:

- Make sure that the older adults you come into contact with are asked, as a matter of course, if they have people caring for them to ensure that carers are identified.

- Ensure that there is clear and easily accessible information for carers, detailing their rights and any local support that is available. This might include anything from information on grants and benefits to details about respite care.

- All assessments relating to the person in need of care should be done in consultation and in partnership with the carer (as long as the person they are caring for consents to this), in line with national and international requirements.

- Raise awareness of the services available for carers, and ensure that this information is available in a number of languages and formats and in places carers may visit, such as community centres, places of worship and GP surgeries, as well as through radio programmes. This provides a variety of opportunities for people to participate in consultations and partnerships to ensure that services understand their needs.

- Promote anti-stigma campaigns and materials which are inclusive of all groups.

- Try to involve older adults and carers in service planning and management structures.

- Be mindful of how gender, age, sexuality and mental health status may be positioned within diverse cultures to ensure that marginalised groups within a community also have a voice and can be involved in the planning and monitoring of services.

- If there is not adequate representation from a particular group (such as, but not limited to, carers from LGBTi groups, carers with learning disabilities, carers from BAME backgrounds, etc.), collaborating with local or national organisations that work with these communities can facilitate greater inclusion.

- Involve service users/experts by experience and carers regularly and as a matter of course in the training of mental health staff in order to ensure that their views and expertise are recognised and embedded in services.

- Ensure that partnerships are real, appropriate, accessible and sustainable, and not tokenistic or pseudo (whereby consultations result in no real changes). Clear, honest and realistic messages need to be given throughout the process.

- Promote or assist with the establishment of self-help groups if this is required.

- Ensure that monitoring of the 'protected characteristics' of the Equality Act 2010 is carried out as a matter of course, and act upon any evidence that certain groups are not using the services. Consultations should be held in places which are not only accessible but feel comfortable for these groups to encourage participation.

- Involve service users and carers in the monitoring and evaluation of services as a matter of principle and not just in specific service user or carer 'projects'.

- All staff should have training on cultural diversity, mental capacity, LGBTi issues and all other elements of diversity, as well as on conducting culturally competent and appropriate assessments.

- Older adults and their carers may not be able to travel easily, and therefore their views can end up being excluded. Ideally, systems should be put in place to ensure that their voices can be heard and to avoid service users or carers feeling that they are either excluded or being given 'different' treatment.

- Consultations or partnerships must ensure that the views of older adults are represented across all service provision and not just in services for older adults. In addition to accessing older adult mental health services, older adults and their carers may be parents and grandparents and may have lived experience of other services.

- Service users and carers should be paid for their time and travel. This is important, respectful and inclusive and should form part of anti-discriminatory practice. Mental health professionals are paid for their time and travel, and service users and carers should be as well.

- Agencies should develop clear strategies to recruit and keep staff from diverse backgrounds and should monitor this.

In summary, this chapter has considered some of the issues which may arise when considering anti-discriminatory practice in relation to carers of older adults with mental health dilemmas. We have examined the definitions and roles of carers as well as relevant legislation and contextual factors. We have identified a range of dilemmas and issues which carers may face, and we have considered how anti-discriminatory practice may need to challenge traditional practices in a variety of situations. This chapter has stressed the importance of ensuring that carers are able to contribute in a range of ways to ensure that service provision is relevant and appropriate to their needs and those of the person they care for. It has also highlighted the importance of ensuring that carers are adequately supported in this vital role in ways which maximise their well-being and that of the person they are caring for. Finally, additional resources, relevant legislation and good practice examples have been provided in a summarised form to help improve anti-discriminatory practice for carers of older people with mental health needs.

Reflective questions

1. Spend a few minutes thinking about what it might be like to be an older adult with a mental health condition who is dependent on a family member as a carer. What does this feel like?

2. What image comes to your mind when you think about a carer? Once you have an image, spend a few minutes thinking and making a list of what issues and challenges might be present for the carer of an older adult with mental health issues.

3. If you were an older adult with mental health issues and were dependent on a carer, what things do you think you would see as important for your well-being?

4. What one thing can you do to ensure that you and the service you work for make an effort to ensure better provision is made for carers of older people with mental health needs?

References

Adamson, J. and Donovan, J. (2005) '"Normal disruption": South Asian and African/Caribbean relatives caring for an older family member in the UK.' *Social Science & Medicine 60*, 1, 37–48.

Age UK (2010) *Invisible but Invaluable: Campaigning for Greater Support for Older Carers.* London: Age UK. Available at www.ageuk.org.uk/en-GB/research/, accessed on 13 May 2014.

Almack, K., Seymour, J. and Bellamy, G. (2010) 'Exploring the impact of sexual orientation on experiences and concerns about end of life care and on bereavement for lesbian, gay and bisexual older people.' *Sociology 44*, 5, 908–924.

BBC News (2007) *Carers save the UK '£87bn a year.* Available at http://news.bbc.co.uk/1/hi/health/7001160.stm, accessed 17 January 2017. Support for carers of older people Independence and well-being 5. London: Audit Commission isbn 186240 482 8

Boen, H., Steffen Dalgard, O. and Bjertness, E. (2012) 'The importance of social support in the associations between psychological distress and somatic health problems and socio-economic factors among older adults living at home: A cross sectional study.' *BMC Geriatrics 12*, 27.

Brodolini, F. (2012) *Long Term Care for the Elderly: Provisions and Providers in 33 European Countries.* Luxembourg: Publications Office of the European Union.

Busby, N. (2011) 'Carers and the Equality Act 2010: Protected characteristics and identity.' *Contemporary Issues in Law 11*, 2, 71–91.

Carers Trust (2015) *Key facts about carers and the people they care for.* Available at https://carers.org/key-facts-about-carers-and-people-they-care, accessed on 3 January 2017.

Carers Trust (2017) *What is a carer?* Available at https://carers.org/what-carer, accessed on 3 January 2017.

Carers UK (2013) *The State of Caring 2013.* London: Carers UK. Available at www.carersuk.org/for-professionals/policy/policy-library/the-state-of-caring-2013, accessed on 6 November 2016.

Carers UK (2014a) *Facts about Carers 2014.* London: Carers UK. Available at www.carersuk.org/for-professionals/policy/policy-library/facts-about-carers-2014, accessed on 6 November 2016.

Carers UK (2014b) *No One Should Have to Care Alone: Break Isolation.* London: Carers UK. Available at www.carersuk.org/news-and-campaigns/alone/breaking-isolation, accessed on 6 November 2016.

Carers UK (2014c) *Caring and Family Finances Inquiry: UK Report.* London: Carers UK. Available at www.carersuk.org/for-professionals/policy/policy-library/caring-family-finances-inquiry, accessed on 6 November 2016.

Carers UK (2015) *State of Caring 2015.* London: Carers UK. Available at www.carersuk.org/for-professionals/policy/policy-library/state-of-caring-2015, accessed on 6 November 2016.

Carersweek *Report In sickness and in Health a survey of 3,400 UK carers about their health and well-being.* London: Carers UK.

Carr, S. (2014) *Social Care for Marginalised Communities: Balancing Self-organisation Micro-provision and Mainstream Support.* Policy Paper 18. Birmingham: Health Services Management Centre, University of Birmingham. Available at www.birmingham.ac.uk/Documents/college-social-sciences/social-policy/HSMC/publications/PolicyPapers/policy-paper-18-sarah-carr.pdf, accessed on 6 November 2016.

Cohen, S. and Willis, T.A. (1985) 'Stress, social support and the buffering hypothesis.' *Psychological Bulletin 98*, 2, 310–357.

Coppel, D.B., Burton, C., Becker, J. and Fiore, J. (1985) 'Relationships of cognitions associated with coping reaction to depression in spousal caregivers of Alzheimer's disease patients.' *Cognitive Therapy Research 9*, 253–266.

Emerson, E. and Hatton, C. (2008) *Estimating the Future Need for Adult Social Services for People with Learning Disabilities in England.* CeDR Research Report, November 2008. Lancaster: Lancaster University Centre for Disability Research.

Fernando, S. (2014) *Mental Health Worldwide: Culture, Globalization and Development.* London: Palgrave Macmillan.

Finch, J. and Groves, D. (1983) *A Labour of Love: Women, Work and Caring.* London: Routledge and Kegan Paul.

Fish, J. (2006) *Hetrosexism in Health and Social Care.* London: Palgrave Macmillan.

Glendinning, C., Mitchell, W. and Brooks, J. (2015) 'Ambiguity in practice? Carers' roles in personalised social care in England.' *Health and Social Care in the Community 23*, 1, 23–32.

Gosman-Hedström, G. and Dahlin-Ivanoff, S. (2012) 'Mastering an unpredictable everyday life after stroke: Older women's experiences of caring and living with their partners.' *Scandinavian Journal of Caring Sciences 26*, 3, 587–597.

Gregory, C. (2010) *Improving Health and Social Care Support for Black and Minority Ethnic Carers.* Briefing Health Report 20. London: Race Equality Foundation.

Heaphy, B., Yip, K. and Thompson, D. (2003) *Lesbian, Gay and Bisexual Lives Over 50.* Nottingham: York House Publications.

Horowitz, A. and Shindleman, L.W. (1983) 'Reciprocity and affection: Past influences on current caregiving.' *Journal of Gerontological Social Work 5*, 5–20.

Institute for Research and Innovation in Social Services (2010) *Improving Support for Black and Minority Ethnic Carers.* Glasgow: IRISS. Available at www.iriss.org.uk/sites/default/files/iriss-insight-7.pdf, accessed on 6 November 2016.

Joint Commissioning Panel for Mental Health (2013) *Guidance for Commissioners of Older People's Mental Health Services: Practical Mental Health Commissioning Guidance for Commissioners of Older People's Mental Health.* Available at www.jcpmh.info/wp-content/uploads/jcpmh-olderpeople-guide.pdf, accessed on 29 August 2015.

Joseph Rowntree Foundation (2008) *What Future for Care?* York: Joseph Rowntree Foundation. Available at www.jrf.org.uk/report/what-future-caresite, accessed on 17 September 2015.

Karlsson, M., Mayhew, L., Plumb, R. and Rickaysen, B. (2006) 'Future costs for long-term care: Cost projections for long-term care for older people in the United Kingdom.' *Health Policy 75*, 187–213.

Kessler, R.C., Price, R.H. and Wortman, C.B. (1985) 'Social factors in psychopathology: Stress, social support and coping processes.' *Annual Review of Psychology 36*, 531–572.

Lane, P. and Tribe, R. (2010) 'Following NICE 2008. A practical guide for health professionals: Community engagement with local black and minority ethnic (BME) community groups.' *Diversity, Health & Care 7*, 2, 105–114.

Mental Health Foundation (2015) *Fundamental Facts About Mental Health 2015.* London: Mental Health Foundation. Available at www.mentalhealth.org.uk/sites/default/files/fundamental-facts-15. pdf, accessed on 6 November 2016.

Mir, G. and Tovey, P. (2003) 'Asian carers' experiences of medical and social care: The case of cerebral palsy.' *British Journal of Social Work 33*, 465–479.

National Black Carers and Carers Workers Network (2008) *Beyond We Care Too: Putting Black Carers in the Picture.* London: Afiya Trust for the National Black Carers and Carers Workers Network. Available at www.southglos.gov.uk/documents/beyond_we_care_too.pdf, accessed on 6 November 2016.

Office for National Statistics (2013a) *2011 Census Analysis: Unpaid Care in England and Wales, 2011 and Comparison with 2001.* Available at www.ons.gov.uk/peoplepopulationandcommunity/ healthandsocialcare/healthcaresystem/articles/2011censusanalysisunpaidcareinenglandand wales2011andcomparisonwith2001/2013-02-15, accessed on 6 November 2016.

Office for National Statistics (2013b) *Full Story. The Gender Gap in Unpaid Care Provision: Is There an Impact on Health and Economic Position?* Available at http://webarchive.nationalarchives.gov. uk/20160105160709/http://www.ons.gov.uk/ons/dcp171776_310295.pdf, accessed on 6 November 2016.

Ott, C., Sanders, S. and Kelber, M.S. (2007) 'Grief and personal growth experience of spouses and adult-child caregivers of individuals with Alzheimer's disease and related dementias.' *The Gerontologist 47*, 6, 798–809.

Pickard, L. (2008) *Informal Care for Older People Provided by their Adult Children: Projections of Supply and Demand to 2041 in England.* Report to the Department of Health and the Cabinet Office. Canterbury: PSSRU. Available at www.pssru.ac.uk/pdf/dp2515.pdf, accessed on 6 November 2016.

Quayhagen, M.P. and Quayhagen, M. (1998) 'Alzheimer's stress: Coping with the care giving role.' *The Gerontologist 28*, 391–396.

Seabrooke, V. and Milne, E. (2009) 'Early intervention in dementia care in an Asian community.' *Quality in Ageing and Older Adults 10*, 4, 29–36.

Shah, A.J., Wadoo, O. and Latoo, J. (2010) 'Psychological distress in carers of people with mental disorders.' *British Journal of Medical Practitioners 3*, 3, 327.

Shipman, B. and Smart, C. (2007) '"It's made a huge difference": Recognition, rights and the personal significance of civil partnership.' *Sociological Research Online 22*, 1.

Smyth, C., Blaxland, M. and Cass, B. (2011) 'So that's how I found out I was a young carer and that I actually had been a carer most of my life.' *Journal of Youth Studies 14*, 2, 145–160.

Tribe, R. (2014) 'Culture, politics and global mental health.' *Disability and the Global South 1*, 2, 251–265.

Tribe, R., Lane, P. and Hearsum, S. (2009) 'Working towards promoting positive mental health and wellbeing for older people within BME communities.' *Working with Older People 31*, 1, 35–42.

Van der Lee, J., Bakker, T.J.E.M. and Duivenvoorden, H.J. (2014) 'Multivariate models of subjective caregiver burden in dementia: A systematic review.' *Ageing Research Reviews 15*, 76–93.

Walker, A. and Walker, C. (1998) 'Normalisation and normal ageing: The social construction of dependency among older people with learning difficulties.' *Disability & Society 13*, 1, 125–142.

Wallcraft, J., Amering, M., Freidin, J., Davar, B. *et al.* (2011) 'Partnerships for better mental health worldwide: WPA recommendations on best practices in working with service users and family carers.' *World Psychiatry 10*, 229–236.

Walsh, K. and O'Shea, E. (2008) 'Responding to rural social care needs: Older people empowering themselves, others and their community.' *Health and Place 14*, 795–805.

Wilson, M., Kellock, C., Adams, D. and Landsberg, J. (2015) *The Scottish Health Survey. Topic Report: Mental Health and Wellbeing.* Edinburgh: Scottish Government. Available at www.gov.scot/Resource/0046/00469088.pdf, accessed on 6 November 2016.

Wirral Carers Strategy (2017) *Wirral Carers Strategy 2014-2017.* Available at info.wirral.nhs.uk/document_uploads/JSNA%202012/CarersDec2012Final.pdf, accessed on 3 January 2017.

World Psychiatric Association (2011) *Madrid Declaration on Ethical Standards for Psychiatric Practice.* Available at www.wpanet.org/detail.php?section_id=5&content_id=48, accessed on 6 November 2016.

Yeandle, S. (2011) 'Why we need to care for the carers.' *Guardian*, 12 December 2011. Available at www.theguardian.com/society/joepublic/2011/dec/12/why-need-care-for-carers, accessed on 6 November 2016.

Yeandle, S., Bennett, C., Buckner, L., Fry, G. and Price, C. (2007) *Managing Caring and Employment, CES Report No 2*. London: Carers UK.

Additional resources

The Institute for Research and Innovation in Social Science (IRISS) provides a toolkit (a set of cards) for people who provide support to older adults, which can be downloaded for free from their website: www.iriss.org.uk/resources/tools/d-cards. These are based on well-being promotion, which helps people think about maintaining and building social and community connections and preventing loneliness.

The following organisations may also be able to offer assistance:

Benefits calculators at www.gov.uk: www.gov.uk/benefits-adviser

Black and Minority Ethnic Carers' Support Service (a provider of services to BAME carers): www.mecopp.org.uk

Mental Health Foundation: www.mentalhealth.org.uk

Mind: www.mind.org.uk, 0300 123 3393 (information is available in multiple languages) The mental health charity, provides information and a range of helpful suggestions about coping as a carer and ensuring that carers' own mental well-being is considered. It also covers such issues as devising a joint crisis plan and developing a strategy to ensure that some of the carers' own needs are met. It provides a range of exercises to assist carers

Mind and Rethink's campaign against the stigma of mental illness: www.time-to-change.org.uk

National Black Carers and Carers Workers Network (regional support networks in the north-west of England, the East Midlands and London): contact through Carers UK

Policy Research Institute on Ageing and Ethnicity (PRIAE; a registered independent charity working to improve pensions, employment, health, social care, housing and quality of life for BAME older adults in the UK and across Europe. The Institute aims to influence national and European policy and increase and encourage good practice in work with BAME older adults): www.priae.org; 0113 285 5990; 31–32 Park Row, Leeds LS1 5JD

Rethink Mental Illness advice line: www.rethink.org; 0300 50000 927

Samaritans: www.samaritans.org, 08457 90 90 90

Specialist Library for Ethnicity and Health (SLEH; aims to select the best available evidence about management of a healthcare service and specific needs in health care for migrant and minority ethnic groups. They only provide guidance on electronically available resources): www.library.nhs.uk/ethnicity

Local carers groups

Local carers groups can be located through the organisations listed below.

Carers UK provides advice on community care and welfare benefits and information to carers: www.carersuk.org; 0207 922 7976; Carers UK, 32–36 Loman Street, London SE1 0EE

The Carers Trust provides support on a range of areas, including respite care, looking after yourself, employment, planning holidays and days out, finances and benefits and getting the most from health professionals, as well as offering a young carers support group and local forums: www.carers.org; 0844 800 4361

Mind: find the contact details for your local branch online at www.mind.org.uk, call 0300 123 3393 or email info@mind.org.uk

NHS Choices Carers Direct: www.nhs.uk/carersdirect

Other charitable organisations also provide support with specific conditions. For example, the RNIB may be able to provide guidance on care for an older adult with a visual impairment.

Relevant legislation and good practice guidelines

Care Act 2014: This came into force in April 2015 and sets out carers' legal rights to assessment and support. Previously this was at the discretion of the local authority. The Act covers a range of matters including wishing to ensure that carers' own objectives are met. It aims to assist in 'putting carers on an equal legal footing to those they care for and putting their needs at the centre of legislation'. The Act relates to England only and replaces the following pieces of legislation: Carers (Recognition and Services Act) 1995; Carers and Disabled Children Act 2000; and Carers (Equal Opportunities) Act 2004. Factsheets and further information can be obtained from the Department of Health (www.gov.uk/government/organisations/department-of-health) or the Carers Trust.

Employment Rights Act 1996: Under this UK-wide legislation, all employees, including carers, have the legal right to request flexible working if they have worked for their employer for at least 26 weeks. Employers are required to deal with requests in a 'reasonable manner'. See ACAS' guide, *The Right to Flexible Working*, available from www.acas.org.uk/index.aspx?articleid=1362.

Equality Act 2010: This UK-wide legislation states that no one should be discriminated against in education, employment or service provision in relation to seven protected characteristics: age, disability, gender reassignment, marital status, race, religion/ belief, and sex or sexual orientation. It also stipulates that a carer cannot be discriminated against on the basis of their association with the person they care for.

Mental Capacity Act 2005: This relates to when someone is deemed to lack the mental capacity to make decisions and how this relates to the individual and their carer. This Act is dealt with in some detail in Chapter 5 of this volume by Ajit Shah.

Your Human Rights: A Pocket Guide for Carers: available to download from www.bihr.org.uk/carersguide.

CHAPTER 7

End of Life Issues and Older People's Mental Health

Pauline Lane and Rachel Tribe

Dying in old age is seen as a natural part of the human condition. However, the individual meanings that we give to both dying and death are influenced by many factors, such as the age of the person who is dying or has died, the way in which he or she died, and our own cultural and spiritual beliefs about death and dying. In the UK, as in many other countries, you have the same rights as everyone else even when you are dying. However, some groups of patients may experience inequalities in accessing appropriate end of life care, and research suggests that many older people receive poor standards of care towards the end of their lives. As professionals, we have both a professional and legal duty to protect and fulfil people's human rights up until their death (Human Rights Act 1998) and to work to eliminate discrimination (Equality Act 2010).

This chapter looks at a range of issues related to dying and how we might maintain anti-discriminatory practice when older people are in the process of dying. It also reflects on some of the issues practitioners face when the person who is dying has diminished capacity. The chapter starts by examining how dying has been portrayed and constructed historically within the UK. It reviews the age at which different groups of people die and questions if there can be such a thing as a 'good death'. The chapter then looks at end of life care (palliative care) and identifies some of the issues that different groups of older people face in trying to access end of life services. Towards the end of the chapter, we address some of the more practical issues concerning advance care plans and power of attorney for older people living with mental health issues. Finally, the chapter addresses ways in which practitioners can promote anti-discriminatory practice in the care of older people living with mental health conditions.

The social context of death and dying

The quality of our lives and the age at which we die are mediated by many factors, including the time and place in which we live as well as the impact of social and economic factors over our lifetime. Records suggest that human life expectancy has increased throughout history. For example, the average life expectancy of stone-age people was probably around 25 years, but following the industrial revolution and the advent of public sanitation in the late 1800s, there was a notable increase in life expectancy to approximately 41 years of age (Cutler, Deaton and Lleras-Muney 2006). Up until the late 1800s, many people died from infectious diseases such as cholera, tuberculosis, typhus and smallpox, with others dying from causes such as malnutrition, childbirth, wounds and infections, as well as the effects of war, poor sanitation and famine. In most Western nations, we have seen a shift from death as largely the province of childhood to death as the province of the old, and in most high-income countries, people are not dying from infectious diseases but rather from long-term conditions (Blauner 1966). For example, in the UK there are approximately 555,000 deaths a year (Office for National Statistics 2015), and while 30 per cent are due to cancer, it is the non-cancerous conditions that account for the majority of deaths today (Dixon *et al.* 2015). As we live longer, we are also more likely to be affected by conditions such as dementia. Indeed, the Alzheimer's Society has suggested that while there are currently 850,000 people living with dementia in the UK, the numbers are set to rise to over 1 million by 2025 and potentially 2 million by 2051 (Alzheimer's Society 2015). Clearly this raises concerns, not only about people's quality of life but also the nature of their care when dying.

Premature mortality

There is a wide variation in death rates among different sections of the population. In the UK, women on average live longer than men, with the average age of death for women being 82.6 years, while for men it is 78.7 (Office for National Statistics 2015). However, gender is not the only factor that might influence our longevity. Research suggests that, on average, people who live in poorer areas are likely to die seven years earlier than those living in the richest areas (Marmot 2010). Furthermore, some social groups are more likely to die at a much younger age than the general population (although, as suggested in the introduction to this book, the social groups outlined below are not mutually exclusive). Research suggests the following:

- People living with a mental illness have a reduced life expectancy and often die around 10 to 15 years earlier than the general population (Walker, McGee and Druss 2015). For example, research suggests that people who have schizophrenia are more likely to face premature death (Brown *et al.* 2010). This could be because some people with mental impairments are less able to recognise their own health needs, but it has also been suggested that health and social care services do not usually manage to offer an integrated response to people with mental and physical healthcare needs (Naylor *et al.* 2012).

- Those who have been disadvantaged throughout their lives usually continue to experience this disadvantage into old age (EuroHealthNet 2010). For example, men aged 25 to 64 from routine or manual work backgrounds are twice as likely to die early than men from managerial or professional backgrounds. These social class differences exist for all the major causes of death, including cancers and heart disease (Office for National Statistics 2015).

- A number of reports have suggested that the healthcare needs of people with learning disabilities are often neglected, and, on average, they will die at between 13 and 20 years younger than the general population (Heslop *et al.* 2013).

- Homeless people tend to die much younger than the general population. Shockingly, the average age of death for a homeless man is 47 years old, and this figure is even lower for homeless women, at 43. Few homeless people live into old age (Thomas 2012).

- Some people in ethnic minority groups die much younger than the average age of death for the dominant White ethnic population. For example, Gypsies and Travellers die between 10 and 12 years younger than the general population (Parry *et al.* 2004).

However, it is notable that there is a lack of data on the death rates of some social groups (Equality and Human Rights Commission 2010). While national data from the UK would suggest that those who are the poorest and most disadvantaged or marginalised are more likely to live in poorer health and die younger, the death rates of many groups of people are also 'invisible' due to a lack of national data. Certainly, society inequality reflects not only the quality of people's health but also the age at which they might expect to die.

The idea of a 'good death'

Throughout history, there has been much debate about what might be considered a 'good death'. Kellehear (2007) has charted how death and dying have been constructed across different periods of history. He argues that when societies changed from hunter-gatherers to settled communities, the idea of a good death became part of a wider moral debate about what it meant to be a good citizen. He suggests that, during early industrialisation, what counted as a 'good death' was a person's moral behaviour during their lifetime as well as how they left their affairs when they died (i.e. not dying in debt). Kellehear suggests that with increasing industrialisation, death started to be managed not by the family but by external professionals such as lawyers, doctors and priests. This meant that a 'good death' included not only moral judgements but also the development of new death 'management structures', such as wills and death certificates. Kellehear also points out that in modern Western society, where we celebrate youth, death is often seen as shameful, and older people who are dying are often hidden in hospitals and care homes. Clearly this is not true of all death: death in war is often portrayed as heroic, as are the early deaths of celebrities, children or young people, and people who 'battle' against certain illness, such as cancer. Yet, interestingly, you rarely hear reports of someone 'battling' against dementia.

Much of the modern debate concerning a 'good death' has emerged from the work of Elizabeth Kübler-Ross, who wrote an influential book in 1969 titled *On Death and Dying*. This book presented conversations between Dr Kübler-Ross and her patients about their reactions to their impending death. The book and later publications generated much debate about how death and dying should be approached.

Kübler-Ross suggested that when people know they are dying, they pass through five different emotional stages. She argued that if patients and doctors could talk openly about dying then a 'good death' would be achievable. From her work, the whole concept of palliative care has developed into care that seeks not only to address a person's physical needs but also to consider wider issues including a person's social and spiritual needs. Professionals have developed palliative care services around her principles of good communication and support for patients and their families. In addition, her work has been very influential in the establishment of the hospice movement in a number of countries and the idea of facing death with dignity and preparedness. However, her philosophy has not been without its critics, and some authors have suggested that the ideology of a 'good death' can mean that professionals frame and shape the experience of dying for their patients, which may actually limit the choices of the individual and how they might like to approach their own death (Hart, Sainsbury and Short 1998).

Although the ideas of a 'good death' and patient choice are often discussed in the literature, in practice, many older people (and especially older people with mental health problems) do not have the same access to palliative care as young people. In promoting anti-discriminatory practice and planning a 'good death' with older people, we need to acknowledge their specific and varying needs and to consider the personal and emotional resources that they have available. As practitioners, we need to recognise that people often have changing care needs, goals and priorities when dying. By learning to listen to a person's needs and by developing person-centred care, we can work towards anti-discriminatory practice.

Palliative care

Palliative care is a multidisciplinary approach to end of life care that seeks to offer the best possible care for a person who is living with a life-limiting illness. For people with low to moderate palliative care needs, services are usually provided by GPs, community nurses, hospital teams and social care agencies. For people with moderate to highly complex palliative care needs, specialist palliative care services are provided. These services are often able to offer specialist advice and support to families, friends and carers, although the overall responsibility for medical care remains with the hospital consultant, if the person is an inpatient, or the GP, if the person is at home or in a care home. Palliative care teams include a wide range of professionals such as:

- palliative care consultants and doctors

- general and specialist nurses including district nurses

- social workers

- occupational therapists and physiotherapists

- other specialist staff such as dieticians and pharmacists

- counsellors, psychologists and psychiatrists

- spiritual leaders

- practitioners offering bereavement support

- volunteers.

These teams of people have expertise in the management or treatment of physical symptoms, and they offer psychological, social and spiritual support for the patient and his or her family. However, it is important to remember that the person with a life-limiting illness must give their consent before a referral is made to a specialist palliative care team. It is also worth reflecting on the fact that not everyone gets access to palliative care. Even when people do die at home, research suggests that it is often the family or close friends who pick up the burden of care, such as managing the logistics, physical tasks, financial costs, emotional burdens, etc. (Rabow, Hauser and Adams 2004).

Ideally, palliative care should enable people to make choices about their end of life care as well as their place of death. Yet the reality is that while most people would prefer to die at home, the majority will actually die in hospital (Ryder 2013). Because of the large number of people dying in hospitals, the Liverpool Care Pathway for the Dying

Patient (LCP) was developed as an approach to improve the quality of end of life care. Despite its best intentions, the Neuberger Review (Department of Health 2013) recommended that the LCP should be phased out due to the fact that the process was often misinterpreted by hospital staff. In its place, individual care plans for the dying have now been brought in to promote a better quality of care in hospitals, and the Leadership Alliance for the Care of Dying People (a coalition of 21 national organisations) has established guidance on caring for people in the last few days and hours of life (Leadership Alliance for the Care of Dying People 2014).

The National Institute for Health and Care Excellence (NICE) (2015) has also developed guidelines for end of life care, in which they promote the idea of shared decision-making. However, the mental capacity to engage in shared decision-making may become limited for many people entering their final days of life. This could be temporary (e.g. as a result of delirium), or it may be a permanent loss of capacity (e.g. dementia or another similar, irreversible condition). The NICE guidelines provide recommendations to help healthcare professionals to navigate the needs of a dying patient with limited mental capacity. In addition, professionals have a clear duty to comply with the Mental Capacity Act 2005 (see Chapter 5 of this volume for more on this).

Mental illness in old age and dying

There is very little research on the experiences of older people who are dying and have a mental health condition. A paper by McGrath and Holewa written in 2004 stated that there was a 'loud silence' (p.107) concerning the research literature on palliative care and hospice services for individuals in the mental health system. Years later, it might still be said that this 'silence' is deafening when looking for research literature on palliative care for older people experiencing mental health problems. The limited research that does exist makes the following suggestions:

- People with a known mental illness are more likely to have reduced life expectancy and generally experience poorer physical health, with physical illness often going undetected for long periods of time (Academy of Medical Royal Colleges 2009).

- Some older people who lack mental capacity might find it hard to recognise that they are ill, or they may find it difficult to communicate their health needs and experiences of pain to others (Talbott and Linn 1978).

- Many older people have more than one medical condition (co-morbidity), and any assessments conducted during a person's terminal illness can be complicated by other underlying conditions as well as by medication taken to relieve the symptoms.

- Some health professionals may ignore or fail to take action in the treatment of physical illness when someone has a known psychiatric disorder, which can result in a delayed diagnosis and a lack of good pain management (Henderson 2004).

With some mental health conditions, it may be difficult to identify when someone is facing the end of their life. Looking, for example, at dementia, the 'dying' process is prolonged and so there it can be difficult to assess when end of life care should be introduced. Research by Sampson, Burns and Richards (2011) suggests that many people living with dementia experience poor end of life care, simply because they are often not perceived to have a terminal illness (despite having symptoms that are similar to those found in the terminal stages of cancer). Consequently, Henderson (2004) suggests that most people with dementia are largely excluded from palliative support as a whole. Other researchers have found that despite often having more profound needs, only a small percentage of terminally ill patients with dementia receive hospice care, as advanced dementia often inhibits the ability to express those needs (Mitchell *et al.* 2007). For family and friends who are carers, their loved one's final journey to death can be especially difficult as they may already be grieving the loss due to dementia of the person they had known for many years.

When working towards meeting the needs of older people living with mental health conditions, it is important to keep in mind that individuals and their families will vary in their capacity to manage a terminal prognosis. Although the person who is dying should ideally be autonomous and make his or her own decisions about care and pain relief at the end of life, in many cases people's lack of capacity prevents them from making informed choices about their own care

(Sjostrand and Helgeson 2008). In these circumstances, the person will require others to act in their best interests under the guidance of the Mental Health Act 2007, and it is therefore important that professionals work with the person's family and other loved ones to promote dignity in dying. We should not assume, however, that an older person who has a mental illness or diminished capacity will necessarily be unable to understand that he or she is dying. Where possible, it is useful to develop advance care planning (see below), as this can help to take into account the person's choices and previously expressed wishes.

Dying and spirituality

While dying can be seen as both a physical and social event, for some people it is also a time of spiritual transformation. People respond in their own unique way to the knowledge that they are dying, and spiritual beliefs are important for many older people as they often help to inform a person's understanding of dying and preparation for death (MacKinlay 2006). Spirituality is hard to define, but it is usually understood as a framework of meaning that may or may not involve a god or other spiritual force or guide. While a person's spirituality may be part of a formal religious practice (such as Hinduism), it may also be a very personal set of spiritual beliefs. Indeed, even if someone does belong to a religious group, he or she may still hold a wide range of different beliefs and practices. Therefore, while it is useful as a practitioner to have some understanding of the beliefs and practices of the religions that are most prevalent in society, it is important to inquire about the specific needs and concerns of the older person you are supporting. For example, at a practical level this may mean ensuring that any home visits are respectful of prayer times and being mindful of appropriate approaches to the care of the dying (Bolliger 2014). It is also important to reflect on the fact that spiritual and cultural practices are not static. For example, although Hindu death rituals include practices that are often conducted for ten days following the death of a loved one, it is important to remember that different families and friends may approach this in different ways and with variations – even if they belong to the same religion – and therefore the focus must be on response to their particular needs.

Some authors have suggested that spirituality can act as a potential resource and comfort for many older people. It may help them to expand their consciousness outside of their own situation and to feel that they are part of something that is much bigger than themselves (Atchley 2009; Manning 2013). Indeed, research also suggests that 'unmet spiritual needs' can negatively impact on a person's capacity to cope with pain and suffering, and spiritual distress can also impact on a person's mental health (Lloyd-Williams 2003). Some practitioners may find it difficult to negotiate the spiritual concerns of the person they are caring for, especially as preregistration training often focuses on the clinical and social issues related to end of life care. Yet NICE (2015) acknowledges in its end of life guidelines that spiritual care is an essential element of good end of life care.

So what might 'spiritual care' look like in practice? Much of the literature on spirituality and end of life care points to the need to develop a shared understanding of the older person's life and his or her spiritual beliefs, which can be referred to later and may help to support future caring practice as the patient's health deteriorates (Atchley 2009; Puchalski 2006). Others have identified the value of continuity of prayer and other spiritual practices, which may help older people to tap into their spiritual memory and can bring comfort to people in distress (Goldsmith 2004). For example, the simple act of placing flowers on a home shrine, reading a spiritual text or listening to chanting or a choir may bring comfort to an older person.

Wherever possible, practitioners should try to take the time to get to know the older person they are caring for and find out what is significant or sacred to him or her. You may feel that it is appropriate to contact a faith leader to conduct any last rites or customs; however, this should only be done in consultation with the older person and his or her family or carers first. Certainly, addressing older people's spiritual needs should form a part of advance care planning (see below), as this will help to ensure that any specific needs and requests about care while dying are met, and any rituals following death are fulfilled.

Equality issues for specific groups

Below is a short discussion concerning older people from different social groups. Please note that the authors are suggesting not that the people within these groups have a single identity but that by using these collective identities it is possible to highlight some of the experiences of exclusion from palliative care services and to identify issues that may impact on professional practice.

Older people from Black, Asian and Minority Ethnic communities

With dramatic demographic changes in the number of older people from different ethnic groups, there is a growing need to rethink how accessible and appropriate end of life care is for people from diverse Black, Asian and Minority Ethnic (BAME) communities (Calanzani, Koffman and Higginson 2013). As suggested in Chapter 3, ethnic minority populations do not form a homogeneous group, and people from different communities and families will hold a variety of beliefs and cultural practices concerning dying and the death of an older family member. However, much of the literature on older people from BAME communities does point to the shared experience of exclusion from palliative care services. Indeed, Calanzani *et al.* (2013) conducted a review of palliative care and found that there was a low uptake of palliative and end of life care services by all BAME groups. The authors identified the following reasons for this:

- lack of referrals, knowledge and information

- religious and family issues in conflict with the palliative care ethos of discussing dying with the patient

- poor communication by professionals and a lack of sensitivity to religious and cultural issues

- lack of advance care planning

- previous negative experiences of care, including racism and a lack of cultural awareness

- geographical location of hospices, with limited or no services in rural areas, leading to a 'postcode lottery'.

Interestingly, in a study conducted in 2015, many older African migrants interviewed stated that:

> their own experiences of working in the care sector strongly shaped their beliefs and attitudes towards palliative and end of life care along

with experiences of racism at work. Their own perceptions of poor standards of care towards elderly and frail patients made many afraid should they have to enter such care themselves in later years. (Smith, Moreno-Leguizamon and Grohmann 2015, p.3)

Clearly, the current evidence indicates that many local palliative care services do not seem to be able to meet the cultural needs of all of their local communities, despite their duty to do so under the Equality Act 2010.

It is useful for practitioners who are developing their own practices of working with BAME elders to read and attend courses to build up their own cultural competence, enabling them to promote more cultural sensitivity in delivering services. However, in practical terms, if a practitioner is unsure about the cultural needs or concerns of a patient in his or her care, it is always better to ask rather than make assumptions.

Lesbian, gay, bisexual, transgender and intersex older people

Research suggests that unless they are dying from AIDS, most lesbian, gay, bisexual, transgender or intersex (LGBTi) people often do not receive the palliative care they need when facing a life-limiting illness. Many LGBTi people fear that health professionals may discriminate against them even at the end of their life (Grace 2005; Harding, Epiphaniou and Chidgey-Clark 2012). Some LGBTi people no longer have contact with their family due to discrimination against them because of their sexual orientation, and therefore it is important to recognise that friends may be their 'chosen family'. There is a need to ensure that these support networks are included in any care planning and that the needs of same-sex carers are recognised. (For a more detailed discussion on this, see Chapter 9 in this volume by Matt Broadway-Horner.) As such, practitioners need to be supportive and sensitive in developing advance care plans and be mindful in the way they talk about issues to ensure the patient's confidentiality.

People with learning disabilities

Although there are approximately 1.5 million people with learning difficulties in the UK (Mencap 2008), research suggests that they and their families often find it difficult to access end of life care services (Jenkins 2005). People with learning disabilities have the same rights as everyone else to access public-sector services, including palliative care. For professionals working with this client group, it is important to remember that a person's learning disability is only one aspect of his or her identity, and it is therefore essential to approach every person as an individual. (See Chapter 8 in this volume for a more detailed discussion on this.)

Until recently, there was very little information on the mental health needs of people with learning disabilities, and NICE (2016) has just published its clinical guidance on 'mental health problems in people with learning disabilities'. Very few studies have looked at the experiences of people with learning disabilities who have a mental illness and are dying. In 2007, Mencap wrote an influential report called *Death by Indifference* following the deaths in NHS care of six people with learning disabilities. A later report in 2012 (Department of Health 2012) suggested that there had been no substantial changes as a result of this report and that people with learning disabilities are still denied equal access to care from the NHS.

Research suggests that people with learning disabilities often have higher levels of unmet health needs than the general population (Michael 2008). They also often have a shorter life expectancy (Alborz, McNally and Glendinning 2005), with the average age at death for people with learning disabilities about 25 years younger than that of the general population (Emerson *et al.* 2011). Furthermore, there is evidence to show that psychiatric disorders are more prevalent in adults with learning disabilities than in the general population, but these disorders frequently go undetected and thus untreated (Deb, Thomas and Bright 2001).

One of the important issues in end of life care for people with learning disabilities is the assessment of health conditions and pain management. While a number of general assessment tools exist, many of these will be inappropriate for people with learning disabilities. Practitioners working in end of life care may have limited experience in providing support for people with learning disabilities, which becomes particularly complex in end of life care. It may be necessary to take a collaborative approach with different professionals involved in caring for the person with learning disabilities in order to better meet his or her needs (Tuffrey-Wijne, Hogg and Curfs 2007). While some people with learning disabilities will be able to communicate their needs, others will find this difficult and may need carers, family or friends to act as advocates for them. However, it is important to observe the Mental Capacity Act 2005, which assumes decision-making capacity unless proved otherwise.

People who are homeless

As mentioned above, homeless people often face a lifetime of exclusion that can lead to chronic health problems and only too often results in an early death. Supporting older homeless people with mental health problems is often challenging, and most homeless services are designed around the needs of young homeless people (see Chapter 11). Consequently, many public-sector services are unsuited to meeting the needs of older homeless people (Crane and Warnes 2000). As homeless people often have little contact with formal services, they are unlikely to seek support for health conditions until long after the symptoms first occurred. Once diagnosed, they need to be informed about the appropriate support available; however, they should remain in control of their choices around the uptake of that support. Practitioners will need to have a discussion with the person about where he or she would like to be cared for and what things he or she might want to do before dying. Practitioners also need to discuss issues such as what should be done with possessions, how to contact family or friends, and whether arrangements for the care of a pet need to be made.

If people are without family or friends, professionals may want to talk about how the dying person might like to be remembered. It may be useful to listen to their past life story to ensure that someone knows about them and to show them that they matter. Professionals will need to work together and more than likely include a wider range of professionals than usual, such as outreach teams and specialist services. Clearly, older homeless people who are mentally ill and in need of end of life care are exceptionally vulnerable. Professional teams may need to act quickly to offer appropriate housing or support. They may also need to work with local homeless charities to facilitate communication with the person's friends and to find out about any funeral arrangements for the person who is dying.

Barriers to providing good palliative care for older people

Research has found that older people and their carers often face a number of barriers in trying to access and receive good end of life care.

Defining the end of life

Part of the problem for older people who are trying to access palliative care services is the very definition of the term 'end of life'. While 'dying' is a biological process, the process of being deemed to 'be dying' is defined and sanctioned by healthcare professionals (Seymour 2007). Palliative care services were originally developed to meet the needs of people dying from cancer, where there is often a more definable 'terminal phase'. However, many older people have co-morbidities (i.e. multiple debilitating conditions) which may lead to uncertainties about the 'final phase' of their life. Consequently, many older people find it difficult to access palliative care services. While one-third of all deaths are of people aged 85 and over, only 15 per cent of those who receive specialist palliative care are in this age group (House of Commons Health Committee 2015). Although many older people wish to die in their own home, they often die in hospital due to the lack of care packages or palliative care services available in the community (Ryder 2013). Indeed, the 'problem' of dying in old age is often marked by extreme disadvantage and discrimination in terms of access to health and social care services (Davies *et al.* 2004).

Lack of staff training

Research suggests that many professionals supporting frail and seriously ill older people have difficulty in recognising the point at which a transition to a palliative care approach would be appropriate (Griffiths *et al.* 2014). Furthermore, professionals often feel inadequately trained to care for cognitively impaired patients, and consequently older people with mental health problems are more likely to experience uncoordinated care across the course of their stay in hospital and often do not have access to the care they need on leaving hospital (Gott *et al.* 2011). Many professionals working with older people with diminished capacity who are dying are also uncertain about what role families should play in decision-making when patients lack decision-making capacity (Ryder 2013).

Responsibility for care

In the UK, many older people die in care homes and nursing homes, which are likely to remain important places for end of life care for the foreseeable future (Froggatt 2001). However, the quality of end of life care in care homes can be very varied. In part, this is due to the fact that many older people live with complex health conditions and co-morbidities that make it difficult for staff to recognise and manage the last days of life (Morrison and Meier 2003). Research by Seymour, Kumar and Froggatt (2011) suggests that the quality of end of life care in care homes is influenced by both clinical and organisational factors, and other researchers have suggested that input from clinical nurse specialists or palliative medicine clinicians is rare and, when it does occur, reactive to crisis situations (Challis *et al.* 2000). Even arranging palliative care for people dying in their own homes can be complex. Research suggests that most people find it difficult to understand all of the different roles of healthcare professionals; carers often have to co-ordinate the collaboration between these different professionals (Oishi and Murtagh 2014). It has been suggested that many hospital admissions could be avoided by offering high-quality care for those who choose to die at home. This rarely occurs, however, as there is a lack of appropriate community-based resources to manage the last stages of a person's life and to provide support to family members and carers (Gott *et al.* 2013).

Advance care planning and legal issues concerning end of life for people with limited mental capacity

As people get older, they often indicate how their assets and possessions should be dealt with by making a will. While this may leave their finances in order, people often do not make plans for the care they would like to receive when they reach the end of their life or lose decision-making capacity. One way of addressing the future needs of older people is through advance care planning (ACP). This is a formal process that aims to help patients set out decisions about their future care if they lose capacity, as set out in the Mental Capacity Act 2005.

(Previously, terminology around ACP had included the concepts of 'living wills' and 'advance directives'.) More details about the Mental Capacity Act 2005 can be found in Chapter 5.

As Macmillan Cancer Support stated in a governmental report: 'if people are not identified as approaching end of life and professionals do not initiate conversations to understand people's needs and preferences, it is far less likely that plans can be put in place to meet those needs' (House of Commons Health Committee 2015, p.24). In other words, part of developing anti-discriminatory practice is to start a conversation as the first step in developing an ACP. ACPs are voluntary, so starting a conversation between family and friends is the first step in developing ACP in case of diminished mental capacity in the future. As part of anti-discriminatory practice, professionals should, where possible, initiate this conversation soon after diagnosis. For example, as dementia is a known degenerative condition, it makes sense to have discussed ACP between practitioners and families in order to agree on decisions before the patient loses capacity. These decisions should also be reviewed regularly while the patient still has capacity and should be used to confirm or amend the care approach.

Case study: Starting a conversation about ACP

George lives with his partner, Josef. They are both in their late eighties but are still mobile. However, they are only able to manage living independently with the support of George's son, who lives in the next town. George knows that he is approaching the end of his life as he has recently been diagnosed with dementia and lung cancer.

George would like to die at home but thinks that he should probably go into a nursing home, as he feels that Josef is not well enough to look after him and his son works long hours some distance away. The issue of dying away from Josef is causing George a great deal of worry, but he has not talked about this with his partner or his son as he does not want to worry them too. He has not asked his GP what support is available locally to help him stay in his own home, or if there are any alternatives to a nursing home available to him.

Initiating ACP would help George and Josef to talk about the options available to them and come to a decision about which would be the best option for everyone. Making this plan together with Josef and his son might also help George to resolve some of his concerns about the prospect of his death.

ACP can be complex and difficult, but Mullick, Martin and Sallnow (2013) have put forward the following points to consider when preparing to have a discussion:

- Patients need time to reflect, and so ACP will often need to extend over several conversations, and it is important that patients understand that plans can be changed and adapted if their needs change.

- Practitioners need to make sure that any outcomes of these discussions are appropriately shared with relevant healthcare teams and updated if any changes are made.

- It is important not to give the patient the impression that it is possible to anticipate and plan for every eventuality.

- Do not assume that other health or social care professionals have already had these discussions – but it is a good idea to check first before starting the conversation.

- Any discussions need to involve the patient's wider family or significant others (with the consent of the patient) in order to avoid conflict if the patient does lose capacity.

ACP can cover both medical treatment and the social aspects of care. However, while ACP is a positive step towards meeting the needs of older people with diminished capacity, currently there is no systematic approach to recording patients' end of life care plans and preferences so that they can be easily accessed by all health and social care staff who treat them (House of Commons Health Committee 2015). Practitioners therefore need to be proactive in sharing information (with the consent of the patient). While the evidence for the effectiveness of ACP is mixed, one retrospective study of 969 deceased hospice patients found that those who did complete ACP spent less time in hospital in their last year of life than those who didn't (Abel *et al.* 2013).

ACP may not suit everyone. A recent study on end of life decisions in Roma families indicated that some Roma are opposed to written end of life plans because the Roma culture is predominantly non-literate and many people do not trust information that is written down (Peinado-Gorlat *et al.* 2015). In terms of promoting anti-discriminatory practice, it is always important to discuss an appropriate approach with patients and their families, friends and significant others.

Developing anti-discriminatory practice in end of life care for older people

The following recommendations may be helpful when developing anti-discriminatory practice in end of life care for older people, particularly those with mental health problems.

Be willing to talk

Having the conversation about what people want at the end of their lives can be difficult and emotional for people who are dying and their families, as well as for the staff who care for them. However, if we are not willing to have a conversation about dying, people may not have the opportunity to say what is important to them at the end of their life.

Work as part of a team

By working in collaboration with others, healthcare professionals can provide effective and person-centred end of life care. Although the patient may be old, the news that he or she is dying may still come as a shock. You will need to work with the patient, family and other professionals to develop a plan that focuses on the needs and concerns of the patient. This plan may need to be reviewed regularly.

Review practice

It is important to identify and challenge any barriers to effective anti-discriminatory practice. For example, is relevant information available in an accessible format for people with learning disabilities; in large print, Braille or audio format for people with visual impairments; or in other languages for non-English-speaking people? It is essential that all members of our community are able to understand the relevant information if they have the mental capacity to do so.

Show understanding and compassion

In most care settings, a person's death may affect staff and other individuals, for example other residents and friends, so issues around end of life care should be approached with understanding and compassion, not just for the patient but for everyone involved in the care process.

Do not make assumptions

When working with people from diverse backgrounds, it is important to avoid assumptions about their identity or relationships. Try to use open language, such as using the word 'partner' rather than 'husband' or 'wife'.

Be open to discussing and supporting people's spiritual needs

Try to be non-judgemental in relation to people's choices and spiritual practices. People construct the process of dying through different cultural frameworks and belief systems. The idea of a pain-free death, for example, is not acceptable for everyone, with many Hindus believing that past transgressions may be redressed through experiencing pain during death (Holloway 2007). It is therefore important for practitioners to be open in discussions about the personal needs of each patient.

Recognise that dying is a process and people's needs change

As practitioners seeking to develop anti-discriminatory practice, it is helpful to discuss the needs and concerns of the patient, as they often change during the final stages of life. It is also important to be sensitive to the needs and concerns of loved ones.

Suggest advance care planning

As suggested above, ACP is important for anyone who has a life-limiting condition. However, it is especially significant if people have been diagnosed with dementia, due to the anticipated deterioration in mental condition and eventual loss of capacity. In these circumstances, health and social care needs will change over time, so ACP should be regularly reviewed.

Look after yourself

Professionals who work with the dying and bereaved are confronted with many emotional challenges, and it is therefore important to learn to look after yourself. This may include asking for professional supervision or counsel from your line manager.

Commission inclusive services

At a time of major change in the UK commissioning environment, it is vital that end of life care and inclusion stay on the agenda. Commissioners planning end of life care services and strategies need to involve people from excluded groups (BAME communities, people with learning disabilities, LGBTi people, homeless people, etc.) to ensure that palliative care services meet the needs of all their local communities. Health and social care organisations need to embed a consideration of diversity into their strategic planning process to help address issues around equality of access, quality of service and the outcomes of palliative care for excluded groups.

Develop and train the workforce

Health Education England and local education and training boards, universities and medical schools need to ensure that they offer effective cultural competency training in end of life care, as well as training in the application of the Mental Capacity Act 2005 and the Deprivation of Liberty Safeguards[15] in palliative care, ensuring that everyone has the dignified death that they deserve.

Final reflections

In this chapter, we have suggested that the idea of a 'natural death' and a 'good death' have been interpreted and constructed in different ways. In Western cultures there is now a strong moral imperative for planning a 'good death' and offering the quality of care that a person wants at the end of their life.

Offering end of life care is always complex and can be even more difficult when offering care to older people with co-morbidities or diminished mental capacity, particularly as the terminal stages of illness are difficult to predict in some mental health conditions (such as dementia). However, it is important to identify when changing the approach to end of life care is appropriate, in collaboration with the patient, family members and other healthcare professionals.

Dealing with end of life issues is always challenging. Practitioners can make end of life issues easier to manage if they are trained and prepared to address some of the key concerns of patients and their families. It is also important for practitioners to acknowledge when they may need to bring in additional help or support, perhaps from the palliative care team, faith leaders, voluntary agencies, or specialists such as the Admiral and Macmillan Cancer Support nurses. Each individual will respond differently to end of life issues, and practitioners should make every effort to act with sensitivity to people's cultural and spiritual needs and to help them to identify what is important to them.

For older people with diminished mental capacity, end of life care is often more challenging. While the Mental Capacity Act 2005 does offer guidance, it is important to discuss advance care planning where possible so that the individual's wishes can be taken into account. Overall, in order to develop effective, anti-discriminatory end of life care for older people with mental health problems, practitioners need to remember that people have different understandings of death and dying and different needs from end of life care. Working in collaboration with the patient, family, friends and other professionals to develop a person-centred approach will help to ensure that care is appropriate and compassionate in the final stages of life.

Reflective questions

1. When you met Mr Gupta he had just been diagnosed with dementia, and now his wife feels she can no longer cope with him as he is wandering and shouting most of the day. His GP considers that he is near to the end of his life, and your manager has found him a place in a care unit for the elderly and severely mentally ill. However, you know that Mr Gupta stated in his advance care plan that he wanted to die at home. Is there anything you can do?

2. You have a good relationship with a local Irish Traveller family who are caring for an elderly aunt who is dying. Although the aunt and her family are happy to talk about her end of life care, they don't want you to write anything down or develop a written advance care plan. Is there anything you can do to ensure that their aunt's wishes are understood by other professionals?

3. Janice has been homeless for most of her life and has recently been diagnosed with terminal cancer. She also has a severe and enduring mental illness. She does not want to die in a hospital as her sister died in one, and she has already told you she is very scared. Janice is talking about getting back on the road again, but her health is deteriorating, and you are worried that she may not have access to the care she needs. With winter coming, she may end up dying on the street. What resources can you use to offer Janice the care she needs?

References

Abel, J., Pring, A., Rich, A., Malik, T. and Verne, J. (2013) 'The impact of advance care planning of place of death, a hospice retrospective cohort study.' *BMJ Supportive and Palliative Care 3*, 168–173.

Academy of Medical Royal Colleges (2009) *No Health without Mental Health: The Alert Summary Report.* London: Academy of Medical Royal Colleges. Available at www.rcpsych.ac.uk/pdf/ALERT%20 print%20final.pdf, accessed on 6 November 2016.

Alborz, A., McNally, R. and Glendinning, C. (2005) 'Access to health care for people with learning disabilities in the UK: Mapping the issues and reviewing the evidence.' *Journal of Health Services Research & Policy 10*, 173–182.

Alzheimer's Society (2015) 'Facts for the media.' Available at www.alzheimers.org.uk/site/scripts/ documents_info.php?documentID=535&pageNumber=2, accessed on 22 September 2016.

Atchley, R.C. (2009) *Spirituality and Aging.* Baltimore, MD: John Hopkins University Press.

Blauner, R. (1996) 'Death and social structure.' *Psychiatry 29*, 4, 378–394.

Bolliger, M. (2014) *What Patients Don't Say if Doctors Don't Ask.* 2nd ed. New York: Influence Publishing.

Brown, S., Kim, M., Mitchell, C. and Inskip, H. (2010) 'Twenty-five year mortality of a community cohort with schizophrenia.' *British Journal of Psychiatry 196*, 116–121.

Calanzani, N., Koffman, J. and Higginson, I. (2013) *Palliative and End of Life Care for Black, Asian and Minority Ethnic (BAME) Groups in the UK: Demographic Profile and the Current State of Palliative and End of Life Care Provision.* London: Marie Curie Cancer Care and Public Health England. Available at www.mariecurie.org.uk/globalassets/media/documents/policy/policy-publications/june-2013/palliative-and-end-of-life-care-for-black-asian-and-minority-ethnic-groups-in-the-uk. pdf, accessed on 22 September 2016.

Challis, D., Mozley, C., Sutcliffe, C., Bagley, H. *et al.* (2000) 'Dependency in older people recently admitted to care homes.' *Age and Ageing 29*, 3, 255–260.

Cutler, D., Deaton, A. and Lleras-Muney, A. (2006) 'The determinants of mortality.' *Journal of Economic Perspectives 20*, 3, 97–120.

Crane, M. and Warnes, A.M. (2000) *Lessons from Lancefield Street: Tackling the Needs of Older Homeless People.* National Homeless Alliance: London.

Davies, E., Higginson, I., World Health Organization and Floriani Foundation (2004) *Palliative Care.* Copenhagen: World Health Organization.

Deb, S., Thomas, M. and Bright, C. (2001) 'Mental disorder in adults with intellectual disability: Prevalence of functional psychiatric illness among a community-based population aged between 16 and 64 years.' *Journal of Intellectual Disability Research 45*, 495–505.

Department of Health (2012) *Six Lives: Progress Report on Healthcare for People with Learning Disabilities.* London: Department of Health. Available at www.gov.uk/government/uploads/system/ uploads/attachment_data/file/212292/Six_lives_2nd_Progress_Report_on_Healthcare_ for_People_with_Learning_Disabilities_-_full_report.pdf, accessed on 6 November 2016.

Department of Health (2013) *More Care, Less Pathway: An Independent Review of Liverpool Care Pathway for Dying Patients.* Review chaired by Baroness Julia Neuberger. London: Department of Health.

Dixon, J., King, D., Matosevic, T., Clark, M. and Knapp, M. (2015) *Equity in the Provision of Palliative Care in the UK: Review of Evidence.* PSSRU Discussion Paper 2894. London: London School of Economics.

Emerson, E., Hatton, C., Robertson, J., Roberts, H. *et al.* (2011) *People with Learning Disabilities in England 2011: Services and Support Report.* Improving Health and Lives, Learning Disabilities Observatory.

Equality and Human Rights Commission (2010) *How Fair is Britain? Equality, Human Rights and Good Relations in 2010. The First Triennial Review.* Manchester: Equality and Human Rights Commission.

EuroHealthNet (2010) *Making the Link: Healthy Ageing and Healthy Equality.* Policy Precis. Available at www.healthyageing.eu/sites/www.healthyageing.eu/files/resources/Equity-Channel-Policy-Precis-Healthy-Ageing.pdf, accessed on 6 November 2016.

Froggatt, K. (2001) 'Palliative care and nursing homes: Where next?' *Palliative Medicine 15*, 42–48.

Goldsmith, M. (2004) *A Strange Land: People with Dementia in the Local Church.* Southwell, Nottinghamshire: 4M Publications.

Gott, M., Gardiner, C., Ingleton, C., Cobb, M. *et al.* (2013) 'What is the extent of potentially avoidable admissions amongst hospital inpatients with palliative care needs?' *BMC Palliative Care 12*, 9.

Gott, M., Ingleton, C., Bennett, M.I. and Gardiner, C. (2011) 'Transitions to palliative care in acute hospitals in England: Qualitative study.' *British Medical Journal 342*, d1773.

Grace, J.A. (2005) *State Initiatives in End of Life Care.* Issue 24. Kansas City, MO: Center for Practical Bioethics.

Griffiths, A., Knight, A., Harwood, R. and Gladman, J. (2014) 'Preparation to care for confused older patients in general hospitals: A study of UK health professionals.' *Age and Ageing 43*, 521–527.

Harding, R., Epiphaniou, E. and Chidgey-Clark, J. (2012) 'Needs, experiences, and preferences of sexual minorities for end of life care and palliative care: A systematic review.' *Journal of Palliative Medicine 15*, 5, 602–611.

Hart, B., Sainsbury, P. and Short, S. (1998) 'Whose dying? A sociological critique of the "good death".' *Mortality 3*, 1, 65–77.

Henderson, M. (2004) 'Mental Health Needs.' In D. Oliviere and B. Monroe (eds) *Death, Dying and Social Differences.* Oxford: Oxford University Press.

Heslop, P., Blair, P., Fleming, P., Hoghton, M., Marriott, A. and Russ, L. (2013) *Confidential Inquiry into Premature Deaths of People with Learning Disabilities: Final Report.* Available at www.bristol.ac.uk/media-library/sites/cipold/migrated/documents/fullfinalreport.pdf, accessed on 22 September 2016.

Holloway, M. (2007) *Negotiating Death in Contemporary Health and Social Care.* Bristol: Polity Press.

House of Commons Health Committee (2015) *End of Life Care: Fifth Report of Session 2014–2015.* London: House of Commons Health Committee.

Jenkins, R. (2005) 'Older people with learning disabilities. Part 2: Accessing care and the implications for nursing practice.' *Nursing Older People 17*, 1, 32–35.

Kellehear, A. (2007) *A Social History of Dying.* Cambridge: Cambridge University Press.

Kübler-Ross, E. (1969) *On Death and Dying.* New York: The Macmillan Company.

Leadership Alliance for the Care of Dying People (2014) *One Chance to Get it Right: Improving People's Experience of Care in the Last Few Days and Hours of Life.* Leadership Alliance for the Care of Dying People.

Lloyd-Williams, M. (2003) *Psychosocial Issues in Palliative Care.* Oxford: Oxford University Press.

MacKinlay, E. (2006) 'Spiritual care: Recognizing spiritual needs of older adults.' *Journal of Religion, Spirituality and Aging 18*, 2–3, 59–71.

Manning, L.K. (2013) 'Navigating hardships in old age: Exploring the relationship between spirituality and resilience in later life.' *Qualitative Health Research 23*, 4, 568–575.

Marmot, M. (2010) *Fair Society, Healthy Lives: The Marmot Review. Strategic Review of Health Inequalities in England Post-2010.* London: The Marmot Review.

McGrath, P. and Holewa, H. (2004) 'Mental health and palliative care: Exploring the ideological interface.' *International Journal of Psychosocial Rehabilitation 9*, 1, 107–119.

Mencap (2007) *Death by Indifference: Following Up the Treat Me Right! Report.* London: Mencap. Available at www.mencap.org.uk/sites/default/files/2016-06/DBIreport.pdf, accessed on 6 November 2016.

Mencap (2008) *Living and Dying with Dignity: The Best Practice Guide to End-of-life Care for People with a Learning Disability.* London: Mencap. Available at www.a2anetwork.co.uk/wp-content/uploads/2010/01/Living-and-Dying-with-Dignity-End-of-life-care_-best-practice-guide-easy-read.pdf, accessed on 23 September 2016.

Michael, J. (2008) *Healthcare for All: Report of the Independent Inquiry into Access to Healthcare for People with Learning Disabilities.* London: Independent Inquiry into Access to Healthcare for People with Learning Disabilities.

Mitchell, S.L., Keily, D., Miller, S., Connor, S., Spence, C. and Teno, J. (2007) 'Hospice care for patients with dementia.' *Journal of Pain and Symptom Management 34*, 1, 7–16.

Morrison, R.S. and Meier, D.E. (2003) *Geriatric Palliative Care.* Oxford: Oxford University Press.

Mullick, A., Martin, J. and Sallnow, L. (2013) 'An introduction to advance care planning in practice.' *British Medical Journal 347.*

Naylor, C., Parsonage, M., McDaid, D., Knapp, M., Fossy, M. and Galea, A. (2012) *Long-term Conditions and Mental Health.* London: The King's Fund. Available at www.kingsfund.org.uk/sites/files/kf/field/field_publication_file/long-term-conditions-mental-health-cost-comorbidities-naylor-feb12.pdf, accessed on 23 September 2016.

NICE (2015) *Care of Dying Adults in the Last Days of Life.* Available at www.nice.org.uk/guidance/ng31, accessed on 23 September 2016.

NICE (2016) *Mental Health Problems in People with Learning Disabilities: Prevention, Assessment and Management.* London: NICE. Available at www.nice.org.uk/guidance/NG54, accessed on 6 November 2016.

Office for National Statistics (2015) *Life Expectancy at Birth and at Age 65 by Local Areas in England and Wales: 2012 to 2014.* Available at www.ons.gov.uk/peoplepopulationandcommunity/birthsdeathsandmarriages/lifeexpectancies/bulletins/lifeexpectancyatbirthandatage65bylocalareasinenglandandwales/2015-11-04, accessed on 6 November 2016.

Oishi, A. and Murtagh, F. (2014) 'The challenges of uncertainty and interprofessional collaboration in palliative care for non-cancer patients in the community: A systematic review of views from patients, carers and health-care professionals.' *Journal of Palliative Medicine 28*, 9, 1081–1098.

Parry, G., Van Cleemput, P., Peters, J., Moore, J. *et al.* (2004) *The Health Status of Gypsies & Travellers in England: Summary of a Report to the Department of Health 2004.* Available at http://leedsgate.co.uk/sites/default/files/media/The-Health-Status-of-GT-in-England.pdf, accessed on 6 November 2016.

Peinado-Gorlat, P., Castro-Martínez, F., Arriba-Marcos, B., Melguizo-Jiménez, M. and Barrio-Cantalejo, I. (2015) 'Roma women's perspectives on end-of-life decisions.' *Journal of Bioethical Inquiry 12*, 3, 409–417.

Puchalski, C. (2006) *A Time for Listening and Caring: Spirituality and the Care of the Chronically Ill and Dying.* Oxford: Oxford University Press.

Rabow, M., Hauser, J. and Adams, J. (2004) 'Supporting family caregivers at the end of life: "They don't know what they don't know".' *Journal of the American Medical Association 291*, 4, 483–491.

Sampson, E.L., Burns, A. and Richards, M. (2011) 'Improving end-of-life care for people with dementia.' *British Journal of Psychiatry 199*, 5, 357–359.

Seymour, J.E. (2007) 'Quality of life to the end: Commentary.' *Communication and Medicine 4*, 117–118.

Seymour, J.E., Kumar, A. and Froggatt, K. (2011) 'Do nursing homes for older people have the support they need to provide end-of-life care? A mixed methods enquiry in England.' *Palliative Medicine 25*, 125–138.

Sjostrand, M. and Helgeson, G. (2008) 'Coercive treatment and autonomy in psychiatry.' *Bioethics 22*, 2, 113–120.

Ryder, S. (2013) *A Time and a Place: What People Want at the End of Life.* Report prepared by Demos. London: Sue Ryder.

Smith, D., Moreno-Leguizamon, C. and Grohmann, S. (2015) *End of Life Practices and Palliative Care among Black and Minority Ethnic Groups.* London: University of Greenwich. Available at www.diversityhouse.org.uk/wp-content/uploads/2016/01/REPORT-End-of-Life-BME-Groups-101115-submitted.pdf, accessed on 23 September 2016.

Talbott, J.A. and Linn, L. (1978) 'Reactions of schizophrenics to life-threatening disease.' *Psychiatric Quarterly 50*, 218–227.

Thomas, B. (2012) *Homelessness Kills: An Analysis of the Mortality of Homeless People in Early Twenty-first Century England.* London: Crisis.

Tuffrey-Wijne, I., Hogg, J. and Curfs, L. (2007) 'End-of-life care for people with intellectual disabilities who have cancer or other life-limiting illness: A review of the literature and available resources.' *Journal of Applied Research in Intellectual Disability 20*, 4, 331–344.

Walker, E., McGee, R.E. and Druss, B.G. (2015) 'Mortality in mental disorders and global disease burden implications: A systematic review and meta-analysis.' *JAMA Psychiatry 72*, 4, 334–341.

Useful resources

General resources

The National Council for Palliative Care explains advance care planning on their website: www.ncpc.org.uk/publication/planning-your-future-care

Policy and laws on ACP vary across England, Scotland, Wales and Northern Ireland, and the Macmillan Cancer Support website has up-to-date details of these regional and legal differences: www.macmillan.org.uk/Cancerinformation/Livingwithandaftercancer/Advancedcancer/Advancecareplanning/Advancecareplanning.aspx

Resources on end of life care for BAME communities

NHS Choices have a large number of resources available in different languages on end of life care (click near the top right of the page on the word 'Translate'): www.nhs.uk/Search/?q=end+of+life

Resources on end of life care for LGBTi people

NHS National End of Life Care Programme report: *The Route to Success in End of Life Care – Achieving Quality for Lesbian, Gay, Bisexual and Transgender People*: www.macmillan.org.uk/Documents/AboutUs/Health_professionals/EndofLifeCare-LGBTRoutetoSuccess.pdf

Stonewall report: *Working with Older Lesbian, Gay and Bisexual People: A Guide for Care and Support Services*: www.stonewall.org.uk/sites/default/files/older_people_final_lo_res.pdf

Resources on end of life care for homeless people

St Mungo's have a resource pack available online on homelessness and end of life care: www.mungosbroadway.org.uk/endoflifecare/resources_section

Resources on end of life care for people with learning disabilities and their families

The British Institute of Learning Disabilities has a number of resources:

>> *About Dementia* in an easy-read format: www.bild.org.uk/our-services/books/health-and-wellbeing/about-dementia

>> Loss, bereavement and end of life care: www.bild.org.uk/information/ageingwell/endoflifecare

Mencap has a number of additional tools that may be helpful, but perhaps the most useful introduction for professionals is their report *Living and Dying with Dignity: The Best Practice Guide to End-of-life Care for People with a Learning Disability*: http://socialwelfare.bl.uk/subject-areas/services-client-groups/adults-disabilities/mencap/1488752008_living_dying_dignity.pdf

The PCPLD Network offers an example put together by Sunderland People First of a pictorial person-centred plan for someone with learning disabilities who is dying: www.pcpld.org/wp-content/uploads/when_i_die_2_0.pdf

Resources on the Mental Capacity Act 2005

The legislation can be accessed online: www.legislation.gov.uk/ukpga/2005/9/contents

Make sure you are looking at the most recent version of the legislation, as amendments are often made. A good place to find resources is the Mental Capacity Law and Policy website: www.mentalcapacitylawandpolicy.org.uk. It includes links to CQC briefings, guidance from the Intensive Care Society, and details of the new (and now live) system for Court of Protection applications from community settings.

PART II

Insights

CHAPTER 8

Ageing and Mental Health Issues for People with Learning Disabilities

Musthafar Oladosu and Rena Kydd-Williams

Introduction and terminology

This chapter looks at people with learning disabilities, the issues they encounter as they get older and some of the barriers they face when accessing services to meet their ongoing physical and mental health needs. It explores key issues in practice, examines accepted definitions and prevalence rates of people with learning disabilities, and then addresses pertinent topics faced by service users and practitioners while incorporating recommendations to enhance anti-discriminatory practice and service provision.

We would like to thank the participants of the POhWER advocacy group, based in Hackney, London, which was set up in 1996 as a charitable organisation. The title of the group is not an abbreviation; it is a take on the word 'power'. The service users, who have various needs as older people with a learning disability, were open and passionate about sharing with us their insights as to what it means to them to get older as well as the concerns they have around mental health issues. The service users selected their own aliases in order to remain anonymous. In this chapter, we have used elements of the interviews conducted with the group to highlight the voices of the service users. Some examples can be found in the following case study.

Case study: Interview with members of the POhWER group

Stick, White and JJ are discussing younger people, getting older, mental health dilemmas, doctors and vulnerability. JJ and White are aware of a housemate who has learning disabilities and mental health problems. However, they seem less sure as to whether he is getting any meaningful help. They are also very aware that he is vulnerable when he goes out alone in the community as the general public might mistake his behaviour for being threatening or abusive.

Stick: Other people can respect us, younger people, so they can understand where we are coming from. In this day and age too many younger people are getting away with murder and stuff and taking the micky out of people that are older than them, so it's about respect.

White: Some people get miserable when they get older!!! [She laughs.] You have to get older; you don't stay the same age every year.

Stick: People will lose their mind; they will say things that they don't mean.

White: When people get older they have lots of things going on up there, like dementia, getting lost, repeating the same questions.

Stick: I think some people with learning disabilities are scared to go to the doctors and they might need help, but they might not be able to understand what the doctor is saying so they stay away... I have worked with People First [an advocacy group] so I know how to stand up for myself, but other people with learning disabilities might not know how to.

JJ: There is a man who lives in our block – he doesn't make any conversation. Staff try to help him but he doesn't shave and he just stares at people. When he goes out he just stares at people at the bus stop and he is vulnerable.

White: I know the same man. He takes tablets and he has mental health problems. He puts the same clothes on all the time and he says bad things to people when he does speak.

The context of care for older people with learning disabilities

The changing landscape of the provision of care in the United Kingdom following the Health and Social Care Act 2012 has had a profound effect on the delivery of services for older people with learning disabilities who require support with mental health and age-related health and social care issues. Historically, people with learning disabilities and their carers have often found it difficult to navigate their way around health and social care (Foundation for People with Learning Disabilities 2015). This has sometimes resulted in poor health outcomes, such as protracted delays in diagnosis, polypharmacy (taking multiple medications, usually five or more) and diagnostic overshadowing (where behaviour or symptoms may be wrongly dismissed as part of the person's learning disabilities). This can potentially lead to a lack of access to treatment and, in the worst scenarios, premature death (Heslop *et al.* 2013). Specialist community-based services for people with learning disabilities have been pivotal in bridging the knowledge and practice gaps while advocating for equitable access and reasonable adjustments to mainstream services for people with learning disabilities.

People with learning disabilities and mental health issues may also suffer double discrimination, or even triple discrimination on account of age, gender, ethnicity or sexuality (Kannabiran *et al.* 2009). We are now experiencing a greater shift from specialised provision for people with learning disabilities to increasing the capacity of mainstream services to meet the needs of people with learning disabilities, in part due to economic restrictions but more so to build more inclusive mainstream services. However, there are concerns that the 'mainstreaming' of services, although conveyed with the best intentions, is still falling short of providing the tailored care that people with learning disabilities require. Concerns have been expressed by advocacy groups such as the Foundation for People with Learning Disabilities (2015), Mencap (2008), People First (2015) and VoiceAbility (2013). Nonetheless, it is possible to find numerous examples of intuitive service provision and good practice, where learning disability and mainstream services have galvanised their resources in order to provide as robust a service as possible.

In light of further radical National Health Service rationalising, restructuring and redistribution of provisions, it is important to be aware of the challenges that ageing people with learning disabilities and mental health concerns face in order to support their particular needs through both practice and the clinical commissioning agenda.

Older people with learning disabilities: Definitions and prevalence

There is often a blurred understanding of what a learning disability is and how it shapes someone's life. Definitions provided by the World Health Organization (1996) and refined by the Department of Health's (2001a) *Valuing People* white paper are well established and quoted in literature:

> A state of arrested or incomplete development of mind characterized by impairment of skills and overall intelligence in areas such as cognition, language, and motor and social abilities. Also referred to as intellectual disability or handicap, mental retardation can occur with or without any other physical or mental disorders. Although reduced level of intellectual functioning is the characteristic feature of this disorder, the diagnosis is made only if it is associated with a diminished ability to adapt to the daily demands of the normal social environment. Mental retardation is further categorized as mild (IQ levels 50–69), moderate (IQ levels 35–49), severe (IQ levels 20–34), and profound (IQ levels below 20).
>
> (Department of Health 2001a; World Health Organization 1996)

Learning disability includes the presence of:

> a significantly reduced ability to understand new or complex information, to learn new skills (impaired intelligence), with:
>
> a reduced ability to cope independently (impaired social functioning),
>
> which started before adulthood, with a lasting effect on development.
>
> (Department of Health 2001a, p.14)

Building upon these definitions and incorporating more socially acceptable terminology, the World Health Organization produced the World Health Organization Disability Assessment Schedule 2.0 (WHODAS 2.0) and the International Classification of Functioning, Disability and Health (ICF), both of which give a global account of disability. Useful assessment tools are available at www.who.int/classifications/icf/whodasii/en (World Health Organization 2014).

At this point it is important to note that the term 'learning difficulty', which is used in the field of education, has also been used to define the client group in question. Despite this interplay between learning disability and learning difficulty among laypersons and professionals outside of the learning disability sphere, learning difficulty relates more specifically to behavioural issues or to learning that has been affected by dyslexia, attention deficit hyperactivity disorder or dyspraxia. More recently, publications have also made reference to the term 'intellectual disability', which is becoming more commonly used. For the purpose of this chapter, we will use the term 'learning disability' and imply the definitions provided by the World Health Organization and the Department of Health.

It is also important for the reader to note that the term 'learning disability' should not cloud the focus to strive for the very best outcome for the individual; the focus should be on empowerment and enablement irrespective of the learning disability, which acts more as a label for service provision and criteria matching. Within this label, people with learning disabilities can fall into one of four categories depending on the severity of their disability, which are outlined in Table 8.1.

Table 8.1 Categories for the severity of learning disabilities (Williams 2013)

Category	Criteria	IQ
Mild learning disabilities	Several self-help skills, can live independently with minimal support, often vulnerable within the community due to 'mate crime'.	50–69
Moderate learning disabilities	Some self-help skills, communication/level of understanding can be limited, may be vulnerable and require some health and social support.	35–49
Severe learning disabilities	Two or more health or physical issues, poor communication and understanding, requires 18–24-hour care.	20–34
Profound learning disabilities	Complex health/physical care needs, subtle communication gestures, requires 24-hour care.	Less than 20

The number of people with learning disabilities in the United Kingdom has been estimated as 1,191,000 (Emerson *et al.* 2011); however, the exact prevalence is not known and thus this figure acts only as a guide. For commissioning purposes, it is accepted that people with learning disabilities make up 2–3 per cent of the population, which translates to 20–30 people per thousand. Emerson and Heslop (2010) predict that the number of adults aged over 70 with learning disabilities who require health and social care services will more than double by 2030. Therefore, future planning for this population is imperative if services are to remain inclusive, progressive and proactive. However, in order to plan effectively for the future, the context of how people with learning disabilities have been treated historically needs to be explored. This is discussed later in this chapter.

Early-onset ageing conditions

The increase in the population of older adults (Office for National Statistics 2014) is receiving much attention through policies and strategies such as the Department for Work and Pensions' (2015) *2010 to 2015 Government Policy: Older People* as well as the Department of Health's (2001b) *National Service Framework for Older People*, which focuses on addressing age-related concerns such as dementia and mental health issues, mobility issues, fall prevention and strokes. People with learning disabilities have also been highlighted within such documents in relation to their specific needs.

People with learning disabilities form a unique populace in that they may experience the early onset of ageing by nature of their predisposing diagnostic condition. Conditions such as Down's syndrome may predispose a person to Alzheimer's-type dementia (Bell, Turnbull and Kidd 2008), with onset of symptoms from as early as age 20 (Cosgrave *et al.* 1999, cited in Hassiotis *et al.* 2003). Despite numerous documents highlighting the connection between Down's syndrome and dementia, service provision and awareness of the needs of this client group can be patchy within mainstream services. As mainstream services are now responding to increased demand from 65–85-year-olds, people with learning disabilities may find these services are not tailored for their premature ageing needs, which may emerge aged 30–40. This lack of provision may be perceived as a form of discrimination in mainstream services against people with learning disabilities with premature ageing needs.

Premature ageing and learning disabilities

It is not uncommon to see people with learning disabilities who are affected by a premature ageing process be placed in a generic nursing home environment where staff are not accustomed to looking after people with learning disabilities and therefore may lack the skills, knowledge and attitude that are required to meet the needs of such individuals. This continues to occur despite the fact that the families of people with learning disabilities have voiced their concerns over the lack of planning for the future of their loved ones. The British Institute of Learning Disabilities (2013) reports that older people with learning disabilities often have little or no choice about where they live and how they are supported. It would appear that due to the lack of planning and the unavailability of appropriate accommodation, older people with learning disabilities are being made to fit into existing service provision regardless of their specific needs. For example, it is not uncommon for people with learning disabilities who are in their forties and have complex health issues to be placed in nursing homes for older people due to the lack of suitable facilities locally. Indeed, Snell (2007) notes that previously active people with learning disabilities in their sixties and even younger are being moved into facilities for people who are much older and less able than them.

People with learning disabilities are generally not consulted or involved in the process of allocation to a particular type of accommodation, which thereby contravenes the Mental Capacity Act 2005 (see Chapter 5 in this volume for more details on the Act). The Act stipulates that there should be clear evidence that individuals consent to decisions that affect their lives, and where individuals lack capacity to consent, a clear process should be followed to demonstrate how a best-interest decision is agreed. The United Nations (2006) directive states that people with learning disabilities should have the opportunity to choose their accommodation and with whom they live and not to be made to live in environments they have not chosen. At this juncture, it is important to note the role of partnership boards that were set up following the *Valuing People* white paper (Department of Health 2001a) to address local social and health needs for people with learning disabilities. We would direct the reader to examine Chapter 7 of the white paper as well as the follow-up document titled *Valuing People Now* (Department of Health 2009).

Chronological age versus entry criteria

Double discrimination is frequently a reality for people with learning disabilities as, often unintentionally, they are excluded from mainstream health and social care services due to the parameters of age and their learning disability (General Medical Council undated). For example, referring agents such as GPs may be left with no other choice but to make requests to neurologists with specialist interests in early-onset dementia, which may not be available or have capacity in every locality. Obtaining entry into a specialist dementia service is often dependent on the relationship between that locality and the commissioned services. Diagnosis will often be managed by the GP and specialist learning disability team through psychology, psychiatry and nursing, while care and support following diagnosis may well be undertaken by the local community's learning disability team, with possible long-arm support from the specialist service. Again, the question for advocates and practitioners alike is whether resources for dementia and other age-related conditions located within mainstream services can be accessed by young and middle-aged adults with learning disabilities and mental health issues. If not, what provisions are being made for such resources to be accessed through specialist learning disability teams?

Historical context of mental health and learning disabilities

Smiley (2005) reports that as recently as the 1980s, people with learning disabilities were deemed to be incapable of developing mental health problems. This argument was based on the perspective that most people with learning disabilities, due to their cognitive disabilities, were incapable of processing and reacting to the same social, cultural and economic factors that are thought to predispose other people to developing mental health problems. There were serious consequences in this simplistic argument for people with learning disabilities. Genuine symptoms of mental illness in this population were at best dismissed as challenging behaviour and dealt with through curtailment of liberty, with the use of various aversive methods such as physical restraints and seclusion. The issue of overprescription of antipsychotic medications to treat behavioural issues in this population has been well documented and is open to much scrutiny (Ahmed *et al.* 2000).

Concern has been raised that these powerful medications have been used as a 'chemical cosh' to quieten those with challenging behaviour (Boseley 2015). However, it is now well established that people with learning disabilities actually suffer a higher risk of mental health problems when compared to those without a learning disability (Cooper 1997; Devine, Taggart and McLornian 2009).

Common life events among people with learning disabilities which may precipitate mental health problems

The British Psychological Society (2015) points out that people with learning disabilities often face a host of challenging life events in their middle age, such as the loss of a parent or long-term carer, moving away from home or the loss of daytime opportunities, such as day services, day centres, one-to-one staff attention, meaningful employment or social activities. The British Psychological Society also identifies abuse and the impact of poor environment as predisposing factors in why baseline functional abilities and behaviour of people with learning disabilities may decline. These factors clearly have the potential to trigger or perpetuate mental health problems, particularly in people with learning disabilities who may be predisposed to developing mental health issues.

Older adults with a learning disability and mental health issues

Life expectancy among people with a learning disability has increased significantly, mainly due to advances in medicine and significant improvements in social care provision, especially since the 1990s. The British Psychological Society (2015) reports that the life expectancy of people with mild learning disabilities is now comparable to that of the general population of a similar socio-economic status. However, they caution that the life expectancy of those with severe learning disabilities remains reduced compared to the general population. Consequently, it is envisaged that the population of people with learning disabilities over 65 years of age will have doubled by 2020 (Janicki and Dalton 2000; McConkey et al. 2006, both as cited in British Psychological Society 2015). In addition, it is estimated that by 2030 there will be a 30 per cent increase in the use of social services by people with learning disabilities aged 50 and over (Turner and Bernard 2014).

Dementia is also prominent in this population, although the definition of dementia as a mental illness is contentious. People with Down's syndrome have long been associated with early-onset dementia and, even when people with Down's syndrome are excluded, the overall prevalence of dementia is still higher among people with learning disabilities than in the general population (Strydom *et al.* 2007). The Alzheimer's Society (2014) reports that when Down's syndrome is excluded, people with learning disabilities aged 50–65 have a one in ten chance of developing dementia, and the risk increases to more than half of that population for those aged 85 or over. This risk is two to three times greater than for the general population. Cooper (1997) lists the following factors as implicated in these rates of prevalence:

- genetic/family history

- physical factors such as illness

- long-term exposure to various psychiatric medications

- psychological issues such as adverse childhood and adult life experiences, including abuse

- social factors, including deprivation, limited opportunities to develop appropriate skills for life and poor social networks.

It is important to note that there is little consistency in the prevalence of mental illness amongst people with learning disabilities, and several of the authors that we refer to have slightly different data. Nonetheless, there is a general consensus that the prevalence of mental health issues is greater in this population irrespective of age group, although different diagnostic criteria and methods used in different studies returned different prevalence rates (Borthwick-Duffy 1994; Smiley 2005). Cooper (1997) reported a staggering figure of 61.9 per cent of psychiatric mortality in adults with learning disabilities who are over 65 years old, while the prevalence is reduced to 11.4 per cent in those who are aged 50–65 years old (when dementia is excluded). Several of the authors cited in this chapter have also consistently highlighted a high prevalence of mental health problems among older adults with a learning disability. It also should be noted that this high prevalence is irrespective of whether issues such as challenging behaviour, autism, Asperger syndrome, Down's syndrome, attention deficit hyperactivity disorder, Rett's syndrome, pica and epilepsy are taken into account.

However, an area that has proven challenging is establishing whether there is any link between the severity of learning disability and prevalence of mental health issues. Reid (1994) observes that it is difficult to determine with any degree of certainty that mental health problems, especially schizophrenia, are present in people with severe and profound learning disabilities. This is because severe communication problems and sensory and postural difficulties are often seen in this population. The detection and diagnosis of mental health problems in people with learning disabilities are in themselves problematic since they often have impaired language, which results in difficulties for practitioners who are attempting to obtain information required for an assessment of mental state (Holland 2000). This may mean that the problem remains unidentified and untreated for a long time, if not always.

The history of services for people with learning disabilities reveals that this population has endured various forms of abuse, especially in long-stay hospitals (University of Glamorgan, Rhondda Cynon Taff People First and New Pathways 2013). Experience of institutional care with its dehumanising consequences may have impacted heavily on older adults with a learning disability, who are more likely to have lived in long-stay hospitals. Recognition of the dehumanising nature of long-stay institutions led to a closure programme which started in the 1980s and gathered pace in the 1990s when the National Health Service and Community Care Act 1990 came into force. The last such hospital closed in April 2009 (Mencap 2009). The traumatic history of abuse suffered by people with learning disabilities in long-stay hospitals has been linked with long-term psychological and mental health consequences, such as post-traumatic stress disorder and behavioural disturbances (University of Glamorgan, Rhondda Cynon Taff People First and New Pathways 2013). The appalling incidence of abuse against a client group at an Assessment and Treatment Unit in Winterbourne View Hospital, Gloucestershire, which thankfully was exposed by the BBC's *Panorama* programme in May 2011, served as a shocking reminder of the poor standards of care received by people with learning disabilities and mental health issues even in some 'specialist' inpatient settings. Although the scandal focused attention on the inpatient care of people with learning disabilities with mental health or behavioural problems (Royal College of Psychiatrists 2013), it is important to note that these failures can be seen across health and social care services.

Lack of appropriate training and skills is one factor that may lead to high stress levels among staff and subsequently poor practices that can put individuals at risk. Therefore, robust training and support for staff, including ascertaining the specific training needs of staff, providing clinical or service-level supervision, and conducting debriefing and counselling are essential for a workforce to be competent and confident in working with people with learning disabilities and mental health issues. Specialist or bespoke training should also target the needs of older people with learning disabilities and middle-aged people with learning disabilities who may develop complex health issues as well as early-onset dementia or other neurological conditions.

People with learning disabilities and mental health problems accessing services

The Joint Commissioning Panel for Mental Health (JCPMH 2013) suggests that a typical GP surgery serving a population area of 2000 people would have 32 adult patients with learning disabilities, out of whom 10–15 would additionally have mental health conditions. However, Radhakrishnan *et al.* (2012, cited in Joint Commissioning Panel for Mental Health 2013) claims that 50 per cent of people with learning disabilities referred to a particular community learning disability service had mental health needs, while the remainder had a high prevalence of autism and/or behaviour perceived as challenging. Attempts have also been made to break down the prevalence of mental health problems in this population into specific mental health diagnostic categories. Smiley (2005) offers the following breakdown of mental health prevalence in the learning disability population: schizophrenia (3%), bipolar affective disorder (1.5%), depression (4%), generalised anxiety disorder (6%), specific phobia (6%), agoraphobia (1.5%), obsessive compulsive disorder (2.5%), dementia at age 65 years and over (20%), and autism (7%). Thorpe (2003) also observed that about 10 per cent of older people with a learning disability experience major mental illness, such as psychotic episodes.

As 98 per cent of the total UK population of people with learning disabilities fall in the range of mild learning disability, it would be interesting to know how many people with mild learning disabilities are not labelled as such and are therefore seen by the mainstream mental health services, especially community mental health services. More work needs to be conducted in this area and, as the authors of *Valuing People* (Department of Health 2001a) argued, people with learning disabilities should have the same access to mainstream health services as anyone else.

Challenges of assessment and diagnosis of mental health problems in older adults with learning disability

Holland (2000) argues that it can be difficult to identify signs of functional decline in people with a learning disability, and any observed behavioural challenges in the person may often be dismissed as part of the person's learning disabilities. A legitimate cry for help with mental health issues may therefore be ignored, resulting in delayed treatment or inappropriate and restrictive measures or interventions imposed on the person to gain conformity. As stated earlier, this is commonly referred to as diagnostic overshadowing. Holland (2000) defines this as a situation whereby changes in someone's behaviour, personality or ability that would be taken very seriously in the general population are dismissed as part of an individual's learning disability profile or diagnosis.

The consequences of missing subtle changes in the individual early on could prove very serious for the individual, carers and others. Many people with learning disabilities rely on others, particularly their carers, to pick up and report their symptoms of ill health and to facilitate access to appropriate health care. The present authors' experiences in practice indicate that the nature and/or severity of cognitive impairment of people with learning disabilities, as well as communication difficulties, can often mean they are unable to describe their own symptoms or report them; this is consistent with the work of Smiley (2005). Help-seeking skills and behaviour are also not well developed in this population. Furthermore, Smiley expressed concerns that carers themselves often lack the skills and knowledge required to reliably assist with this as they may not be familiar with the symptoms and labelling of mental health problems. For instance, the British Psychological Society (2015) points out, with regard to recognising early dementia among people with a learning disability, that because signs and symptoms can be subtle and can only be recognised through careful observation, they may be missed by families and carers who are so close to the person that minor, yet important, changes in behaviour go unnoticed.

Problems may then be left unreported and untreated until greater distress, frustration and more severe behavioural changes occur in the individual concerned. Anecdotal evidence from practice suggests that the majority of referrals to learning disability psychiatry are made during crises and when the stress level of the carers has reached breaking point, or when the individual's behaviour is affecting others.

Apart from communication difficulties that are seen in people with learning disabilities, their manifestation and presentation of mental health symptoms often follow unusual and atypical patterns. The individual concerned also lacks insight or understanding into their conditions. The picture may be compounded by the fact that common psychiatric symptoms, such as social withdrawal, excessive agitation, a lack of concentration, stereotyped movement disorders or abnormal sleep, can be an expression of underlying brain damage or distress rather than symptoms of an illness. It is therefore important to have a clear premorbid picture with which any observed change in behaviour can be compared. The challenge faced by psychiatrists is establishing that a change has occurred and that the baseline has altered (Cooper and Holland 2007). For a person with severe/profound learning and physical disabilities, social withdrawal may be even harder to detect as often the person relies on others to be taken from place to place. Social withdrawal could therefore present as long periods of sleep, non-communication, prolonged lack of eye contact, or the burying of the head into the torso or lap. McGillivray and McCabe (2010) also stress that it can be difficult for clinicians and carers to establish and diagnose depression as its manifestation may be masked by other, more prominent behaviours.

Case study: Detecting mental health problems in people with learning disabilities

A middle-aged man with mild to moderate learning disabilities was suspected also to have mental health problems due to his rocking behaviour, which was thought to be a habitual movement or a sign of mental distress. However, after a full and detailed history was taken, the rhythmical rocking turned out to be an interpretation of his memory of praying with his family as a child. This information had been lost through his various placements, and little attention had been paid to his cultural beliefs and norms, leading to a misinterpretation and misattribution of his rocking behaviour.

Cooper (1997) stresses that as psychopathology and presentation of mental health problems among people with learning disabilities are different, the assessment process must be flexible enough to capture the unique behaviours but robust enough to aid clinical judgement. It is therefore important to gather a good history from the carer and those who know the individual well and would be able to report what was 'normal' for the individual, with full inclusion of the person in question, irrespective of whether the person can contribute vocally or not. People with learning disabilities are more likely to give compliant answers, depending on their language acquisition, or agree with the last item when presented with more than one answer. (For example, the question 'Are you happy or sad?' is likely to yield an answer of 'sad', whereas 'Are you sad or happy?' is likely to yield an answer of 'happy'.) Cooper (1997) also reports that people with learning disabilities often find it difficult to report different emotional states or to find the vocabulary to do so.

Cooper (1997) stresses the importance of completing a developmental history, which would include the nature of the individual's learning disabilities, to gain insight into the individual's current level of functioning. Early childhood history, including how the individual and the family came to terms with the person's learning disabilities and any coping mechanisms that had been tried in the past, may also help in prescribing developmentally appropriate treatments. The other major area of difference is the process of the mental-state assessment. According to Cooper (1997), mental health symptoms in this population can be 'labile', meaning that a person with learning disability with depression may be able to laugh, smile and even joke, and it may appear during the short mental-state assessment interview as if nothing is wrong, but they may not be able to sustain this over a long period of time. Episodes of instability or intermittent distress may be signs of the onset of depression or dementia, and therefore time, patience and creative thinking are of high value in reaching a meaningful diagnosis when working with people with learning disabilities.

Knowing the communication style and vocabulary of older adults with learning disabilities can be particularly helpful for avoiding the problems of compliant answers and suggestibility when carrying out mental state assessments, although it is important to remember that the process of ageing in itself can also bring about many of the changes that might be associated with mental health problems. When dealing with people with a different linguistic upbringing, it is important for practitioners to be aware of cultural phrases or words in an individual's mother tongue that are intertwined with the English language, so interpretation is key. A number of tools have been developed that are specific to this population; some are tailor-made, and others have been developed through the adaptation and modification of existing general psychiatric diagnostic tools (Flynn and Gravestock 2010).

According to colleagues in practice in the London Borough of Hackney (personal communication), these tools are used by specialists in learning disability, although there is no evidence that mainstream psychiatry, including services for older adults, use them when people with a learning disability come to their clinics. Identification and detailed discussion of these tools are outside the scope of this chapter. However, availability of appropriate assessment process and intervention has led to debate on whether older adults with learning disabilities are better served by specialist learning disability services or should be seen by services for older adults (Benbow *et al.* 2010).

Specialist vs generic service provision

People with learning disabilities face barriers to accessing mainstream mental health services, and when they do gain access they may be met with services that do not always understand their needs or know how to respond to those needs. Evidence shows that people with learning disabilities and mental health problems have more complex needs than those with the same mental health issues in the general population.

Also, Bouras *et al.* (2004, as cited in Hemmings 2010) observes that despite advances in mainstream mental health services, such as the development of various innovative community services like Assertive Outreach, Crisis Resolution Teams and Home Treatment Teams, people with learning disabilities and mental health problems have not always enjoyed the benefits of these advances. This population is predominantly restricted to accessing specialist services, and this is particularly the case for older adults with mental health problems who face exclusion from general old-age psychiatry because of their learning disability. Chaplin (2004, as cited in Hemmings 2010) argues that there is no evidence to demonstrate that either specialist learning disability services or older adult psychiatry services are better in meeting the needs of older adults with learning disabilities. What is not in doubt, however, is that older adults with a learning disability have many of the same needs as other older adults in the general population and will need the same kind of support with a reasonably adjusted approach to suit the individual concerned. While specialist learning disability services have expertise in dealing with a wide variety of learning disabilities, generic old-age psychiatry also brings expertise about the ageing process and associated mental health issues, including how to treat and respond to these issues.

Benbow *et al.* (2010) observe that there is no clarity on what quality of care and equality of service provision for older people with learning disabilities and mental health problems should look like. The report points out that services for this population are patchy: there appears to be no consistency in quality or quantity of service provision, especially with regard to the provision of memory clinics, which are scarce and often are not linked in with other specialist learning disability services where available. The report also identifies that although older adult services may be able to see older adults with mild learning disabilities, they lack the skills, knowledge and experience required to assess those with moderate to severe learning disabilities. It concludes that neither specialist old-age psychiatry services nor specialist learning disability services are equipped to fully meet the needs of this population. It suggests a collaborative approach, with clear local pathways stating the referral processes for each service, and the running of joint clinics rather than setting up yet another separate service for a relatively small population of older adults with learning disabilities. The present authors would also suggest that joint training and skill sharing opportunities among health and social care professionals in both services would be the way forward.

Case study: Good practice in collaborative and joint services

A good practice example in the London Borough of Hackney is an epilepsy clinic for local people with learning disabilities who have epilepsy, which has been jointly set up and run by a consultant psychiatrist in learning disabilities and the consultant neurologist from the local hospital. The clinic is also attended by learning disability and epilepsy specialist nurses. A similar collaborative approach is also being trialled at a clinic in Hackney where a specialist learning disability service and old-age psychiatrists are targeting people with dementia in the borough.

Meeting needs and providing services

The publication of a number of reports, including *Death by Indifference* (Mencap 2007), *Healthcare for All* (Michael 2008) and the *Confidential Inquiry into Premature Deaths of People with Learning Disabilities* (CIPOLD; Heslop *et al.* 2013), as well as the 2011 Winterbourne View scandal, have led to increased awareness among health and social care providers of the health needs of people with learning disabilities. Each of these publications reveals the tragic failure of health services in meeting the needs of this population. They also highlight the failure of health and social care services to communicate effectively with each other, share information, and agree shared strategies and care pathways for meeting the health needs of people with learning disabilities in all phases of ill health. However, while physical health issues attract attention and headlines, mental health issues among people with learning disabilities in general, and older adults in particular, are hardly recognised. When mental health issues in older adults are identified, there is often no clarity as to which service should take the lead in treatment and care, resulting in a delay to appropriate treatment and support.

Social exclusion and isolation are real issues for those who live on their own and who may have very limited social networks. It has been noted by the British Institute of Learning Disabilities (2013) that two-thirds of adults with learning disabilities live with their families, mainly parents who are also in their old age and may be frail and have their own health issues. This leads sometimes to a role reversal, with the person with a learning disability adopting the role of a carer. Ward (2012) points out that as individuals with learning disabilities and their carers grow older together, the risk of social isolation increases. This is due to them having to stay at home more, either because of a reduced level of support to go out and engage in activities or feelings of obligation to stay at home for the sake of their parent(s). Considering this lack of social support and the care needs and/or roles of older people with learning disabilities, Benbow *et al.* (2010) highlight the fact that there is a need to develop a range of services, such as inpatient provision for people with dementia and functional disorders, community support that is available 24 hours a day and works flexibly around individuals, crisis support services, short break provisions, and residential or nursing care homes.

Prevention of falls

Already at a higher risk of mental health problems, older adults with learning disabilities also have the additional burden of failing physical health. One physical indicator of ageing is the frequency of falls, and the prevention of falls and secondary injuries is a worldwide concern (World Health Organization 2007). In isolation, an increase in falling may not trigger a concern for a person with a learning disability or his or her carer, but it can be an indicative symptom of dementia (occurring due to increased wandering or cognitive decline) or age-related physical ailments (Age UK 2014; NHS Choices 2015).

In the general elderly population, the likelihood of a fall occurring rises in the first week after a person's transition from a place of familiarity, such as his or her family home, to somewhere unfamiliar, such as a care home or purpose-built retirement home (CNA 2012). For people with learning disabilities, such transitions between places of care can be more frequent across their lifespan and may at times be more protracted. Furthermore, people with learning disabilities may not be referred to targeted projects run by FallSafe nurses (Sutton and Windsor 2014) or have access to falls champions. Thus the inclusion of people with learning disabilities within the National Falls Prevention Campaign does not seem to have been implemented effectively. This may be more pertinent for older females, who are more susceptible to osteoarthritis during and after the menopause, meaning that even the gentlest fall can be very serious (NHS Choices 2015).

Conversely, national initiatives such as Health Facilitation for People with Learning Disabilities – which facilitates nurses experienced or trained in learning disability to work at strategic and local levels to upskill referring agents on the needs of the client group – have made improvements in access to targeted projects for people with learning disabilities. They are a very useful resource and should be a point of contact for primary care clinicians and social services.

Carers of older people with learning disabilities

Clinical clues of progressing dementia in a person with learning disabilities may not be noticed until severe behavioural or health-related changes occur. This may have an emotional impact on the carer, who may interpret the interventions suggested by specialist services to be restrictive, disempowering or even derogatory. Consider the following example: an interprofessional assessment identifies that the swallow reflex of an individual is deteriorating, as well as the ability to self-feed. Recommendations may include special eating utensils, enhanced body positioning, thickening the consistency of food, changing the eating environment, and further investigation in relation to enteral feeding in order to maintain safe eating and drinking and prevent dysphagia (problems with swallowing) (Ball *et al.* 2012). The National Patient Safety Agency (2007) states that dysphagia is a risk factor for people with learning disabilities and can lead to premature death. However, the carer may well see this advice as disabling, especially if the normalisation of mealtimes is one of the enjoyable moments for the person with a learning disability and something that the whole family can partake in. Such changes also highlight that progressive deterioration of functioning ability may require yet more adaptations to the family and/or carer's lifestyle, which may have remained somewhat stable for a period of time.

Roberts (2010) highlights the idea that practitioners may perceive carers to be obstructive if they are not engaging with the process of intervention, and this may lead professionals to attach labels such as 'non-compliance' and 'non-engaging' to carers in relation to healthcare goals. Meanwhile, legislation and policy place great emphasis on collaboration between professionals and carers, recognising that carers are invaluable (James 2013). However, practitioners have to strive to balance the needs of the client, their capacity to consent, the use of the least restrictive intervention, promotion of a good quality of life, maintainance of the family unit and consideration of the carer. This is no easy task in light of heavy caseloads and budget restrictions. Health professionals are bound by a duty of care (Department of Health 2013), yet increasing scrutiny of their safeguarding competencies may lead them to develop a risk-averse approach to their work, which could be interpreted as restrictive and disempowering for service users – particularly in the eyes of carers. However, the seriousness of dysphagia in the older person with learning disabilities is greatly evidenced. With this in mind, healthcare professionals should endeavour to discuss the potential deterioration of life skills with carers early on in the relationship, before signs and symptoms become apparent, and in parallel with seeking the wishes of the individual.

Case study: Good practice in healthcare planning

An example of good practice can be found in the Haringey Learning Disability Team, who have created a pictorial 'complex needs health pathway' for people with learning disabilities, titled *My Health Pathway*. The leaflet is pan-London and can be used by carers and professionals alike to facilitate useful planning conversations. The leaflet can be accessed online: www.housingandsupport.org.uk/documentdownload.axd?documentresourceid=345.

Recommendations

In the light of the points raised in this chapter, the following recommendations are made:

- Targeted training or awareness-raising events around common mental health issues are required for paid/unpaid carers of people with learning disabilities. These would aid carers in spotting subtle changes in mental health.

- A person-centred approach needs to be developed and embedded in collaborative joint service provision in order to become more inclusive of people with learning disabilities. This includes drawing on specialist knowledge.

- The use of an interprofessional approach in memory clinics for people with learning disabilities at the local level would ensure greater accessibility and more appropriate care.

- Healthcare providers should consider the choice of diagnostic tools being used in relation to their adaptability and suitability for people with learning disabilities.

- Specialist learning disabilities services should share their register of people with learning disabilities – before the client group approaches old age – with older adult services and agree or commission for a clearer pathway of services.

- The criteria for accessing older adult services should be more flexible in order to include those more susceptible to early-onset disorders.

- Clinical Commissioning Groups (CCGs) need to look at the needs of people with learning disabilities and early-onset ageing and mental health problems in relation to what provision is needed within each locality. Greater emphasis on joint funding would enable a smoother delivery of services.

- Routine screening for fall prevention should take place from the age of 65, but should possibly be introduced earlier for people with learning disabilities. This is particularly important before a person with learning disabilities moves to a new home environment.

- Targeted exercise programmes should be offered to all people with learning disabilities in older age to maintain bone strength and co-ordination (Merom *et al.* 2012).

- Social support arrangements need to be flexible and fluid but underpinned by appropriate models of health and social care to ensure a 'seamless service'. They must not be governed by red tape and contracture.

Reflective questions

1. Think about your own life and some of the many freedoms that you have enjoyed as an independent adult (such as parties, relationships, work, children, etc.). How different do you think your life would have been if you had a moderate learning disability?

2. Think about your closest friends and how you confide in them with some of your deepest secrets. How do you think it would feel if you had a moderate learning disability and your closest friends may actually be your parents or carers?

3. Think about some of the major life choices you have made (such as where to live, choice of partner, who you socialise with, etc.). How do you think it would feel if those major life choices had been made by someone else based on certain criteria?

4. Imagine you are 35 years of age with a learning disability and you wish to go on a supported holiday with your peers. However, due to your complex health conditions, the only options available to you are for people aged 65 and over. How would this experience of exclusion and double discrimination make you feel?

5. Imagine you have a headache but are unable to verbally communicate your pain to others. What kind of gestures would you make to indicate where the pain is? How do you think you would feel if these gestures were being ignored or pacified or if you were given medication that had no pain-relieving properties? How do you think your gestures would be interpreted by the following people who do not know you very well?

   a. GP

   b. adult nurse (non-specialist)

   c. agency care worker

Acknowledgements

A special thanks to the following people, who contributed to this chapter by sharing their knowledge and insight:

- The POhWER advocacy group and their facilitator, Jo. (This group did not have any representation from people with severe physical disabilities; therefore we recommend that further interviews should be held with family and carers who represent this client group.)

- Dr Sanjay Nelson, consultant psychiatrist, Hackney Learning Disabilities Services.

- Dr John Rowe, consultant clinical psychologist, Hackney Learning Disabilities Services.

References

Age UK (2014) *Staying Steady – Keep Active and Reduce Your Risk of Falling.* London: Age UK.

Ahmed, Z., Fraser, W., Kerr, M.P., Kiernan, C. *et al.* (2000) 'Reducing antipsychotic medication in people with a learning disability.' *British Journal of Psychiatry 176*, 1, 42–46.

Alzheimer's Society (2014) *Younger People with Dementia.* London: Alzheimer's Society. Available at www.alzheimers.org.uk/Younger_People_with_Dementia, accessed on 28 May 2014.

Ball, S.L., Panter, S.G., Redley, M., Proctor, C.A. *et al.* (2012) 'The extent and nature of need for mealtime support among adults with intellectual disabilities.' *Journal of Intellectual Disability Research 56*, 4, 382–401.

Bell, D., Turnbull, A. and Kidd, W. (2008) 'Differential diagnosis of dementia in the field of learning disabilities: A case study.' *British Journal of Learning Disabilities 37*, 56–65.

Benbow, S.M., Kingston, P., Bhaumik, S., Black, S., Gangadharan, S.K. and Hardy, S. (2010) *Travelling Alone or Travelling Together? The Interface between Learning Disability and Old Age Psychiatry.* Staffordshire University and Older Mind Matters Ltd.

Borthwick-Duffy, S.A. (1994) 'Epidemiology and prevalence of psychopathology in people with mental retardation.' *Journal of Consultant Clinical Psychology 62*, 1, 17–27.

Boseley, S. (2015) 'Fears that antipsychotic drugs being used as "chemical cosh" in disability care.' *Guardian*, Tuesday 1 September. Available at www.theguardian.com/society/2015/sep/01/antipsychotic-drugs-may-be-used-as-chemical-cosh-to-control-behaviour, accessed on 23 September 2016.

British Institute of Learning Disabilities (2013) *Supporting Older Families.* Available at www.bild.org.uk/information/ageingwell/olderfamilies, accessed on 5 September 2015.

British Psychological Society (2015) *Dementia and People with Intellectual Disabilities: Guidance on the Assessment, Diagnosis, Interventions and Support of People with Intellectual Disabilities Who Develop Dementia.* Leicester: The British Psychological Society.

CNA (2012) *Fall Prevention.* Available at www.advanced-healthcare.com/wp-content/uploads/2011/07/April-2012-Inservice.pdf, accessed on 5 September 2015.

Cooper, S. (1997) 'Learning disabilities and old age.' *Advances in Psychiatric Treatment 3*, 312–320.

Cooper, S. and Holland, A. (2007) 'Dementia and Mental Ill-health in Older People with Intellectual Disabilities.' In N. Bouras and G. Holt (eds) *Psychiatric and Behavioural Disorders in Intellectual and Developmental Disabilities.* 2nd ed. Cambridge: Cambridge University Press.

Department for Work and Pensions (2015) *2010 to 2015 Government Policy: Older People.* London: DWP.

Department of Health (2001a) *Valuing People: A New Strategy for Learning Disability for the 21st Century.* London: Department of Health.

Department of Health (2001b) *National Service Framework: Older People.* London: Department of Health. Available at www.gov.uk/government/publications/quality-standards-for-care-services-for-older-people, accessed on 5 September 2015.

Department of Health (2009) *Valuing People Now: A New Three Year Strategy for People with Learning Disabilities.* London: HMSO.

Department of Health (2013) *The NHS Constitution – The NHS Belongs to Us All.* London: Department of Health.

Devine, M., Taggart, L. and McLornian, P. (2009) 'Screening for mental health problems in adults with learning disabilities using the Mini PAS-ADD.' *British Journal of Learning Disabilities 38*, 252–258.

Emerson, E. and Heslop, P. (2010) *A Working Definition of Learning Disabilities.* London: Department of Health.

Emerson, E., Hatton, C., Robertson, J., Roberts, H. *et al.* (2011) *People with Learning Disabilities in England 2011: Services & Supports.* Available at www.improvinghealthandlives.org.uk/publications/1063/People_with_Learning_Disabilities_in_England_2011, accessed on 5 September 2015.

Flynn, A. and Gravestock, S. (2010) 'Assessment, Diagnosis and Rating Instruments.' In N. Bouras and G. Holt (eds) *Mental Health Services for Adults with Intellectual Disability: Strategies and Solutions* New York: Psychology Press.

Foundation for People with Learning Disabilities (2015) *Learning Disability A–Z.* Available at www.learningdisabilities.org.uk/help-information/learning-disability-a-z/h/health, accessed on 5 September 2015.

General Medical Council (undated) *Discrimination.* Available at www.gmc-uk.org/learningdisabilities/200.aspx, accessed on 16 April 2015.

Hassiotis, A., Strydom, A., Allen, K. and Walker, Z. (2003) 'A memory clinic for older people with intellectual disabilities.' *Aging and Mental Health 7,* 6, 418–423.

Hemmings, C. (2010) 'Service Use and Outcomes.' In N. Bouras and G. Holt (eds) *Mental Health Services for Adults with Intellectual Disability: Strategies and Solutions.* New York: Psychology Press.

Heslop, P., Blair, P., Fleming, P., Hoghton, M., Marriott, A. and Russ, L. (2013) *Confidential Inquiry into Premature Deaths of People with Learning Disabilities: Final Report.* Available at www.bristol.ac.uk/media-library/sites/cipold/migrated/documents/fullfinalreport.pdf, accessed on 22 September 2016.

Holland, A.J. (2000) 'Ageing and learning disability.' *British Journal of Psychiatry 176,* 26–31.

James, N. (2013) 'The formal support experiences of family carers of people with an intellectual disability who also display challenging behaviour and/or mental health issues: What do carers say?' *Journal of Intellectual Disabilities 17,* 1, 6–23.

Joint Commissioning Panel for Mental Health (2013) *The Mental Health Clustering Tool for People with Severe Intellectual Disability.* London: Joint Commissioning Panel for Mental Health.

Kannabiran, M., McCarthy, J., Hemmings, C., Mir, G. and Bouras, N. (2009) 'People with intellectual disabilities and mental health problems: Effects of ethnicity on experiences of services.' *Policy and Practice 6,* 2, 121.

McGillivray, J. and McCabe, M. (2010) 'Detecting and treating depression in people with mild intellectual disability: The views of key stakeholders.' *British Journal of Learning Disabilities 38,* 1, 68–76.

Mencap (2007) *Death by Indifference.* London: Mencap.

Mencap (2008) *Health and Social Care Reform Comments by Mencap.* Available at https://old.mencap.org.uk/sites/default/files/documents/2008-11/081911Mencap%20response%20DH_2.pdf, accessed on 30 December 2016.

Mencap (2009) *Housing for people with a learning disability.* Available at http://www.glh.org.uk/wp-content/uploads/2013/04/2012.108-Housing-report_V7.pdf, accessed on 30 December 2016.

Merom, D., Pye, V., Macniven, R., Ploeg, H. *et al.* (2012) 'Prevalence and correlates of participation in fall prevention exercise/physical activity by older adults.' *Preventive Medicine 55,* 613–617.

Michael, J. (2008) *Healthcare for All: Report of the Independent Inquiry into Access to Healthcare for People with Learning Disabilities.* London: HMSO.

National Patient Safety Agency (2007) *Problems Swallowing? Resources for Clients and Carers.* London: NPSA.

NHS Choices (2015) *Falls.* Available at www.nhs.uk/Conditions/Falls/Pages/Introduction.aspx, accessed on 6 November 2016.

Office for National Statistics (2014) *Older People.* Available at https://www.ons.gov.uk/peoplepopulationandcommunity/populationandmigration/populationestimates/bulletins/annualmidyearpopulationestimates/2015-06-25, accessed 30 December 2016.

People First. Available at http://peoplefirstltd.com/ , accessed on 17 January 2017.

Reid, A.H. (1994) 'Psychiatry and learning disabilities.' *British Journal of Psychiatry 164,* 613–618.

Roberts, J. (2010) 'Dysphagia: The challenge of managing eating and drinking difficulties in children and adults who have learning disabilities.' *Tizard Learning Disability Review 15,* 1.

Royal College of Psychiatrists (2013) *People with Learning Disability and Mental Health, Behavioural or Forensic Problems: The Role of In-patient Services.* London: Royal College of Psychiatrists.

Smiley, E. (2005) 'Epidemiology of mental health problems in adults with learning disability: An update.' *Advances in Psychiatric Treatment 11,* 3, 214–222.

Snell, J. (2007) 'Learning disabilities: Elderly people face loss of independence in disability.' *Community Care,* 3 October. Available at www.communitycare.co.uk/2007/10/03/learning-disabilities-elderly-people-face-loss-of-independence, accessed on 5 September 2015.

Strydom, A., Livingston, G., King, M. and Hassiotis, A. (2007) 'Prevalence of dementia in intellectual disability using different diagnostic criteria.' *British Journal of Psychiatry 191,* 150–157.

Sutton, D. and Windsor, J. (2014) 'A care bundle approach to falls.' *Nursing Times 110,* 20, 21–23.

Thorpe, L. (2003) *Geriatric Psychiatry: Mental Health Issues of Older People with Intellectual Disabilities.* Canada: CPA Bulletin de l'APC.

Turner, S. and Bernard, C. (2014) *Supporting Older People with Learning Disabilities: A Toolkit for Health and Social Care Commissioners.* Birmingham: British Institute of Learning Disabilities.

United Nations (2006) *Convention on the Rights of Persons with Disabilities.* Available at www.un.org/disabilities/convention/conventionfull.shtml, accessed on 5 September 2015.

University of Glamorgan, Rhondda Cynon Taff People First and New Pathways (2013) *Looking into Abuse Research Team: Research by People with Learning Disabilities.* Wales: University of Glamorgan, Rhondda Cynon Taff People First and New Pathways.

VoiceAbility (2013) *The Care Act.* Available at www.voiceability.org/the_care_act, accessed on 5 September 2015.

Ward, C. (2012) *BILD Factsheet: Older People with a Learning Disability.* Kidderminster: British Institute of Learning Disabilities.

Ward, C. (2012) *Perspectives on Ageing with a Learning Disability.* York: Joseph Rowntree Foundation. Available at www.jrf.org.uk/report/perspectives-ageing-learning-disability, accessed on 5 September 2015.

Williams, R. (2013) 'The Challenges for Children and Young People with Learning Disability from Black Asian Minority Ethnic (BAME) Background.' In C. Thurston (ed.) *Essential Nursing Care for Children and Young People: Theory, Policy and Practice.* Abingdon: Routledge.

World Health Organization (1996) *ICD-10 Guide for Mental Retardation.* Geneva: WHO. Available at www.who.int/mental_health/media/en/69.pdf, accessed on 23 September 2016.

World Health Organization (2007) *Global Report on Falls Prevention in Older Age.* Geneva: WHO. Available at www.who.int/ageing/publications/Falls_prevention7March.pdf, accessed on 23 September 2016.

World Health Organization (2014) *WHO Disability Assessment Schedule 2.0 (WHODAS 2.0).* Available at www.who.int/classifications/icf/whodasii/en, accessed on 5 September 2015.

Further reading

Age Concern (2007) *Working with Older People with Learning Disabilities: Lessons from an Age Concern Pilot Programme Research Briefing.* London: Age Concern. Available at www.ageuk.org.uk/documents/en-gb/for-professionals/equality-and-human-rights/16_0208_working_with_older_people_with_learning_disabilities_lessons_from_an_age_concern_pilot_programme_2008_pro.pdf?dtrk=true, accessed on 23 September 2016.

Bhaumik, S., Gangadharan, S., Hiremath, A., Swamidhas, P. and Russell, S. (2011) 'Psychological treatments in intellectual disabilities: The challenges of building a good evidence base.' *British Journal of Psychiatry 198,* 6, 428–430.

Bigby, C. (2002) 'Ageing people with lifelong disability: Challenges for the aged care and disability sectors.' *Journal of Intellectual and Developmental Disability 27,* 4, 231.

Bouras, N. and Holt, G. (2010) 'Service Use and Outcomes.' In C. Hemmings (ed.) *Mental Health Services for Adults with Intellectual Disability: Strategies and Solutions.* New York: Psychology Press.

British Psychological Society (2013) *Classification of Behaviour and Experience in Relation to Functional Psychiatric Diagnoses: Time for a Paradigm Shift. DCP Position Statement.* Leicester: The British Psychological Society.

Brown, H. (2004) 'A rights-based approach to abuse of women with learning disabilities.' *Tizard Learning Disability Review 9*, 4, 41–44.

Buys, L., Boulton-Lewis, G., Tedman-Jones, J., Edwards, H., Knox, M. and Bigby, C. (2008) 'Issues of active ageing: Perceptions of older people with lifelong intellectual disability.' *Australian Journal on Ageing 27*, 67–71.

Chinn, D., Abraham, E., Burke, C. and Davies, J. (2014) *IAPT and Learning Disabilities Research Report, October.* London: King's College.

Department of Health (2008) *Making It Happen for Everyone.* London: HMSO.

Foundation for People with Learning Disabilities (2012) *Learning Difficulties and Ethnicity: Updating a Framework for Action.* London: Foundation for People with Learning Disabilities. Available at www.learningdisabilities.org.uk/content/assets/pdf/publications/Equalities_framework_-_final_combined_report_170512.pdf?view=Standard, accessed on 5 September 2015.

Joint Commissioning Panel for Mental Health (2015) *Learning Disability Services.* London: Joint Commissioning Panel for Mental Health. Available at www.jcpmh.info/good-services/learning-disabilities-services, accessed on 5 September 2015.

Looking into Abuse Research Team (2013) *Looking into Abuse: Research by People with Learning Disabilities.* Wales: University of Glamorgan, Rhondda Cynon Taff and People First and New Pathways.

McCarthy, J. (2001) 'Post-traumatic stress disorder in people with learning disability.' *Advances in Psychiatric Treatment 7*, 163–169.

Office for National Statistics (2012) *Population Ageing: Statistics.* Available at http://researchbriefings.files.parliament.uk/documents/SN03228/SN03228.pdf, accessed on 5 September 2015.

Shaw, K., Cartwright, C. and Craig, J. (2011) 'The housing and support needs of people with an intellectual disability into older age.' *Journal of Intellectual Disability Research 55*, 9, 895–903.

Strydom, A. (2015) *Dementia in Individuals with Intellectual Disabilities – Epidemiology.* Available at www.bps.org.uk/system/files/user-files/DCP%20The%20Faculty%20for%20People%20with%20Intellectual%20Disabilities/public/andre_strydom_-_dementia_in_individuals_with_intellectual_disabilities_-_epidemiology.pdf, accessed on 5 September 2015.

World Health Organization (2001) 'Burden of Mental and Behavioural Disorders.' In *World Health Report 2001 – Mental Health: New Understanding, New Hope.* Geneva: WHO. Available at www.who.int/whr/2001/chapter2/en/index4.html, accessed on 5 September 2015.

Chapter 9

Ageing, Sexual Orientation and Mental Health: Lesbian, Gay, Bisexual, Transgender and Intersex Older People

Matt Broadway-Horner

Introduction

Discrimination against lesbian, gay, bisexual, transgender and intersex (LGBTi)[16] people can often mean they are denied the basic human right to live the life they are born to lead (Kimmel *et al.* 2006). Traditionally, LGBTi people have often had to live in secret, hidden from the dominant heterosexual society, and many older people are still worried about disclosing their sexual identity (Kimmel *et al.* 2006). In this chapter I will explore some of the many issues facing older LGBTi people. The chapter starts with a brief overview of the history of the LGBTi communities and how they have been treated as 'invisible citizens' through mechanisms of the law and the medicalisation of the 'homosexual' (Jennings 2007). Then I examine some of the fears and concerns held by members of LGBTi communities when accessing services, and this is discussed in relation to issues of sexuality, mental health and ageing. It is my hope that in reading this chapter you will gain a deeper understanding of the issues raised and then think of areas of application for your own development as a non-discriminatory practitioner, as well as identifying needs for further service development.

Absent from history: LGBTi people in the UK

LGBTi people have often been absent from the writing of history. Evidence suggests that same-sex relationships existed before the emergence of Christianity, as far back as the Celts, and at certain times in history LGBTi people were commonly seen as unremarkable (Ellis 2004). However, over time the category of heterosexuality developed as the dominant sexual value in society, especially in relation to the family, and consequently other experiences of sexuality became constructed as 'abnormal'. The criminalisation of homosexual sex apparently came about because of its growing visibility in the Victorian era amongst (though not limited to) the upper and aristocratic classes (Cook 2011). In order to prevent the visibility of homosexuality in all forms, there was a movement to stop what was viewed as 'indecency in private' as well as in public (Jennings 2007). In 1886 in England, the Criminal Law Amendment Act outlawing sexual relations between men (but not between women) was given Royal Assent by Queen Victoria. As most British colonies at the time had been forced to give up their own legal systems and operate under the British legal system instead (Tiwari 2013), this law was also enacted across the British colonies. The Offences Against the Person Act 1861 was amended to remove the death sentence for 'buggery'; however, the penalty became imprisonment of between ten years and life (Licata and Petersen 2013). Unfortunately, trans and intersex people often got persecuted under the same law, which is typical of the tendency to place transgender and intersex people under the label of sexuality and not in their rightful place under the label of gender (Green *et al.* 2011).

Prior to colonisation by the Europeans, many cultures and countries had LGBTi practices that were considered normal as part of a continuum of sexuality and gender (Tiwari 2013). As a result of the British colonial mechanisms of power and the regulation of homosexuality, many minorities from member states of the Commonwealth of Nations are still more likely than not to keep their sexuality or gender private, for fear of a cultural backlash (Amory 1997). It is argued that this continues to have a profound effect on many Black and minority ethnic LGBTi people in the UK, who often have to struggle with cultural tensions about sexuality/gender as well as the racism that can occur within LGBTi communities in the UK today (Varney 2012). For example, in Sri Lanka, where people often have arranged marriages, the expectation is that a person will marry for the honour of the family, which may cause difficulties when sexuality or gender does not match. Therefore, some married men or women are not enjoying a full marriage because they have been forced to marry, for 'family honour', a gay, lesbian or trans person (Equal Ground *et al.* 2014).

Many of the worst examples of state killings of lesbian and gay people came during the Nazi atrocities of the Second World War, when almost 1 million gay men and women living in Berlin disappeared and 100,000 known gay and lesbian people were sent to the death camps. This has left a historical legacy that should never be repeated (Herzog 2004). However, in many countries heterosexuality continues to be viewed as the 'normal' way of living, and this is backed up by legislation; consequently, many LGBTi people continue to find themselves persecuted or prosecuted by the state. This is the case in at least 82 countries (Stocks 2015), including Russia, Turkey, Uganda and the Gambia (Thompson 2014).

So far, I have shown how LGBTi people have historically received prejudicial treatment, and it may be suggested that as a consequence of this many people from LGBTi communities are likely to be hesitant in trusting both state-provided and private health services. This may be particularly true for older people who remember and may have direct experiences of this persecution. In the next section, I look at some of the state reforms that have impacted upon the lives of LGBTi people in the UK. I then discuss how the law dominated lives in such a way that LGBTi people have historically gone 'underground' and become invisible rather than be prosecuted or persecuted, which I argue may have muted the conversation between healthcare services and LGBTi people.

State reforms in the UK

The retelling of LGBTi history is often constructed as a story of 'progressive enlightenment' in which LGBTi people emerged into liberation (Chauncey 1989). However, while these stories of resistance are valuable, many others present experiences of shame and, with it, a life of silence and secrecy for fear of judgement by others (Stonewall 2011). Knocker (2012) investigated the perspectives of older LGBTi people and interviewed a cross-section of older people including Patrick, whose experiences were similar to the many who lived in fear, having seen their friends taken into the care of psychiatric services just because they were gay. Patrick states:

> You just tried to lead a normal life as a 'bachelor'. People used to say about me, 'He's very shy!' I just closed off my sexual life. I would joke with other people and be a bit anti-gay myself, which I feel sad about now. (Knocker 2012, p.5)

In the same study, Adam described how he felt like an invisible man, as the only way to encounter other gay or bisexual men was to meet in communal areas like parks or public toilets. Meetings like these were eventually described with the term 'cottaging', which became a criminal offence. Undercover policemen would try to entrap gay and bisexual men through these meetings in order to control their behaviour, which turned the meetings into a dangerous risk. Those who were arrested would suffer humiliation and future difficulties, especially if the arrest resulted in a police record, making the prospect of applying for jobs or indeed getting married problematic. Many people also found the persecution of their sexuality traumatic as, if identified, they were recorded on the sex offenders register alongside convicted paedophiles and rapists (Knocker 2012). Many LGBTi people were vilified as sexual deviants, which was consistently confused with being a sex offender. As such, many LGBTi people would seek heterosexual marriages to 'feel normal' or to hide their sexuality so they did not 'stand out' (Kimmel *et al.* 2006).

This discriminatory stance overflowed into the care of children, and as recently as 1988, section 28 of the Local Government Act stated that that no local authority shall 'promote homosexuality' nor the 'acceptability of homosexuality as a preferred family relationship'. This further exacerbated the idea of LGBTi people as deviant, although it is notable that no local authority has ever been charged or prosecuted under section 28. The LGBTi charitable organisation Stonewall argues that fear of the effects of section 28 did hinder the work of local authorities in providing services and support to LGBTi communities, and it was not until 2003 that section 28 was finally taken off the statute books (Stonewall 2012).

Many older people will still remember the Wolfenden report (1957) which recommended that 'homosexual acts between consenting adults' should be decriminalised, and in 1967 the Sexual Offences Act came into force in England and Wales, decriminalising homosexual acts between two men over 21 years of age 'in private'. In 1980, male homosexuality was also decriminalised in Scotland. The European Commission ruled unanimously that the British government was guilty of breaching article 8 of the European Convention on Human Rights by refusing to legalise consenting homosexual behaviour in Northern Ireland, and in 1982 male homosexuality was decriminalised in Northern Ireland with the passing of law reform in the House of Commons (Stonewall 2012).

Like gay, bisexual and trans people, lesbians have also suffered the humiliation of being arrested, suffering equally devastating, but notably different, discrimination and abuse (Stocks 2015). For example, a research study reported the atrocities that happened to a participant called Jo, who recalled losing her girlfriend to a stabbing in a violent street attack after they had both been raped (Knocker 2012). Jo believes that the police were heavily biased by the fact that the women were lesbians, and, as a consequence, no one was charged for the murder. One policeman had apparently said to her that if they had not been lesbians then the crime would not have occurred. Unsurprisingly, Jo felt completely unsupported by the police and felt that they were blaming her and her 'lifestyle' for the tragedy, despite her devastation at the death of her partner (Knocker 2012).

Psychiatry and LGBTi experiences

Along with the legal system, mental health services have traditionally failed to accept the diversity of human sexuality, and indeed they have played a role in the punitive treatment of LGBTi people (Bayer 1987). Prior to 1974, many LGBTi persons would have been treated for their sexual preferences with abusive treatments such as electroconvulsive therapy, frontal lobotomy, isolation, aversion therapy and drug therapies, all of which effectively dehumanised them and stripped away their individuality as well as their rights as a citizen (Stocks 2015). For many, being defined as 'mentally ill' due to their sexual preferences or gender also meant that they could not buy a house, obtain a loan or apply for a mortgage (Bayer 1987). It was only in 1974 that the American Psychiatric Association removed homosexuality as a psychiatric diagnosis in its revision of its *Diagnostic and Statistical Manual* (DSM-II). However, the World Health Organization did not remove it from its classification manual, *International Statistical Classification of*

Diseases and Related Health Problems, until its tenth edition (ICD-10) in 1990 (Herek 1990).

Insight

I remember, when I first worked on acute admission wards, meeting a lady who was in a psychiatric crisis. She had been under the treatment of the local mental health team for the last 40 years, and, when able, she told me a little of her life story. Her initial contact with services started because her mother was concerned about her lesbian affairs and so enrolled her on an LSD treatment programme in the 1950s to try to change her into a straight (heterosexual) woman.

LSD treatment involved the use of hallucinogenic drugs to induce hallucinations, with the underlying theory that people were more suggestible while hallucinating and mental health practitioners would thereby be able to induce behavioural changes, in this case changing sexual preference from homosexuality to heterosexuality. This treatment was commonly used alongside lobotomy, hypnotherapy and electroconvulsive treatments in psychotherapy to help change unwanted behaviour, until LSD treatments were discontinued in the 1970s (Falco 1991).

Needless to say, the LSD treatment did not change her sexual preference and sadly caused her many more problems, leading to additional diagnoses and hospitalisations. She has longed for the touch of the woman who loved her all those years ago, but because of her treatment she now believes lesbianism to be morally wrong. This is just one of the ways that medicine and the state tried to control female sexuality.

Another interview by Knocker (2012) tells the story of a man called Leslie, who described being medically and psychologically brutalised when undergoing aversion therapy. Leslie was encouraged to rehearse his self-hatred and sexual fantasies over and over again to a doctor. These fantasies were then replayed to Leslie via a recorder as he was given an injection to induce vomiting. The damages from this so-called therapy cost him many years of recovery and coming to terms with the fact that his sexuality is not abnormal. In this area, vast progress has been made; in the USA, for example, President Obama put a stop to 'conversion therapies' (Fredriksen-Goldsen *et al.* 2014), which had been used to impose heterosexual values on to LGBTi people.

It would be nice to think that control practices and discrimination based on human sexuality and gender have now ended, but research suggests that it continues in many places, with LGBTi people finding it incredibly hard to live life as they would like to. According to Fredriksen-Goldsen *et al.* (2014), many trans people change their name at least once in their lifetime, which can itself cause difficulties. Services have not got used to the idea that someone may want to change gender, and so procedures are not yet in place to help these people (Stocks 2015). In the UK, many trans people are not on the electoral register because of the requirement to be assessed for a Gender Recognition Certificate (GRC) (Ellis, Bailey and McNeil 2015). This is a process of being assessed by a professional as to whether the gender ascribed to the individual should be changed, a decision which follows strict criteria. It has been argued by Stocks (2015) that these assessors may or may not understand the issues at stake, leading to sexist and/or transphobic treatment.

The assessment process for gender reassignment is reportedly not the most pleasant of experiences, and according to Ellis *et al.* (2015), getting the certificate is a long, drawn-out process, which keeps the trans population silent and invisible, especially in older age. Society assigns gender in so many important aspects of our daily lives: on birth certificates, passports, legal papers, utility bills and job contracts. There seems to be no escape for the person who needs to be the other gender in order to be a visible and fully functioning citizen. On the other hand, there is a widespread availability of medical procedures in Britain to help people make the transition from one gender to another. According to Meikle (2015), the NHS performs 3000 of these operations each year. Meikle suggests, however, that trans people are treated as 'second-class citizens' due to the long waiting lists and the many GPs who are reluctant to refer people on to specialists. According to Ellis *et al.* (2015), the process of gender change can take 2–5 years due to the stages involved, including the initial psychiatric evaluation.

The psychiatric assessment is a complex process in which, ultimately, the trans person has to agree to the diagnosis of gender dysphoria before proceeding to the hormone treatment stage. They then move on to the social gender role transition stage, lasting 2 years, before the penultimate stage of the surgical procedures. Social gender role transition is the process of living in the needed gender and immersing themselves completely in this life for two years by experiencing the hormonal treatments and dressing and interacting as the needed gender type with friends and family. All aspects of life are to be experienced and engaged in fully while receiving counselling to aid the transition (Ellis *et al.* 2015).

What about the mental health needs of older LGBTi people?

Considering the legislation, medicalisation and discrimination that has controlled the lives of LGBTi people, it is important to explore the impact that this has had on them as they grow older. According to Stonewall (2012), Wallace *et al.* (2011) and Van Wagenen, Driskell and Bradford (2013), there are many fears and concerns from the LGBTi community about growing older and how the services offered to older people may erode their sense of freedom and independence. LGBTi people may not have children or family to help look after them in old age, and they are more likely than their straight peers to live alone. Being reliant on services brings with it the fear that they may experience the discrimination that has historically been characteristic of public services, or even that care may be made unavailable to them (Van Wagenen *et al.* 2013).

A poll carried out by Stonewall (2012) measured perceptions of the care and treatment that straight (heterosexual) and LGBTi populations may receive in old age. Among LGBTi people, 72 per cent were concerned about losing their independence and worried about whether they would receive adequate care and how this would be made available to them. In comparison, the straight community were also concerned about these issues, but on average the figures came in at 10–12 per cent lower, suggesting that they were not as fearful as their LGBTi counterparts (Stonewall 2012). In light of this, further research is necessary to address the service needs of older LGBTi people, including those with mental health problems. In addition, concerns in practice about the attitudes of staff and their acceptance of people's sexual and gender identities need to be addressed in an active and directive manner.

Many care institutions have a tendency to take a 'one size fits all' approach, which may overlook different sexualities and genders. Health professionals may not have any particular knowledge or understanding of LGBTi history and may therefore fail to look through the lens of various sexualities and gender to provide validation and acceptance as part of a holistic approach to care and well-being. For example, Knocker (2012) investigated gay issues and how they were handled in care homes, but found that a common response was 'You won't find anyone gay here' (Knocker 2012, p.4). For many older LGBTi people, having friends or life partners visit was a particular concern; they were worried about showing affection or holding hands at the bedside for fear of recrimination or that this could have a negative impact on the care provided. As such, many older people struggle with informing others about their sexuality and spoke about needing reassurance from services that an LGBTi-friendly person was caring for them (Knocker 2012). Herein lies the contradiction: according to Stonewall (2012) and Stocks (2015), LGBTi people are more likely to seek help from public-sector services than their straight counterparts, yet they are much more concerned about being met with discrimination. More needs to be done to collect data about their experiences and improve their prospects in order to alleviate the concerns of these communities.

A number of authors have explored the influences of gender identity, sexual orientation, histories of coming out, marital status and friendship networks on people. Similar to the straight community, the issues include the fundamental needs of self-acceptance, having a purpose in life, the presence of a life partner and financial security, and these are all predictors of a good quality of life for older LGBTi people (Heaphy, Yip and Thompson 2004; Hughes, Harold and Boyer 2011; Schope 2005). In contrast, the experience of a lifetime of discrimination can impact upon LGBTi people's mental health in many different ways, and I turn now to some of the research evidence of challenges for and resilience to this.

Challenges

A number of authors have examined the mental health challenges faced by some LGBTi people. For example:

- Cahill (2003) argues that prolonged stress due to being stigmatised and marginalised also has a negative impact on mental health, with many people living in shame and being excluded by their loved ones because of their sexuality and gender identification.

- King *et al.* (2008) conducted a meta-analysis of 25 studies investigating mental health issues such as suicide and self-harm and found that there were twice as many LGBTi people compared to the straight community involved in suicide attempts and significantly higher rates of depression, anxiety and alcohol dependence in LGBTi communities.

- Indeed, Stonewall (2012) found a 7 per cent increase in several disorders such as anxiety and depression in the LGBTi communities compared to another study by King *et al.* (2008) focusing on the straight population.

- Maguen and Shipherd (2010) found that 41 per cent of trans-men and 20 per cent of trans-women reported suicide attempts. In addition, factors such as school and workplace bullying and homophobic attacks were cited as reasons for these attempts, and the subsequent use of drugs and alcohol was mentioned as a way of coping.

- Farquhar, Bailey and Whittaker (2001), King and McKeown (2003), Robertson (1998) and Van Wagenen *et al.* (2013) have all found a significantly higher incidence of mental health problems and distress within the LGBTi communities compared to straight communities.

- Stonewall (2013) report that the main reasons LGBTi people seek therapy and treatment are anxiety and depression, and some studies have found higher rates of tobacco, drug and alcohol use in these communities in older age compared to the straight population (Gruskin *et al.* 2007; Valanis *et al.* 2000).

- McCann *et al.* (2013) surveyed LGBTi people aged 55 years plus living in Ireland. Of 444 participants, one-third described having a mental illness at some point in their life or were currently taking medication prescribed for treatment of a mental health condition. Fifty-two per cent had thought seriously about ending their life, and 27 per cent had self-harmed. Illicit drug use was reported at 5 per cent, which is significantly higher than the figure of 0.5 per cent in the straight population. One-quarter of the sample had suffered violence, and one-fifth reported having been punched and beaten because of their sexual identity.

- In LGBTi adults over the age of 70, D'Augelli and Grossman (2001) found a strong correlation between previous experience of violence and victimisation and a greater incidence of mental health conditions such as depression, low self-esteem and internalised homophobia. Older LGBTi people who had not experienced violence reported higher self-esteem and less internalised homophobia or suicidal ideation.

- Otis and Skinner (1996) have suggested that LGBTi people often face double victimisation, not only in the initial attack but also in reporting it to authorities such as the police or housing services. This is reflected in Stonewall's (2013) *Gay British Crime Survey* finding that a quarter of those who experienced hate crime subsequently changed their behaviour in an attempt not to be perceived as gay in order to avoid being victimised again. These changes went beyond simple body posture and looking confident to potential changes in identity and being told by services to look 'more straight'.

Resilience

While the above studies have highlighted some of the many challenges that LGBTi people face and the negative effects of homophobia, transphobia, biphobia and interphobia, it is also important to consider any positive outcomes that have emerged from these challenges for the respective communities. Some theorists suggest that LGBTi communities have built solidarity and resilience in response to their oppression and persecution. For example, according to Gabbay and Wahler (2002) and Jones and Nystrom (2002), many LGBTi people become adept at dealing with discrimination and adjusting to hostile and non-inclusive environments. In addition, a number of studies have shown that LGBTi people have a wide range of responses and many are very resilient (Hughes 2008; Orel 2004; Woolf 2000).

It is also interesting to note that when measuring adjustment to age, the straight population scored lower in their ability to adjust to ageing than LGBTi communities, and research suggests that many

LGBTi people are more successful at ageing, embracing it rather than ignoring it (Bradford, Ryan and Rothblum 1994; Brotman, Ryan and Cormier 2003; Orel 2004). It would appear that the coming-out process is beneficial to coping with crisis, and, according to Kimmel (1978), this may act as a buffer for adapting to any crisis situation that is encountered, including growing older. In this way, the resilience of LGBTi people facilitates healthy and successful ageing despite the concerns and mental health problems discussed previously.

LGBTi people as service users

The discussion so far has raised a number of relevant questions regarding the current issues surrounding the mental health and well-being of older LGBTi people. First, are LGBTi people seeking help from public services, and if so, in what ways do they access and present themselves to services? Second, are LGBTi people using other services that aim to support their specific needs, such as GUM clinics that provide counselling for sexuality issues within which depression is often included? Third, are LGBTi people receiving support from other, more informal networks within the LGBTi 'family' or community, and if so, what kind of support is most useful? Varney (2012) states that we do not know the answers to these questions because services in the UK do not monitor sexuality (unlike in America). One problem with the lack of inclusion of sexual orientation and gender identity in routine UK data collection is that few studies have a large enough sample to enable the analysis of differences between sub-groups within LGBTi populations. This therefore limits the ability to understand and compare the impact of multiple identities on health outcomes. Varney (2012) proposes systematic collection of data to facilitate a deeper knowledge of LGBTi health outcomes, which would require Clinical Commissioning Groups to encourage services to move away from heteronormativity and towards more inclusive services by ensuring these issues are part of the mandatory criteria for funding bids.

Queer theory, ageing and sexuality

By looking through the lenses of ageing and sexuality and the interaction between the two, we can gain a better understanding of the complexities of the LGBTi experience of ageing. Many studies in

LGBTi theory have centred on identity politics, which is often disputed by Queer theory. Identity categories are designed to identify the 'sexed subject' and place individuals within a single restrictive sexual orientation. In contrast, Queer theory is concerned with exploring the categories of gender and sexuality and what constitutes identity. Queer theorists propose that identities are not fixed and consist of so many varied components that categorising and labelling identities and people based on just one characteristic would be wrong (Warner 1999). Queer theory suggests that there is an interval between what a subject 'does' (role-taking) and what a subject 'is' (the self). So despite its title, Queer theory's goal is to destabilise and deconstruct identity categories and look beyond what is visible, which requires us to rethink the issue from the starting block of homonormativity.

So what has this got to do with ageing? Many studies show that not only do LGBTi people adjust well to ageing but they often have increased tolerance to others, a greater sense of control over the type of family they want, and more flexibility in gender roles and identification (Dorfman *et al.* 1995; Sandberg 2008). Furthermore, studies by Grossman (2006) and Masini and Barrett (2008) found that many LGBTi people have established a 'chosen family', often formed of friends gathered over a lifetime who provide networks for both social engagement and support in distressing situations. In this way, LGBTi people may have had greater opportunity to construct their own identity in comparison to their straight counterparts.

Queer theory conceptualised the notion of 'embracing the shame', which has been adopted by and given strength to the communities involved in LGBTi politics. It acts as a mechanism to move from being classed as 'deviant' citizens in the marginal, excluded parts of society, to becoming acknowledged within the mainstream. In addition to LGBTi politics, the concept of embracing the shame holds well for ageing as it looks at the cultural negativity of ageing and opens up discussions on the idea of the norm of gender and sexuality, bringing more attention to developing individual expression in opposition to societal pressure for traditional ideas (Sandberg 2008). Queer theory aims to move away from the traditional and stereotypical ideas of gender, sexuality and reproduction and instead offers a way of looking at the individual in the context of self and the roles desired to be undertaken. It looks at embracing the negative aspects of ageing and moving forward into the next phase of life with a positivity that comes from breaking the mould of social expectations and the social reconstruction of the authentic self.

According to Rowe and Kahn (1987), successful ageing reduces the risk of younger generations believing stereotypical ideas of older people, and instead highlights the contribution that older people can make as vibrant, active participants in society. This benefit has the potential to reproduce itself in younger generations as older people who exemplify successful ageing may become role models for health and may encourage younger people to make necessary lifestyle changes for themselves. However, this theory has not been without critics, and Featherstone and Wernick (1995) suggest that it is oversimplistic and overlooks other factors, such as class, ethnicity and accessibility to work and services, which also contribute to 'successful' ageing. Other authors have also acknowledged that lower socio-economic groups are often unable to afford the same benefits as wealthier groups.

Deacon *et al.* (1995) have argued that there is a need to aid successful ageing by revisiting and dispelling myths around ageing, including ideas such as 'sexual expression is just for the young', 'older people are unattractive' or 'older people should be asexual', or otherwise they are labelled a 'sexual deviant'. Yet Bretschneider and McCoy (1988), Kinsey, Pomeroy and Martin (1948), Masters and Johnson (1966) and Spiegelhalter (2015) have all shown that people who are sexually active when young will often still be sexually active in older age (60–94 years). Research by Masters and Johnson (1966) suggested that the preferred sexual activity when younger may change with age, and those who are ageing successfully adapt to these changes, with many remaining sexually active until the end of their lives. Across these points, Queer theory offers individuals a way of reclaiming their life by not conforming to the normative stereotype but instead creating a space for themselves and their 'chosen family'. Indeed, this may prove useful for many people from diverse backgrounds in terms of culture and other characteristics protected under the Equality Act 2010 who are working to break the stereotypes of ageing, mental health and sexuality.

Applications of non-discriminatory practice

So far, this chapter has looked at the history of LGBTi people, the mental health needs of older LGBTi people, and Queer theory in relation to sexuality and ageing. I now turn to applications in practice and offer some recommendations for LGBTi-inclusive service provision.

Trust can only be developed if you deliver what you promise

Many LGBTi people will read about the inclusivity and openness of service provision in marketing literature before accessing your service. If a promise of inclusivity is broken in the first face-to-face encounter, it is unlikely that the individual will return. Acceptance and inclusion needs to be explicit, as is evident in this interview with Anwar, aged 63, in London:

> I don't think the larger society has fully accepted gay people and services for older people still lack infrastructures and sensitivity specific to older gay people. (Stonewall 2012, p.29)

Examine your own attitudes

A good place to start is to reflect on your own attitudes towards older LGBTi individuals, especially if you are from a background that does not affirm the LGBTi orientation. Hillman and Hinrichsen (2014) argue that there is room to both be an effective practitioner and hold private personal and religious views; you may need to make a clear distinction between the two. Let us always remember to look at the individual rather than a label.

Remember the codes of practice and conduct

It is important to note that all professions will be judged by what they say and how they act, but also in what they don't say and their inaction. Codes of conduct are there not only to protect the public but also to protect professionals and ensure we are providing a good service. We have a duty of care to those people who are accessing the service, and our job is to offer compassion and understanding, not to deny this according to our prejudice and personal beliefs. Personal belief systems are for the personal life of the care professional, not for public attention.

Mind your language

Language is of huge importance as it carries with it meaning and context, as Rowena states:

> Just as it is important to have someone speak English or the same language as you, so you can communicate, I need someone who can 'speak lesbian!' Our culture is different and we have different ways of doing things. It is a bit indefinable, but really important. (Knocker 2012, p.11)

For instance, rather than asking a woman 'Do you have a husband?', it is more appropriate to alter the language to 'Do you have a partner?'. Similarly, when talking to children about their parents, it is preferable to talk about 'parent 1', 'parent 2', 'parent 3' and so on, rather than referring to the nuclear family model of 'Mum and Dad', in order to help recognise and include blended and extended families as 'normal'. Another point concerns the term 'next of kin', which should be replaced with a nominated person 'in case of emergency'. This simple advice makes it easier for services to identify the right person. Objective and sexuality-neutral terms like 'acknowledged family' or 'permitted visitors' also cater for a plethora of family arrangements that deserve equal status.

Refrain from making assumptions

It is important not to assume that LGBTi people do not have children, as many do have their own birth children from other relationships, and others adopt or foster children. As we have seen, many older people may have hidden their LGBTi identity and lived a 'traditional' lifestyle that includes children and grandchildren, so do not fall into the trap of stereotyping people by using your own preconceptions, ideas and language (Hillman and Hinrichsen 2014).

Friends are the family in most cases

The LGBTi community is a strong force fighting many battles together and standing in solidarity. According to Stonewall (2011), many people express a difficulty in maintaining links with birth families due to stigma and isolation caused by homophobia, biphobia and transphobia. It would seem reasonable to allow a change in formal procedures in inpatient care settings from visits by 'just family' to visits by 'significant others' to allow for a broader range of support. Allowing a legitimate and legal role for friends to support older individuals may reduce distress and also reduce the risk of poor treatment by family members and/or services. For example, I recall a story of a 74-year-old gay patient in a hospital ward whose family denied him contact with his LGBTi friends, despite the fact that the family had not seen their gay relative in 35 years.

Legal mechanisms to consider

Not everyone will have relatives or loved ones to help them in older age, and so it is important to ask about and encourage your client to make advance decisions or arrange lasting power of attorney regardless of whether or not he or she is married or in a civil partnership. Indeed, due to the risk of discriminatory practice, these legal mechanisms are even more important for older people from LGBTi communities to ensure that their needs and wishes are respected in the event of the loss of mental capacity.

Older mentally ill LGBTi people still enjoy sex

People's sexuality seems to 'disappear' in services for older people due to assumptions that the sex drive of older people has disappeared into thin air. Consequently, the sexual needs of older people are ignored, which can be particularly difficult for older generations whose sexual needs had previously been oppressed.

Opportunities for monogamous couples

For many years prior to the Marriage Act 2013, same-sex partners were not able to get married and therefore did not have the same options as their straight counterparts in areas such as insurance, mortgages, company benefits and hospital visiting times. Although this is changing, there is still a lot to be done to allow LGBTi people the same freedoms and opportunities. Health and social care settings ought to be void of judgement about sexuality and should offer an open environment that allows simple human contact between life partners during times of illness (Stonewall 2011).

Open relationships and what people want

Open relationships are an area that is often met with retaliation and resistance from the heterosexual majority. In an open relationship, an individual may have a 'life partner' with whom they have made a long-term commitment. However, within this loving relationship the individual may also engage with other sexual partners who are casual or permanent fixtures of a different expression of love or lust that meets different needs, such as a more active sex drive or an exploration of sexuality. Most open relationships are happy ones, with rules that provide transparency and clarity of communication (Spiegelhalter 2015). In the past, this was frowned upon by many mental health professionals, who even attached psychopathological labels to this life choice (Licata and Petersen 2013). There is now a greater acceptance that human beings as a species may not be fully programmed to be in monogamous relationships and that additional sexual partners can be perfectly natural (Spiegelhalter 2015). Indeed, the topic of open relationships has been much more prevalent in recent years, especially in the media, which is a different story to that of 10 years ago. However, many older people may still be reluctant to discuss issues around open relationships, so it is important to build trust and be understanding and non-judgemental if the topic is raised.

Older people and sex workers

Some older people may be in contact with legalised sex workers in order to satisfy their sexual needs. As a practitioner, this topic should be approached with discretion and with anti-discriminatory values. As an additional consideration, practice should include meeting the needs of the sex workers as well, who are often vulnerable to violence and exploitation. Everyone should be treated equally and non-judgementally, recognising and respecting a person-centred approach and diversity (UK Network of Sex Work Projects 2008).

Professional development and training

Stonewall (2011) has highlighted many recommendations for services inclusive of older LGBTi people, but the need for more training for professionals about meeting the diverse needs of LGBTi communities and the need to consult LGBTi communities in service development and delivery are particularly compelling. This is vital for building trust and equality (Hillman and Hinrichsen 2014).

Final thoughts

The following are my personal recommendations for establishing an inclusive, non-discriminatory service for older LGBTi people:

- Actively bring in LGBTi people as non-executive board members to be part of the decision-making processes of the health and social care trust or third-sector organisation.

- Promote your anti-discriminatory practices that work with LGBTi communities publicly in the media so as to make the wider community aware of developments.

- Services have to be clear that they are in the public and not the religious domain; therefore public displays of affection are to be expected in hospital wards and you need to be quietly respectful and accepting.

- In the words of psychologist Albert Ellis, 'Acceptance is not love. You love a person because he or she has lovable traits, but you accept everybody just because they're alive and human' (Jones 2009, p.136).

Case study: Mary-Beatrice

You have been seeing 74-year-old Mary-Beatrice, who has come into the care of the medical ward. Mary-Beatrice lived in a care home but needed to be assessed by the NHS and social services as she was experiencing confusion and disorientation and had had a number of falls.

In hospital, Mary-Beatrice quickly deteriorated and lost weight. She has a son who comes to look after his mother on the ward due to the fact that she was not eating and the hospital staff were not paying this enough attention. The visiting policy is 'only relatives at visiting times', so her son is not allowed to stay all day to make sure she eats. He feels that the staff are not looking after his mother well.

At the end of your last ward round, Mary-Beatrice is in pain and is found shouting for help when her son arrives for a visit. As you explore this further, you find that the son has complained about the treatment of his mother, and on the medication charts it can be seen that no medications have been prescribed or given for pain. The son is requesting to see a doctor, but it will be two weeks before he has the chance to speak with a doctor.

Mary-Beatrice's personal history includes her being a lesbian, and her partner died ten years ago. She suffers from bipolar I disorder, and the only treatment she has received on the ward is psychiatric medication.

Questions:

1. What would you do about this case where screams of pain are being ignored and misinterpreted? How would you assess Mary-Beatrice's needs through the four lenses in a non-discriminatory way?

2. What are the potential implications of your assessment, and what action would you take to implement your care plan?

3. In hindsight, what are the learning points to ensure this does not happen again? What would you consider in developing a care package where Mary-Beatrice is the central focus?

Case study: Rudi

You have been seeing 94-year-old Rudi for two weeks since he came into the care of the medical ward. Rudi lives alone and needs to be assessed by health and social care services. His life partner died 20 years ago, but since then he has had three lovers with whom he meets for sex and companionship. Recently, Rudi has been complaining of pain in his stomach, and it is clear from his hospital admission paperwork that he has been suffering from this for three weeks. In hospital, Rudi wants to see his friends and lovers but not his family, who have ignored him for most of his life. The problem is that the hospital ward's visiting policy states 'only relatives', and so he has to endure seeing his relatives again.

At the end of your last ward round, Rudi states that he is feeling depressed and that he thinks it would be better if he 'ended it all'. As you explore this further, it is clear that Rudi is missing his gay friends and lovers, and he asks to see them. Rudi states clearly that he doesn't want to upset his relatives, but he does not enjoy seeing them; he prefers to see his 'gay family'.

Questions:

1. What would you do in this situation? Can hospital visiting policy be changed? It may be a juggling act to try to meet the

needs of the patient and negotiate your way through 'next of kin' and citizenship rights.

2. What issues will you need to consider if you go with or against Rudi's known wishes?

3. What are the potential implications of your actions?

4. Looking at aftercare, what issues would you need to consider in developing a care package where Rudi is the central focus?

Appendix: Timeline of relevant key events since 1967

Timeline provided with permission by Stonewall.

1967. The Sexual Offences Act came into force in England and Wales and decriminalised homosexual acts between two men over 21 years of age and 'in private'.

1974. The Campaign for Homosexual Law Reform (Northern Ireland) appealed to the European Court of Human Rights to force the UK to extend the 1967 Sexual Offences Act there.

The APA no longer recorded homosexuality as a psychiatric condition in the seventh edition of DSM-II.

1977. Lord Arran's bill to reduce the gay age of consent to 18 was defeated in the House of Lords.

1980. Male homosexuality decriminalised in Scotland.

The European Commission ruled unanimously that the British government was guilty of breaching article 8 of the European Convention on Human Rights by refusing to legalise consenting homosexual behaviour in Ulster.

1982. Male homosexuality was decriminalised in Northern Ireland with the passing of law reform in the House of Commons.

1986. London Borough of Haringey's Lesbian and Gay Unit wrote to all school head teachers in the borough urging them to promote positive images of homosexuality to their pupils. A vicious backlash was provoked.

1988. Section 28 of the Local Government Act, preventing the 'promotion' of homosexuality by local authorities, came into force on 24 May with backing from Minister for Local Government Michael Howard. Protests number 10,000 people in London and 15,000 in Manchester.

1996. Stonewall produced 'Queer Bashing' report and survey results.

Lisa Grant challenged South West Trains for employment discrimination.

The Inland Revenue published new guidelines recognising same-sex partners in pension schemes.

1998. Two British Labour MPs, David Borrow and Gordon Marsden, came out as gay. An overwhelming majority of 336 MPs in the House of Commons voted for an equal age of consent for homosexual and heterosexual people.

Gregory Woods was appointed the first Professor of Lesbian and Gay Studies in the UK.

Nick Brown MP became the first British Cabinet minister to come out publicly as gay while in post.

1999. The House of Lords ruled that same-sex partners should be treated as family and had the right to succeed a tenancy.

The Law Commission proposed that partners of same-sex couples should be able to claim damages in fatal accident cases.

The first Bi Visibility Day was held on 23 September to celebrate bisexual people and challenge biphobia.

2000. The UK government lifts the ban on lesbian women and gay men serving in the armed forces.

2001. Age of consent was reduced to 16.

2004. The Civil Partnership Bill was introduced.

The Sexual Offences Act abolished the crimes of 'buggery' and 'gross indecency'.

Stonewall set up partnerships with Friends and Families of Lesbians and Gays (FFLAG) and Lesbian & Gay Youth Scotland to discuss homophobic bullying in schools.

The Civil Partnership Act was passed in November, giving same-sex couples in civil partnerships the same rights and responsibilities as married heterosexual couples.

2011. The Department of Health lifted the lifetime ban on gay men donating blood. It is now possible for gay men who have not had sex in the last year to donate.

2013. The Marriage (Same-Sex Couples) Act was passed in England and Wales.

Daniel Kawczynski became the first MP in Britain to come out as bisexual.

Stonewall sent rainbow laces to all the professional football clubs in the UK to encourage players to show their commitment to stamping out homophobia from the sport.

Stonewall released research showing that one in six lesbian, gay and bi people in Britain have experienced a hate crime based on their sexual orientation.

Olympic diver Tom Daley came out as being in a same-sex relationship, becoming a YouTube sensation.

References

American Psychiatric Association (1987) *Diagnostic and Statistical Manual of Mental Disorders*. 3rd ed., rev. (DSM-III-R). Arlington, VA: American Psychiatric Association.

Amory, D.P. (1997) '"Homosexuality" in Africa. Commentaries in African Studies: Essays about African social change and the meaning of our professional work.' *A Journal of Opinion 25*, 1, 5–10.

Bayer, R. (1987) *Homosexuality and American Psychiatry: The Politics of Diagnosis*. Princeton, NJ: Princeton University Press.

Billingham, S.E. (2013) *Teach the Children Well: Young Adult Literature and Queer Content*. Working paper, University of Nottingham, Nottingham.

Bradford, J., Ryan, C. and Rothblum, E.D. (1994) 'National lesbian health care survey: Implications for mental health care.' *Journal of Consulting and Clinical Psychology 62*, 228–242.

Bretschneider, J.G. and McCoy, N.L. (1988) 'Sexual interest and behaviour in healthy 80–102 year olds.' *Archives of Sexual Behaviour 17*, 109–129.

Brotman, S., Ryan, B. and Cormier, R. (2003) 'The health and social service needs of gay and lesbian elders and their families in Canada.' *The Gerontologist 43*, 192–202.

Cahill, S., Battle, J. and Meyer, D. (2003) 'Partnering, parenting, and policy: Family issues affecting Black lesbian, gay, bisexual, and transgender (LGBT) people.' Race and Society, 6, 2, 85–98.

Chauncey, G. Jr (1989) 'From Sexual Inversion to Homosexuality: The Changing Medical Conceptualization of Female "Deviance".' In K. Piess and C. Simmons (eds) *Passion and Power: Sexuality in History*. Philadelphia, PA: Temple University Press.

Cook, M. (2011) *A Gay History of Britain: Love and Sex Between Men Since the Middle Ages.* London: Praeger Publishing.

D'Augelli, A. and Grossman, A. (2001) 'Disclosure of sexual orientation, victimization, and mental health among lesbian, gay and bisexual older adults.' *Journal of Interpersonal Violence 16*, 10, 1008–1027.

Deacon, S., Minichiello, V. and Plummer, D., (1995) 'Sexuality and older people: Revisiting the assumptions.' *Educational Gerontology: An International Quarterly*, 21, 5, 497–513.

Dorfman, R., Walters, K., Burke, P., Hardin, I. *et al.* (1995) 'Old, sad and alone: The myth of the aging homosexual.' *Journal of Gerontological Social Work 24*, 29–44.

Ellis, H. (1901) *Studies in the Psychology of Sex: Volume 2: Sexual Inversion.* Philadelphia, PA: F.A. Davis.

Ellis, P.B. (2004) *The Celts: A History.* London: Caroll & Graf.

Ellis, S.J., Bailey, L. and McNeil, J. (2015) 'Trans people's experiences of mental health and gender identity services: A UK study.' *Journal of Gay & Lesbian Mental Health 19*, 1, 4–20.

Equal Ground, Center for International Human Rights of Northwestern University School of Law and Heartland Alliance for Human Needs & Human Rights, Global Initiative for Sexuality and Human Rights (2014) *Human Rights Violations Against Lesbian, Gay, Bisexual, and Transgender (LGBT) People in Sri Lanka: A Shadow Report.* Report submitted for consideration at the 100th session of the Human Rights Committee, March 2014, Geneva, Switzerland.

Fae, J. (2015) 'Changing your name should be a joyous moment, but for many it's a nightmare.' *Guardian*, 19 May. Available at www.theguardian.com/commentisfree/2015/may/19/changing-your-name-nightmare-trans, accessed on 24 September 2016.

Falco, K.L. (1991) *Psychotherapy with Lesbian Clients: Theory into Practice.* New York: Routledge.

Farquhar, C., Bailey, J. and Whittaker, D. (2001) *Are Lesbians Sexually Healthy? A Report of the lLesbian Sexual Behaviour and Health Survey.* London: South Bank University.

Featherstone, M. and Wernick, A. (1995) Images of aging: Cultural representations of later life. Taylor & Francis: US.

Foucault, M. (1990) *The History of Sexuality – Volume I: An Introduction.* Trans. Robert Hurley. New York: Vintage Books.

Fredriksen-Goldsen, K.I., Cook-Daniels, L., Kim, H.-J., Erosheva, E.A. *et al.* (2014) 'Physical and mental health of transgender older adults: An at-risk and underserved population.' *The Gerontologist 54*, 3, 488–500.

Freud, S. (1905) 'Three Essays on the Theory of Sexuality.' In J. Strachey (ed. and trans.) *The Standard Edition of the Complete Psychological Works of Sigmund Freud* (Vol. 7, pp.123–245). London: Hogarth Press.

Gabbay, S. and Wahler, J. (2002) 'Lesbian ageing: Review of the growing literature.' *Journal of Gay and Lesbian Social Services 14*, 3, 1–21.

Grant, J.M., Mottet, L.A. and Tanis, J. (2011) *Injustice at Every Turn: A Report of the National Transgender Survey.* Washington, DC: National Gay and Lesbian Task Force and National Center for Transgender Equality.

Green, J., McGowan, S., Levi, J., Wallbank, R. and Whittle, S., (2011). 'Recommendations from the WPATH consensus process for revision of the DSM diagnosis of gender identity disorders: Implications for human rights.' *International Journal of transgenderism*, 13, 1, 1–4.

Gross, G. and Blundo, R. (2005) 'Viagra: Medical technology constructing aging masculinity.' *Journal of Sociology and Social Welfare 12*, 1, 85–97.

Grossman, A.H. (2006) 'Physical and Mental Health of Older Lesbian, Gay and Bisexual Adults.' In D. Kimmel, T. Rose and S. David (eds) *Lesbian, Gay, Bisexual and Transgender Aging: Research and Clinical Perspectives.* New York: Columbia University Press.

Gruskin, E.P., Greenwood, G.L., Matevia, M., Pollack, L.M. and Bye, L.L. (2007) 'Disparities in smoking between the lesbian, gay and bisexual population and general population in California.' *American Journal of Public Health 97*, 8, 1496–1502.

Heaphy, B. Yip, A.K. and Thompson, D. (2004) 'Aging in a non-heterosexual context.' *Ageing and Society 24*, 881–902.

Herek, G.M. (1990) 'The context of anti-gay violence: Notes on cultural and psychological heterosexism.' *Journal of Interpersonal Violence 5*, 3, 316–333.

Herek, G.M., Gillis, J.R., Cogan, J.C. and Glunt, E.K. (1997) 'Hate crime victimization among lesbian, gay and bisexual adults: Prevalence correlates, and methodological issues.' *Journal of Interpersonal Violence 12*, 195–215.

Herzog, D. (ed.) (2004) *Sexuality and German Fascism*. New York: Berghahn Books.

Higgins, A., Sharek, D., McCann, E., Sheerin, F. *et al.* (2011) 'Visible lives: Identifying the experience and needs of older lesbian, gay people' narratives on health and aged care.' *Journal of Gay and Lesbian Social Services 20*, 167–186.

Hillman, J. and Hinrichsen, G.A. (2014). 'Promoting an affirming, competent practice with older lesbian and gay adults.' *Professional Psychology: Research and Practice*, 45, 4, 269.

Home Office (2014) *Hate Crimes, England and Wales, 2013/14* (HOSB: 02/14). London: Home Office.

Hooker, E. (1957) 'The adjustment of the male overt homosexual.' *Journal of Projective Techniques 21*, 18–31.

Hughes, A.K., Harold, R.D. and Boyer, J.M. (2011) 'Awareness of LGBT aging issues among aging services network providers.' *Journal of Gerontological Social Work 54*, 659–677.

Hughes, M. (2008) 'Imagined futures and communities: Older lesbians and gay people's narrative on health and aged care.' *Journal of Gay and Lesbian Social Services 20*, 167–186.

Jennings, R. (2007) *A Lesbian History of Britain: Love and Sex Between Women Since 1500*. London: Praeger Publishing.

Jones, D.W. (2009) *The Psychology of Jesus: Practical Help for Living in Relationship*. New York: Eveready Letter & Advertising Incorporated.

Jones, E. (1957) *Sigmund Freud: Life and Work (Vol. 3)*. London: Hogarth.

Jones, T.C. and Nystrom, N.M. (2002) 'Looking back, looking forward: Addressing the loves of lesbians 55 and older.' *Journal of Women and Aging 14*, 59–76.

Kimmel, D.C. (1978) 'Adult development and aging: A gay perspective.' Journal of Social Issues 34, 3, 113–130.

Kimmel, D., Rose, T., Orel, N. and Greene, B. (2006) 'Historical Context for Research on Lesbian, Gay, Bisexual and Transgender Aging.' In D. Kimmel, T. Rose and D. Steven (eds) *Lesbian, Gay, Bisexual and Transgender Aging*. New York: Columbia University Press.

King, M. and McKeown, E. (2003) *Mental Health and Social Wellbeing of Gay Men, Lesbians and Bisexuals in England and Wales*. London: Mind.

King, M., Semlyen, J., Tai, S.S., Killaspy, H. *et al.* (2008) 'A systematic review of mental disorder, suicide, and deliberate self harming lesbian, gay and bisexual people.' *BMC Psychiatry 8*, 1, 1–17.

Kinsey, A.C., Pomeroy, W.B. and Martin, C.E. (1948) *Sexual Behaviour in the Human Male*. Philadelphia, PA: WB Saunders.

Knocker, S. (2012) *Perspectives on Ageing: Lesbians, Gay Men and Bisexuals*. York: Joseph Rowntree Foundation.

Krafft-Ebing, R. (2013) *Psychopathia Sexualis: The Classic Study of Deviant Sex*. New York: Skyhorse Publishing.

Licata, S. and Petersen, R.P. (2013) *The Gay Past: A Collection of Historical Essays*. Abingdon: Routledge.

Maguen, S. and Shipherd, J. (2010) 'Suicide risk amongst transgender individuals.' *Psychology and Sexuality 1*, 34–43.

Masini, B.E. and Barrett, H.A. (2008) 'Social support as a predictor of psychological and physical wellbeing and lifestyle in lesbian, gay and bisexual adults aged 50 and over.' *Journal of Gay and Lesbian Social Services 20*, 1/2, 91–110.

Masters, W.H. and Johnson, V.E. (1966) *Human Sexual Response*. Boston: Little, Brown.

McCann, E., Sharek, D., Higgins, A., Sheerin, F. and Glacken, M. (2013) 'Lesbian, gay, bisexual and transgender older people in Ireland: Mental health issues.' *Aging and Mental Health 17*, 3, 358–365.

Meikle, J. (2015) 'NHS treats transgender people as second-class citizens, says watchdog.' *Guardian*, 20 May. Available at www.theguardian.com/society/2015/may/20/nhs-treats-transgender-people-as-second-class-citizens-says-watchdog, accessed on 22 June 2015.

Orel, N.A. (2004) 'Gay, lesbian and bisexual elders: Expressed needs and concerns across focus groups.' *Journal of Gerontological Social Work 43*, 57–77.

Otis, M.D. and Skinner, W.F. (1996) 'Prevalence of victimization and its effects on mental well-being among lesbian and gay people.' *Journal of Homosexuality 30*, 3, 93–121.

Robertson, A.E. (1998) 'The mental health experiences of gay men: a research study exploring gay men's health needs.' *Journal of Psychiatric and Mental Health Nursing,* 5, 1, 33–40.

Robinson, P. (1976) *The Modernization of Sex.* New York: Harper & Row.

Rowe, J. and Kahn, R. (1987) 'Human aging: Usual and successful.' *Science 237,* 143–149.

Sandberg, L. (2008) 'The Old, the Ugly and the Queer: Thinking old age in relation to queer theory.' *Graduate Journal of Social Science 5,* 2, 117–138.

Schope, R.D. (2005) 'Who's afraid of growing old? Gay and lesbian perceptions of aging.' *Journal of Gerontological Social Work 45,* 23–39.

Skinner, W. and Otis, M. (1996) 'Drug and alcohol use among lesbian and gay people in a southern U.S. sample: Epidemiological, comparative, and methodological findings from the Trilogy Project.' *Journal of Homosexuality 30,* 3, 59–92.

Spiegelhalter, D. (2015) *Sex by Numbers: What Statistics Can Tell Us about Sexual Behaviour.* London: Profile and Wellcome Collection.

Stocks, T. (2015) 'To what extent have the rights of transgender people been underrealized in comparison to the rights of lesbian, gay, bisexual, and queer/questioning people in the United Kingdom?' *International Journal of Transgenderism 16,* 1, 1–35.

Stonewall (2011) *Working with Older Lesbian, Gay and Bisexual People.* Available at www.stonewall.org. uk/sites/default/files/older_people_final_lo_res.pdf, accessed on 24 September 2016.

Stonewall (2012) *Lesbian, Gay and Bisexual People in Later Life.* Available at www.stonewall.org.uk/ sites/default/files/LGB_people_in_Later_Life__2011_.pdf, accessed on 19 June 2015.

Stonewall (2013) *Homophobic Hate Crime: The Gay British Crime Survey 2013.* Available at www. stonewall.org.uk/documents/hate_crime.pdf, accessed on 19 June 2015.

Thompson, D. (2014) 'Why persecuting homosexuals is all the rage in the developing world.' *Telegraph,* 31 January. Available at http://blogs.telegraph.co.uk/news/damianthompson/100257632/ why-persecuting-homosexuals-is-all-the-rage-in-the-developing-world, accessed on 22 June 2015.

Tiwari, G. (2013) 'LGBT rights: Colonization and international human rights standards.' *A Contrario ICL,* 31 December. Available at http://acontrarioicl.com/2013/12/31/lgbt-rights-colonisation, accessed on 15 May 2015.

Twigg, J. (2000) *Bathing: The Body and Community Care.* London: Routledge.

UK Network of Sex Work Projects (2008) *Good Practice Guidance. Working with Sex Workers: Outreach.* Available at www.uknswp.org/wp-content/uploads/GPG2.pdf, accessed on 24 September 2016.

Valanis, B.G., Bowen, D.J., Bassford, T., Whitlock, E., Charney, P. and Carter, R.A. (2000) 'Sexual orientation and health: Comparisons in the women's health initiative sample.' *Archives in Family Medicine 9,* 9, 843–853.

Van Wagenen, A., Driskell, J. and Bradford, J. (2013) '"I'm still raring to go": Successful aging among lesbian, gay, bisexual and transgendered older adults.' *Journal of Aging Studies 27,* 1, 1–14.

Varney, J. (2012) *Minorities within Minorities – The Evidence Base Relating to Minority Groups within the LGB&T Community.* London: GLADD and Public Health England.

Wallace, S.P., Cochran, S.D., Durazo, E.M. and Ford, C.L. (2011) *The Health of Ageing Lesbian, Gay and Bisexual Adults in California.* Los Angeles, CA: UCLA Center for Health Policy Research.

Warner, M. (1999) *The Trouble with Normal: Sex, Politics and the Ethics of Queer Life.* Cambridge, MA: Harvard University Press.

Woolf, L.M. (2000) 'Agism.' In P. Roberts (ed.) *Aging.* Pasadena, CA: Salem Press.

Chapter 10

Understanding the Lives of Older Gypsies and Travellers and the Impact of Inequality on their Mental Health

Siobhan Spencer and Pauline Lane

Introduction

This chapter seeks to offer the reader an understanding of the context of the lives of older Gypsies and Travellers and examine some of the key issues that may impact on their mental health. The chapter has been co-written by Siobhan Spencer, who is from the Gypsy community and is in the final stages of her PhD, and Pauline Lane, who is not a Gypsy herself but has worked with community members as a researcher for many years.

As a quick introduction to Gypsy health issues, the authors and Redmark Films have made a short film that you can view here: https://vimeo.com/19265453.

Terminology

Please note that in the UK the term Gypsy is used to describe Romany Gypsies, and this is how the community defines itself, although the word Gypsy (with a capital G) should only be applied to Romany Gypsies (of English, Scottish or Welsh origin). Romany Gypsies and Irish Travellers are both recognised as ethnic groups under British law (see the 1989 ruling on *Commission for Racial Equality v Dutton*);

however, within these ethnic groups each community has its own distinct culture and community languages.

Interestingly, in all European Community documentation the term 'Roma' is used to describe a wide range of communities *including* Gypsies, Travellers and Roma people (European Commission 2012). However, in the UK context, the Roma are usually considered to be more recent migrants, while Gypsies and Travellers have lived in the UK for hundreds of years and have evolved a distinct culture in their own right.

It is important to recognise that although many older Romany Gypsies and Travellers are likely to share similar experiences of social exclusion and discrimination, all elders should be treated as individuals.

Romany Gypsy and Traveller populations in the UK

Studies have estimated that the UK population of Gypsies and Travellers is between 270,000 and 360,000 people (Commission for Racial Equality 2006), with an estimated population of 200,000 Roma people (Brown, Scullion and Martin 2013). In 2011, the national census invited Gypsies and Irish Travellers to identify their ethnicity for the first time, but only 58,000 people identified themselves as belonging to these ethnic groups (Office of National Statistics 2014). These figures are generally considered to be a gross underestimate of the total Gypsy and Traveller population in the UK, as many nomadic community members would not have been offered a census form and, of those who were, many community members would not want to identify their ethnicity for fear of further discrimination (Irish Traveller Movement in Britain 2013).

The impact of government policy on Gypsy and Traveller life

It is impossible to understand the health and social care needs of older Gypsies and Travellers without understanding the context of their lives. The social determinants of their health include the conditions into which they are born and their life experiences, as well as those forces and systems that shape their daily life. For older Gypsies and Travellers, these determinants of health usually include a lifetime of discrimination and social exclusion from the wider settled community, as well as exclusionary policy measures imposed by the state (Equalities and Human Rights Commission 2009; Lane, Spencer and McCready 2012). Historically, being nomadic has always been an important part of Gypsy and Traveller identity, and this way of life continues to play an important role in their families, work and culture today. However, while travelling is part of their cultural heritage, not all Gypsies and Travellers actually travel; many now live on permanent trailer (caravan) sites or in housing. This is not always by choice and is often forced on to people due to issues such as the lack of legal stopping places and/or ill health (Lane, Spencer and Jones 2014).

For centuries, nomadic Gypsies and Travellers have moved around the UK, traditionally using common land as lawful stopping places, but successive governmental laws and policies have reduced access to common land across the UK. Consequently, Gypsies and Travellers have been prevented from stopping at traditional resting places. Historically, the Highways Act 1959 and other legislation uprooted many families from their winter resting quarters, and as a result more Gypsies and Travellers were forced on to the road all year round with very few places to stop legally. In 1968, the Labour government did try to redress the virtual outlawing of Gypsy and Traveller life (Taylor 2013) with the Caravan Sites Act, which required local authorities to provide sites. However, these sites were often located in areas that were unsafe for families – for example, near rubbish dumps, motorways and industrial sites (Commission for Racial Equality 2005; Greenfields 2009; Scottish Parliament 2013).

Sadly, anti-Gypsyism has returned to government policy, and today Gypsy and Traveller families find that there are very few legal places to stop. Many people are forced to resort to unauthorised encampments or simply pulling up on the roadside or in other unsuitable places (Cemlyn *et al.* 2009). This is not good for family life and is especially detrimental for children and for older frail people; roadside stopping offers no facilities (such as running water), and the continued instability and trauma of evictions can often become part of daily life, impacting on mental and physical health (Lane *et al.* 2012). Furthermore, even authorised sites are still not fit for purpose today, and many community members report that they are forced to live in conditions that would not be tolerated for any other sections of society (Hodges and Cemlyn 2013; Lane *et al.* 2014). This clearly has an impact on the health and well-being of older Gypsies. Many older Gypsies and Travellers find that they are no longer able to continue their traditional nomadic life and are often forced into housing (Greenfields and Ryder 2010). For many Gypsies and Travellers (old and young), this can have a serious psychological effect on their mental health (Greenfields and Smith 2010).

In response to government-induced marginalisation, some Gypsies and Travellers have tried to purchase their own land, but evidence shows that this is usually refused:

> [Gypsies' and Travellers'] attempts to obtain planning permission almost always met with failure: statistics quoted by the European Court [found that] 90% of applications made by Gypsies had been refused whereas 80% of all [other] applications had been granted. (Commission for Racial Equality 2005)

In 2015, the government introduced a new policy paper ('Planning Policy for Traveller Sites 2015') that aims to 'redefine who Gypsies or Travellers are for planning purposes' (The Traveller Movement 2015, p.2). The policy states that if a Gypsy or Traveller stops travelling permanently, even due to poor health or old age, they will cease to be considered a Gypsy or Traveller (under planning law), and they will not be eligible to apply for planning permission for a Traveller site. These changes to planning policy will make it harder for Gypsies and Travellers to get planning permission and will force them to travel for periods of the year in order to qualify to live on a permanent authorised Traveller site. The Traveller Movement (2015, p.2) has suggested that this 'will result in an increase in unauthorised encampments and potentially have a detrimental impact on the elderly, disabled, those in poor health, community members' work opportunities and children's education'. So ironically, just at a time when there has been a decrease in local authority site provision and there are few other places to stop, the government is forcing more Gypsies and Travellers on to the road in order to qualify for planning permission. However, it is expected that this policy will be challenged in the High Court (The Traveller Movement 2015).

Social determinants of older Gypsies' and Travellers' health

Older Gypsy and Traveller people have always played an active role in the economic and social lives of their families, and the concept of retirement is not familiar in their culture (Lane *et al.* 2012). Traditionally, working roles might change as people get older, rather than old age being the end of their working life altogether (although this would depend on the nature of work and the health of the person). However, changes to land laws and the lack of stopping places mean that while some elders are still managing to work, there are now very limited opportunities for employment for those forced to live on a permanent site or in bricks-and-mortar accommodation. It is also notable that because of their traditional employment practices (usually casual and seasonal labour), most older Gypsies and Travellers are unlikely to have made sufficient national insurance contributions to enable them to draw a full pension; women in particular are unlikely to have made sufficient contributions towards retirement as their caring roles mean they are likely to have had only casual employment throughout their lifetimes (Equality and Human Rights Commission 2009). Sadly, the Equality and Human Rights Commission (2009) has suggested that due to the high mortality rates in Gypsy and Traveller communities, it is likely that only a few Gypsies and Travellers will become old enough to draw a state pension, and research suggests that Gypsies and Travellers tend to die between 10 and 12 years younger than the general population (Commission for Racial Equality 2004; Parry *et al.* 2004).

Many older Gypsies and Travellers will have faced a lifetime of poverty, social exclusion and racism (Equality and Human Rights Commission 2010), and these factors often impact on their mental and physical health in old age. It is widely recognised that the accumulated conditions and experiences of a person's lifetime (the social determinants of health) can have a serious impact on their health and well-being (Zaidi 2014). For example:

- There is evidence to show that forced evictions can also reduce older Gypsies' and Travellers' access to health care, and the lack of continuity of care can contribute to late diagnosis, poor follow-up and management of chronic illness, as well as exclusion from health promotion and screening programmes (Gill *et al.* 2013; Lane and Tribe 2010). Many older Gypsies and Travellers will face serious issues related to their accommodation; for example, many sites are isolated, which can create problems for older Gypsies and Travellers who might need to access health and social care services (Jones 2010).

- Many Gypsies and Travellers have low levels of literacy (Dawson 2004; Greenfields 2008), and this can make it very difficult for older people to navigate the health and social care systems. Older people may need support with filling in forms, and they may benefit from advocacy services as they are often unfamiliar with medical processes and terminology.

- Many Gypsies and Travellers report that they find it difficult to access health services because they do not have proof of identity or a permanent address. GP surgeries will often only register them as temporary patients, which can have an impact on the continuity of care as well as health screening (Lane *et al.* 2014). As a consequence, many Gypsies and Travellers are forced to access the NHS through hospital accident and emergency departments (Hall, Sadouni and Fuller 2009).

Before moving on to look more specifically at mental health issues, it is important to recognise that in addition to discrimination by the state, most Gypsies and Travellers will have faced a lifetime of racial discrimination (Lane *et al.* 2014). A number of small studies have highlighted some horrific incidents of racism, such as arson and gang attacks (London Gypsy and Traveller Unit 2001), and widespread discrimination and racist abuse from neighbours (Shelter 2007). However, it is important to recognise that racism against Gypsies and Travellers is not just a small local issue. Both the European Court of Human Rights (2016) and the Council of Europe (2011) have drawn attention to the fact that, right across the UK, Gypsies and Travellers routinely face discrimination that can involve violent and even fatal physical attacks (Equality and Human Rights Commission 2009). The European Commission (2013) has also noted that the UK media often acts as a catalyst for intolerance and discrimination and has a significant impact on the public understanding of Gypsy and Traveller communities. As ethnic groups, Gypsies and Travellers are often subject to personal racist attacks, community-level racist attitudes as well as institutional racism (Lane *et al.* 2014), and clearly this can have an impact on their mental health. Yet as Sashidharan (1993) suggests, when looking at the correlation between ethnic groups and mental illness there is risk of pathologising ethnic groups rather than looking at the inequality in power and the racism that are inherent in many societies. Therefore, when considering older people's mental health issues, it is important to reflect on the context of their life and experiences as well as any organic causes of mental illness.

Meeting the mental health needs of older Gypsies and Travellers

Before discussing older people's mental health needs, it is important to note that the Department of Health does not collect any ethnic data on Gypsies and Travellers, so they are not represented in national or local health statistics (despite being legally recognised ethnic groups). Consequently, there is no national data on the mental health of older Gypsies and Travellers and only very few studies on the mental health of Gypsies and Travellers in general. The mental health needs of older people are rarely mentioned in the literature.

Clearly, the social determinants that impact on a person's physical health can also influence their psychological health. Research suggests the following:

- Gypsy and Traveller communities are believed to have rates of anxiety and depression many times greater than the population average, and with this they have higher suicide rates (Equality and Human Rights Commission 2009; Goward *et al.* 2006).

- Bereavement is a very common precipitating factor in depression for Gypsies and Travellers, which perhaps is not surprising due to the high mortality rates in these communities. Excessive alcohol consumption is sometimes reported alongside depression following bereavement (Parry *et al.* 2004).

- In some Gypsy and Traveller communities, drug dependency is also found to be an increasingly serious problem, which is often exacerbated by social exclusion (Fountain 2006).

- Without a permanent address, many older Gypsies and Travellers (in common with other family members as mentioned) will face challenges in accessing mental health services through a GP. Even if they are registered, many older people will still find it difficult to trust professionals and talk about mental health concerns. There is often a fear among Gypsies and Travellers that service providers will not respect their culture and concerns (Jones 2010). A number of studies have reported hostility or prejudice from healthcare providers, and clearly this can have an impact on the families' help-seeking behaviour (Greenfields 2008; Lane *et al.* 2014; Van Cleemput *et al.* 2007).

- Most Gypsies and Travellers will have little knowledge of mental health services and will often be unaware of talking therapies (Derbyshire Gypsy Liaison Group 2008). There is often a reluctance to contact outside agencies for help, which is hardly surprising given their past negative experiences with authorities. Mental health services are often perceived as only for those who have 'completely lost it', and they are frequently viewed with suspicion (Bristol Mind 2008, p.1). Research also suggests that the 'rules' set up by many health and social care professionals (i.e. that the patient should turn up on time, and that people should attend appointments on their own and not with the whole family) mean that mental health services and particularly talking therapies are often not seen as appropriate for their cultural needs (Goward *et al.* 2006).

- Most mental health services seem to be constructed around the needs of the individual rather than families or communities (Goward *et al.* 2006), which means that services often fail to meet the needs of Gypsy and Traveller people, who tend to live in extended families and depend on each other (Lau and Ridge 2011). Individual therapy also fails to address the multiple levels of social exclusion experienced by many older Gypsies and Travellers, where the social context of their lives need to be challenged in order to address many of the social causes of mental health problems.

Within most Gypsy and Traveller families, in common with many other cultural groups, mental health issues are often seen as difficult to discuss, and, culturally, it is more acceptable to use the term 'nerves' rather than mental health (Derbyshire Gypsy Liaison Group 2008). Research suggests the following:

- While individual Gypsies and Travellers may hold different health beliefs, in general these health beliefs tend to be fairly fatalistic (Van Cleemput *et al.* 2007), and this may mean that older people delay seeking help for mental health concerns (Parry *et al.* 2004).

- There is also a strong element of self-reliance and stoicism in many Gypsy and Traveller families, born outside or on the fringes of a hostile society (Atterbury and Bruton 2011). This can be a positive trait, but it may also delay families in seeking help or support for mental health problems (Treise and Shepherd 2006). This can result in late diagnosis and treatment, which can have an impact on people's recovery journey.

Taking people's health beliefs and practices into account is important in delivering anti-discriminatory practice. In the following, Spencer, Page and Dawson (2009) offer a good example of how small things can make a difference to the health and comfort of older Gypsies and Travellers.

Culture and hygiene

It might be useful for practitioners to have some understanding of the concept of *Mochadi*. This Gypsy concept is similar to issues concerning cleanliness and cultural taboos in Kosher law in the Jewish community, as it relates to many aspects of daily life. For example, many Romany Gypsy people will not use a toilet or sink in a caravan, and many older Gypsy people will not tolerate a toilet being located inside the trailer (caravan) due to cultural taboos. Even if they are extremely frail, they will endure the struggle to use the facilities outside. However, many older people will not want to discuss toilet-related aids, as this will be seen as a personal and private issue, so it might be useful to have a discussion with a community advocate first.

This issue of hygiene is also important in hospital care. One of the authors of this chapter (Siobhan Spencer) reflects on her experience of an old Gypsy man who nearly starved in hospital because of hygiene concerns. During his stay, the nurse would often place his bedpan on the bedside table and a few minutes later his food would arrive and be placed on the same table. Consequently, he refused hospital food and would only eat what his wife and daughters brought into the hospital. (Adapted from Spencer *et al.* 2009.)

Bricks-and-mortar accommodation and the impact on mental health

One of the biggest issues that can have an impact on the mental health of older Gypsies and Travellers is a change of accommodation from living in a trailer (caravan) to living in bricks-and-mortar accommodation. This change may be prompted by a number of factors, but for many older people it is caused by poor health itself or a lack of suitable stopping places. Yet research by Parry *et al.* (2004) details how Gypsies and Travellers report that those who live in houses have significantly higher levels of anxiety symptoms compared with those who live in trailers. Moving into bricks-and-mortar accommodation or a care home often means that older Gypsies and Travellers have to move away from their extended family, community and familiar living site. While some people do adapt to living in bricks and mortar, for others, this significant change and social isolation from their loved ones leads to distress, including severe depression and occasionally suicide (Cullen, Hayes and Hughes 2008). Most bricks-and-mortar accommodation is not designed to meet the cultural needs of Gypsies and Travellers. For example, the location of sleeping areas, kitchens and toilets all have cultural taboos associated with them, and a failure to address these concerns may mean that the older person is not able to settle in (Derbyshire Gypsy Liaison Group 2008).

Certainly there may be times when an older family member needs to move into a care home (e.g. in the case of severe and advanced dementia). However, this can have a deep impact on the families who have to make that decision. Many families may not talk about the fact that they have had to access help or place their relative in a care home as they may feel that they have failed that relative. Families may try to remain living near to their older relative, but stopping laws and the lack of trailer sites often prevent this from happening.

Case study: A Gypsy family adapting to the cultural needs of older relatives who now live in bricks-and-mortar accommodation

One Gypsy family was caring for two elderly aunts who were now living in a house because one aunt had dementia and the other was very frail. However, the aunts found it difficult to settle in the house having spent all of their lives on the road. The family managed to meet their needs by locating a trailer (caravan) in the garden of the house. The older ladies slept in the house, but during the day they lived in the trailer in the garden, and this made them feel much happier. In this way the family were able to maintain the mental and physical health needs of their aunts and also meet their cultural needs.

If older people are moving into bricks-and-mortar accommodation, it may be useful to have some understanding of the Romany Gypsy belief in the *Muller Mush*. The *Muller Mush* is the belief that, after a person dies, their spirit lingers in this world until the personal belongings of the deceased person are destroyed. This usually happens through burning their belongings, though traditionally it involved burning the person's caravan with its contents inside. Belief in the *Muller Mush* is very strong in the older generation, who often find themselves forced into bricks-and-mortar accommodation. Romany Gypsy elders often believe that bricks-and-mortar housing could have a ghost of the previous tenant living in it, who has not yet been put to rest as the belongings have not been destroyed. This belief can manifest itself very strongly and can be very real to the person involved, but it is often misunderstood by health professionals who assume that the person is suffering from hallucinations or psychosis (Derbyshire Gypsy Liaison Groups 2008). The situation can often be relieved by telling the residents about who has been living in the house before them. However, this does not always alleviate the distress, and practitioners should be understanding of this belief and the need to move out of the accommodation. An additional consequence of this belief is that when a family member dies in a house, some Gypsy or Traveller families will feel that they need to move out as quickly as possible. For practitioners working with Gypsy families, it may be useful to discuss this with the family before an older family member is moved into new accommodation.

The resilience of older Gypsy and Traveller people

Older people play an important role in the family and community, and sharing their experiences can be particularly important for the young, as most older adults have a lifetime of practice in managing racism and discrimination and learning how to stand up for their rights. A report on the experiences of older Gypsies (Lane *et al.* 2012) suggests that while many older people do reflect on their experiences of discrimination over their lifetime, they also reflect on their resilience. For example, two older Gypsies describe their experiences and reflections:

> It is not always easy being a Gypsy; we have times when we have had to barricade to protect ourselves. I remember once they came

with a bulldozer and dogs but we managed to stop them because we were living there legally. (Uncle Sam, Gypsy elder, cited in Lane *et al.* 2012, p.7)

Sometimes they even take your trailer, your home. It is because there is nowhere to go. It is just not safe to stop. They think we have no rights and they think we don't know about rights. When you talk to different people they seem shocked that we know that we have rights. (Aunt Mary, Gypsy elder, cited in Lane *et al.* 2012, p.7)

Research suggests that many families from minority communities help their young people to develop protective strategies against discrimination by teaching them how to anticipate and cope with discrimination (Demo and Hughes 1990). They argue that this approach may protect their young people from the associated negative psychological consequences of discrimination (Phinney and Chavira 1995) and so the experience of older Gypsies and Travellers is usually valued in the community. In addition, older family members are the guardians of family histories and community values, and their role may therefore become increasingly significant as many younger Gypsies and Travellers are now denied the opportunity to travel freely and experience life on the road as lived by their ancestors.

Caring and intergenerational reciprocity

The kind of access that we have to social support systems can influence our health outcomes. It has been suggested that one of the advantages of living in communities is that they offer high levels of social capital, such as mutual dependency, high reciprocity and caring (Putnam 1995), and this may protect against many social stressors (Kawachi and Berkman 2001). Certainly, Gypsies and Travellers traditionally prefer to live in extended family settings, and it is well documented that younger family members generally offer care and support to older relatives; this is a source of pride for many older people as it acts as a demonstration of cultural values of reciprocity and respect (Clark and Greenfields 2006; Jesper, Griffiths and Smith 2008).

In the past, when the whole family was mobile, older Gypsies and Travellers would have been able to make more choices about how they lived their lives, but now many elders are stuck living on permanent sites. Consequently, many older people feel trapped and unable to return to their nomadic life, yet they are also unable to live together with extended families as many of the permanent sites are very small. However, Gypsies and Travellers have always offered each other a high level of intergenerational support, and so loneliness and isolation are not common features of ageing in Gypsy and Traveller families (Lane *et al.* 2012). However, it is notable that in most families it is usually the women (particularly unmarried or single women) who provide most of the practical support to their older family members.

Significantly, while research suggests that site availability restrictions can affect people's ability to offer or receive support (Cemlyn *et al.* 2009), data from the last national census (Office for National Statistics 2014) indicated that Gypsies and Travellers provide some of the highest levels of unpaid care in England and Wales, with 4 per cent providing an average of 50 hours per week or more of unpaid care work compared to 2 per cent for the region as a whole. Research also suggests that most of these family carers have little or no knowledge of how external agencies can help to organise packages of care for their older adults, and many carers do not know how to search for support or navigate the referral pathways (Minority Ethnic Carers of Older People Project in Scotland 2013). One local study suggests that many Gypsy and Traveller carers struggle on very low incomes:

> In one family the husband was partially sighted, diabetic and had heart problems. His wife was his carer, but she was also caring for her mother who has dementia, who lives in a trailer a few doors up. Their 16-year-old son is a young carer for his grandmother at night and sleeps in her trailer and does jobs for her in the day when he can before and after school. They did not know what financial benefits or other services were available to them. (West Sussex Local Involvement Network 2010, p.5)

Greenfields and Ryder (2010) also suggest that many Gypsy families design their working lives around the needs of their elders 'so that parents and grandparents are supported at all times' (p.103). However, many family members find that planning laws impact on how they can organise care and support for their relatives as they are often not allowed to stay on the same site or even on sites near to their relatives due to planning restrictions (Home and Greenfields 2006).

So in terms of promoting anti-discriminatory practice, it is possible that initiatives such as direct payment and personal budgets may have the potential to offer greater choice and flexibility to older Gypsies and Travellers and their carers. However, due to low levels of literacy and a lack of understanding of how social care support works, it is unlikely that Gypsy and Traveller older people and their carers are aware of any potential sources of support (Equality and Human Rights Commission 2009).

Case study: Choice and control – Using personal budgets

Hester (76) and her husband, Jake (77), had moved from their trailer into housing as a result of serious health problems. The adjustment was difficult, and the couple missed having their grandchildren and other family around them. Because Jake had a disability and Hester had a chronic health condition, they were assessed as needing home care support. However, the couple were very unhappy with the agency carers as different people seemed to come through the door every day and no one seemed to have any insight into their needs as Gypsies, particularly concerning issues around personal care, such as washing.

Hester started to become more withdrawn and quiet. Eventually, Jake mentioned this to their social worker and admitted that he was worried that Hester was having trouble with her nerves (i.e. mental health). The social worker talked with them for a while, and he told them about personal budgets and helped them to fill out the forms. They were able to use their personal budget to employ a Gypsy friend to come and be their carer instead of using a care agency. Hester's mental health improved, as the new carer not only met their cultural care needs but also kept them in touch with local Gypsy news.

While there is very limited research on the mental health of Gypsies and Travellers (and almost none of the mental health needs of older Gypsies and Travellers), the message from the literature is nonetheless clear: the most significant social determinant for mental health, and the biggest threat to social inclusion, is the issue of accommodation and access to safe stopping places for older Gypsies and Travellers. Many of the inequalities that older Gypsies and Travellers face originate in the wider political issue of land ownership, land enclosure and governmental planning policies, as well as racism and other forms of social exclusion. All of these factors can have profound effects on older people's physical and mental health.

Insight: Aunt Louisa May in conversation with Siobhan Spencer

This case study has the permission of the participant, but her name and some identifying features have been changed.

Louisa May has lived on a local authority site for over 15 years, and she has not been able to travel due to her own and her husband's ill health. Now aged 72, Louisa May lost her husband nine years ago. Sadly, she had only just managed to obtain a carer's allowance after struggling to care for him for eight years. He had been trying to keep working but had developed a type of diabetes that was extremely hard to manage, along with other complications. After passing away unexpectedly, there was an autopsy, which the family did not want because it delayed the funeral, and Louisa May found this very stressful. (It was instilled into us as children that burial should happen on the fourth day after death and not later.) She has two daughters; one lives over 200 miles away, but luckily she has her other daughter on site with her. Her two daughters-in-law are also very good to her. (In the Gypsy tradition, wives often join their husbands' families.) They help Louisa May's daughter with her own care needs as she herself had previously suffered two heart attacks.

Talking about her life, Louisa May reflected on her days on the road compared with life on the site:

> I gets lonely on here. I don't see the people I used to see. Drives me mad looking at that gateway all day. I remember a time when we could pull into a fresh green field, you could smell the freshness of the grass, now look where we end up. Still, it is somewhere to stop. I'm lucky I've got my gal here but a few years ago I was very depressed, very, very depressed, after everything that happened, you know, don't you?

Louisa May often made reference to her husband's death and how it had come out of the blue and had not been expected. She would not qualify exactly what she meant by using his name. I was always brought up with the belief that you did not mention the name of anyone who had passed away unless the family specifically brought up the person's name. So I just nodded as she spoke, and she went on to reflect on life on the site: 'These sites to me are like the reservations, just like the Indians, but we've got to have 'em.'

I had a general chat with Louisa, and we both agreed that things were better years ago, but life was stressful for other reasons. Some families have recently been struggling with their youngsters dabbling in drugs. The 'psychedelic' period of the 1960s and 1970s passed the Romany Gypsy people by; we were happy, but now it seems that drugs have got hold of some of the young people with a vengeance.

Talking with Louisa May, it seemed that there were many things in her pot:

- bereavement, which happened suddenly and came as a shock to all the family even though her husband had not been very well

- the passing of the old way of life that appeared better (although on reflection there were bad things in the past as well!)

- worry over the modern lifestyle, modern influences and loss of the old ways (and this is no different to any household in the UK)

- concern about young people and drugs in our community (many community members will not talk about it, as our community is already discriminated against and there is a fear of being viewed as being in a 'lower than the low' position, and so the problems are often not addressed).

Recently, Louisa May had disability adaptations made to her plot, and this has made her daily life a bit easier. This is a positive aspect of paying to live on a local authority site; however, other Gypsy people with private sites have often found it difficult to access funding for disability adaptations, and there is a lack of knowledge around this subject in the community. In terms of resilience, Gypsy people have always adapted, and Louisa May has her family around her, and she has some social life in going out to the 'ladies-only night' at the local bingo club. Occasionally she will go to a Born Again Christian meeting. Spiritual beliefs can often help people deal with life stresses. Some community members have got a lot out of the Born Again church – it has assisted with tackling alcoholism and other social ills – but others decry it, saying that it has eroded Gypsy culture. However, Louisa once said to me:

> You know, my gal, that *rashai* [preacher] was really good last night. It was a good sermon. You know it's a sin to do *dukkerin* [fortune telling], you know that's the *butsi* [work] of the *beng* [devil] that! But I'm alright, sister, cos I'm a prophet.

Wonderfully adapted, I feel. So Louisa May manages to adapt as life throws her fresh challenges.

Questions:

1. What do you think are the key challenges that Louisa May is facing in her daily life?

2. If Louisa needed to be moved into a care home due to failing health, what practical steps could you take with the staff to make sure the transition into bricks and mortar was made easier for her?

3. Self-awareness is often seen as an integral part of many cultural competence frameworks. How can you develop more cultural competence about the mental health needs of older Gypsies and Travellers?

4. In recent years there has been a deepening understanding of institutional racism. Are there any processes or structures in the organisation that employs you that might continue to promote discrimination against older Gypsies and Travellers?

Promoting anti-discriminatory practice in mental health services for older Gypsies and Travellers

Understanding the underlying determinants of health and inequities among older Gypsies and Travellers is important. While many local public-sector services 'include' the needs of Gypsies and Travellers in their policy documents (such as their Joint Strategic Needs Assessments), in practice these needs are often neglected, and the voices of older Gypsies and Travellers are very rarely heard. They are often an invisible population within an already marginalised community (Equality and Human Rights Commission 2009). Older Gypsies and Travellers will be living in your area, and 'just because they are not using your services does not mean that they are not there' (Jones 2010, p.7). In terms of promoting anti-discriminatory practice, there are many things that professionals can do, and some of these are outlined below.

Offering appropriate accommodation

As suggested above, poor living conditions and environmental factors are the single most influential contributing factor to the poor health status of all Gypsies and Travellers. This makes partnership working between the different agencies really important, including the Clinical Commissioning Groups, local authorities, Housing and Environmental Health, and Gypsy and Traveller organisations.

Working in partnership with Gypsy and Traveller community groups

Gypsy and Traveller community groups have a very valuable role as they can often speak *for* their communities as well as *about* them. They also represent a substantial body of expertise. Consulting and working in partnership with local groups is important in both sharing cultural knowledge and information and developing appropriate services. Good communication can help to build trust between agencies and Gypsy and Traveller communities. Local Gypsy elders are 'experts by experience' and they can help to shape and improve local services.

Including Gypsy and Traveller elders in the public sector Equality Duty

The effective use of equality legislation can also help to ensure that older Gypsies and Travellers gain access to public-sector services as well as to welfare benefits (such as Attendance Allowance or Carer's Allowance). The Equality Act 2010 requires local authorities to take steps to ensure that the views of Gypsy and Traveller older people (and others with protected characteristics) are heard and are part of any Equality Impact Assessment when developing or reviewing policies. The public sector Equality Duty (2011) means that local authorities must eliminate discrimination and victimisation, advance equality of opportunity between persons, and foster good relations between people. Health and social care professionals have an important role in ensuring that this is happening.

Working with the family, not just the individual

Practitioners can help older Gypsy and Traveller people by acknowledging that they belong to communities with great cultural and family resources as well as individually having assets of resilience that can be built on. The role of the practitioner is to enable older Gypsy and Traveller people to continue to live the kind of life that they value, and this will usually involve the whole family, not just the individual.

Using direct payments to support cultural needs

With the development of self-directed support and the personalisation agenda, professionals can explore different ways to provide appropriate care for older people from Gypsy and Traveller communities. This means that there is some potential for Gypsy and Traveller groups to develop and commission their own services, which would be more culturally appropriate. However, due to low levels of literacy and a lack of understanding of how social care support works, most families will need support from practitioners in applying for personal budgets.

Improving access to mental health services

Planning laws and the lack of adequate stopping places mean that many Gypsies and Travellers find it difficult to register with GP surgeries without a permanent address. GP surgeries have a legal duty not to discriminate against individuals with characteristics protected under the Equality Act 2010, and they should therefore adapt their systems to accommodate better access.

Professional development

Education, information and training are required to reduce discrimination and increase existing support to meet the mental health needs of Gypsies and Travellers. Many national Gypsy and Traveller organisations are able to arrange cultural trainers to work with practitioners.

Supporting the practical needs of older Gypsies and Travellers

Trailer sites and houses often need adaptations and disability access to take into account the needs of older Gypsies and Travellers and to help to maintain personal care. However, many older people will not be aware of what is available or how to apply for adaptations, and practitioners may need to explain the process and offer help with filling in the appropriate forms.

Developing culturally appropriate health information

Gypsy and Traveller communities need more information, support, training and advice on mental health issues, especially concerning the mental health of older people (including information on recognising dementia). A high proportion of community members have very low levels of literacy, so there is a need for materials to be developed in partnership with community organisations to ensure that information is culturally appropriate. It is useful to use neutral language in leaflets, such as 'memory problems' rather than 'dementia', and 'nerves' rather than 'mental health' or 'mental illness'. Due to low levels of literacy across the community, there is also a need for accessible materials, such as DVDs.

The Derbyshire Gypsy Liaison Group have produced a number of easy-read health resources for community members, available here: www.dglg.org/health-publications.html. They also have a publication on older people entitled *Shoon te o Puri Folki* (Listen to the Elders) (Derbyshire Gypsy Liaison Group 2009).

The Traveller Movement have developed an online video about mental health, available here: www.youtube.com/watch?v=WcDK9ZLZg-k

Developing inclusive services

The Health and Wellbeing Boards need to ensure that Gypsies and Travellers are included as local stakeholders. These boards will be relying on the local Joint Strategic Needs Assessments to inform their work. It is therefore critical that local Gypsy and Traveller health assessments are conducted and that these communities are fully involved in this process.

Gill *et al.* (2013) have developed an evidence-based commissioning guide, which emphasises best practice in delivering services to Gypsies and Travellers, available here: http://bit.ly/JDCK75.

Leeds GATE have produced a short film, *Dying at Fifty*, that looks at the life expectancy of Gypsies and Travellers: www.youtube.com/watch?v=iScu8ywM0nQ

Addressing discrimination

While the UK government has adopted policy measures to eliminate hate speech, a clearer strategy is needed to take action against the media or individuals that incite discrimination and racism against Gypsy and Traveller communities and individuals. Any media outlet that incites direct or indirect discrimination, hatred or violence against these communities should be condemned, and legal action should be taken.

Building community capacity

Although many Gypsy and Traveller community groups are starting to build their expertise, a lot of these groups will need some support from non-Gypsy/Traveller professionals, especially in areas of welfare advice (such as applying for Universal Credits or Personal Independence Payments). Some local Gypsy support groups give mental health support by phone and drop-ins. This is undertaken in a holistic way; for example, the Derbyshire Gypsy Liaison Group has a good-to-talk phone line and signposting service.

Commissioning for mental health to include older Gypsies and Travellers

A recent cost–benefit analysis demonstrated that an improved health and social care pathway not only offers clear benefits to Gypsy and Traveller people themselves but delivers greatly reduced costs to health and social care services (Leeds GATE 2013). Commissioners should ensure that non-discriminatory practices are included in commissioning contracts.

References

Atterbury, J. and Bruton, L. (2011) *DRE West Sussex Black and Ethnic Minorities CDW Service.* OFFT Final report, January 2011.

Bristol Mind (2008) *Do Gypsies, Travellers and Show People Get the Support They Need with Stress Depression and Nerves? Findings from a Research Project by Bristol Mind.* Presentation to the West of England Gypsy, Traveller and Show People Forum, February 2008.

Brown, P., Scullion, L. and Martin, P. (2013) *Migrant Roma in the United Kingdom: Population Size and Experiences of Local Authorities and Partners.* Salford: University of Salford. Available at www.salford.ac.uk/__data/assets/pdf_file/0004/363118/Migrant_Roma_in_the_UK_final_report_October_2013.pdf, accessed on 24 September 2016.

Cemlyn, S., Greenfields, M., Burnett, S., Matthews, Z. and Whitwell, C. (2009) *Inequalities Experienced by Gypsy and Traveller Communities: A Review.* Research Report 12. Manchester: Equality and Human Rights Commission.

Clark, C. and Greenfields, M. (2006) *Here to Stay: The Gypsies and Travellers of Britain.* Hatfield: University of Hertfordshire Press.

Commission for Racial Equality (2004) *Gypsies and Travellers: A Strategy for the CRE 2004–2007.* London: CRE.

Commission for Racial Equality (2005) 'Gypsies and Travellers: Britain's forgotten minority.' *European Human Rights Law Review 10,* 335–343.

Commission for Racial Equality (2006) *Common Ground: Equality, Good Race Relations and Sites for Gypsies and Irish Travellers. Report of a CRE Inquiry in England and Wales.* London: CRE. Available at www.lancsngfl.ac.uk/projects/ema/download/file/commonground_report.pdf, accessed on 6 November 2016.

Council of Europe (2011) *Human Rights in Europe: No Grounds for Complacency.* Strasbourg: Council of Europe. Available at www.coe.int/t/commissioner/source/prems/HR-Europe-no-grounds-complacency_en.pdf#page=46, accessed on 6 November 2016.

Cullen, S., Hayes, P. and Hughes, L. (2008) *Good Practice Guide: Working with Housed Gypsies and Travellers.* London: Shelter. Available at http://england.shelter.org.uk/__data/assets/pdf_file/0010/57772/Working_with_housed_Gypsies_and_Travellers.pdf, accessed on 6 November 2016.

Dawson, R. (2004) *Literacy Levels amongst 300 Travelling People.* Blackwell: Derbyshire Gypsy Liaison Group.

Demo, D.H. and Hughes, M. (1990) 'Socialization and racial identity among Black Americans.' *Social Psychology Quarterly 53,* 364–374.

Derbyshire Gypsy Liaison Group (2008) *'I Know When It's Raining': Report of the Community-Led Research Project Focussing on the Emotional Health and Well-Being Needs of Romany Gypsies and Irish Travellers in the East Midlands Region.* NIMHE Mental Health Programme.

Derbyshire Gypsy Liaison Group (2009) *Shoon te o Puri Folki* (Listen to the Elders). Matlock: Robert Dawson.

Equality and Human Rights Commission (2009) *Inequalities Experienced by Gypsy and Traveller communities: A Review.* Research Report 12. Manchester: Equality and Human Rights Commission.

Equality and Human Rights Commission (2010) *Assessing Local Authorities' Progress in Meeting the Accommodation Needs of Gypsy and Traveller Communities in England and Wales.* Research Report 68. Manchester: Equality and Human Rights Commission.

European Commission (2012) *Communication from the Commission to the European Parliament, the Council, the European Economic and Social Committee and the Committee of the Regions National Roma Integration Strategies: a First Step in the Implementation of the EU Framework.* Available at http://eur-lex.europa.eu/legal-content/EN/ALL/?uri=CELEX:52012DC0226, accessed on 6 November 2016.

European Court of Human Rights (2016) *Factsheet – Roma and Travellers.* Available at www.echr.coe.int/Documents/FS_Roma_ENG.pdf, accessed on 6 November 2016.

Fountain, J. (2006) *An Overview of the Nature and Extent of Illicit Drug Use amongst the Traveller Community: An Exploratory Study.* Dublin: National Advisory Committee on Drugs.

Gill, P., MacLeod, U., Lester, H. and Hegenbarth, A. (2013) *Improving Access to Health Care for Gypsies and Travellers, Homeless People and Sex Workers: An Evidence-based Commissioning Guide for Clinical Commissioning Groups and Health & Wellbeing Boards.* London: RCGP/Inclusion Health. Available at http://bit.ly/JDCK75, accessed on 24 September 2016.

Goward, P., Repper, J., Appleton, L. and Hagan, T. (2006) 'Crossing boundaries: Identifying and meeting the mental health needs of Gypsies and Travellers.' *Journal of Mental Health 15,* 315–327.

Greenfields, M. (2008) 'Accommodation needs of Gypsies/Travellers: New approaches to policy in England.' *Social Policy and Society 7,* 1, 73–89.

Greenfields, M. (2009) 'Reaching Gypsies and Travellers.' *Primary Health Care 19,* 8, 26–27.

Greenfields, M. and Ryder, A. (2010) '"Being with Our Own Kind": The Contexts of Gypsy–Traveller Elders' Social and Leisure Engagement.' In B. Humberstone (ed.) *Third Age and Leisure Research: Principles and Practice.* Eastbourne: Leisure Studies Association.

Greenfields, M. and Smith, D. (2010) 'A question of identity: The social exclusion of housed Gypsies and Travellers.' *Research, Policy and Planning 28*, 3.

Hall, V., Sadouni, M. and Fuller, A. (2009) *Gypsies' and Travellers' Experience of Using Urgent Care Services within NHS Brighton and Hove Boundaries: April 2008–August 2009*. Brighton: University of Brighton. Available at www.gypsy-traveller.org/wp-content/uploads/2012/02/fft_ae_report. pdf, accessed on 25 September 2016.

Hodges, N. and Cemlyn, S. (2013) 'The accommodation experiences of older Gypsies and Travellers: Personalisation of support and coalition policy.' *Social Policy and Society 12*, 2, 205–219.

Home, R. and Greenfields, M. (2006) *The Dorset Gypsy, Traveller, Accommodation and Other Needs Assessment (GTAA)*. Chelmsford: Anglia Ruskin University.

Irish Traveller Movement in Britain (2013) *Gypsy and Traveller Population in England and the 2011 Census*. London: ITMB. Available at www.travellermovement.org.uk/wp-content/uploads/2014/03/ Gypsy-and-Traveller-population-in-England-policy-report.pdf, accessed on 25 September 2016.

Jesper, E., Griffiths, F. and Smith, L. (2008) 'A qualitative study of the health experience of Gypsy Travellers in the UK with a focus on terminal illness.' *Primary Health Care Research and Development 9*, 2, 157–165.

Jones, A. (2010) *Working with Older Gypsies and Travellers: A Briefing for Local Age UKs/Age Concerns*. London: Age UK.

Kawachi, L. and Berkman, L. (2001) 'Social ties and mental health.' *Journal of Urban Health 78*, 3, 458–467.

Lane, P. and Tribe, R. (2010) 'Towards an understanding of the cultural health needs of older Gypsies.' *Working with Older People 14*, 2, 23–30.

Lane, P., Spencer, S. and Jones, A. (2014) *Gypsy, Traveller and Roma: Experts by Experience. Reviewing UK Progress on the European Union Framework for National Roma Integration Strategies*. Chelmsford: National Federation of Gypsy Liaison Groups and Anglia Ruskin University.

Lane, P., Spencer, S. and McCready, M. (2012) *Perspectives on Ageing in Gypsy Families*. York: Joseph Rowntree Foundation Trust.

Lau, A. and Ridge, M. (2011) 'Addressing the impact of social exclusion on mental health in Gypsy, Roma, and Traveller communities.' *Mental Health and Social Inclusion 15*, 3, 129–137.

Leeds GATE (2013) *'Gypsy and Traveller Health – Who Pays?' Health Pathways: Cost-Benefits Analysis Report*. Leeds: Leeds Gypsy and Traveller Exchange (GATE).

London Gypsy and Traveller Unit (2001) *Housed Irish Travellers in North London*. London: London Gypsy and Traveller Unit.

Minority Ethnic Carers of Older People Project in Scotland (2013) *Hidden Carers, Unheard Voices: Informal Caring within the Gypsy/Traveller Community in Scotland*. Edinburgh: Minority Ethnic Carers of Older People Project in Scotland.

Office for National Statistics (2014) *2011 Census Analysis: What Does the 2011 Census Tell Us about the Characteristics of Gypsy or Irish Travellers in England and Wales?* London: ONS. Available at www.ons.gov.uk/peoplepopulationandcommunity/culturalidentity/ethnicity/articles/what doesthe2011censustellusaboutthecharacteristicsofgypsyoririshtravellersinenglandandwales/ 2014-01-21, accessed on 6 November 2016.

Parry, G., Van Cleemput, P., Peters, J., Walters, S., Thomas, K. and Cooper, C. (2004) *The Health Status of Gypsies and Travellers in England*. Report of Department of Health Inequalities in Health Research Initiative Project 121/7500. Sheffield: University of Sheffield.

Phinney, J.S. and Chavira, V. (1995) 'Parental ethnic socialization and adolescent coping with problems related to ethnicity.' *Journal of Research on Adolescence 5*, 31–53.

Putnam, R.D. (1995) 'Bowling alone: America's declining social capital.' *Journal of Democracy 6*, 1, 65–78.

Sashidharan, S.P. (1993) 'Afro-Caribbeans and schizophrenia: The ethnic vulnerability hypothesis re-examined.' *International Review of Psychiatry 5*, 129–144.

Scottish Parliament (2013) *Equal Opportunities Committee 1st Report, 2013, Session 4: Where Gypsy/ Travellers Live*. Edinburgh: Scottish Parliament.

Shelter (2007) *Good Practice Guide: Working with Housed Gypsies and Travellers*. London: Shelter.

Spencer, S., Page, B. and Dawson, R. (2009) *An Improved Path to a Better Road: An Information Booklet for Health Care and Other Professionals*. Derbyshire Gypsy Liaison Group. Available at www.dglg.org/health-publications.html, accessed on 6 November 2016.

Taylor, B. (2013) *A Minority and the State: Travellers in Britain in the Twentieth Century*. Manchester: Manchester University Press.

The Traveller Movement (2015) *Government Changes to Planning Policy for Traveller Sites*. London: The Traveller Movement. Available at www.travellermovement.org.uk/wp-content/uploads/2015/09/New-Government-changes-to-Planning-Policy-for-Traveller-sites-September-20151.pdf, accessed on 25 September 2016.

Treise, C. and Shepherd, G. (2006) 'Developing mental health services for Gypsy Travellers: An exploratory study.' *Clinical Psychology Forum 163*, 16–19.

Van Cleemput, P., Parry, G., Thomas, K., Peters, J. and Cooper, C. (2007) 'Health-related beliefs and experiences of Gypsies and Travellers: A qualitative study.' *Journal of Epidemiology and Community Health 61*, 205–210.

West Sussex Local Involvement Network (2010) *Health and Social Care Needs of Gypsy and Traveller Families and Communities in West Sussex*. Billingshurst: West Sussex Local Involvement Network.

Zaidi, A. (2014) *Life Cycle Transitions and Vulnerabilities in Old Age: A Review*. New York: UNDP. Available at http://hdr.undp.org/sites/default/files/hdr_2014_zaidi_final.pdf, accessed on 6 November 2016.

Chapter 11

Social Exclusion and Anti-discriminatory Practice: The Case of Older Homeless People

Peter Cockersell

Introduction

I have long been interested in homeless and other socially excluded people. When I was a teenager, I sometimes used to sleep out on the streets or in the parks or stations in central London (even though I had a bed in my parents' home in Harrow, north-west London), and I met some fascinating homeless people. I remember an old (to me, anyway) man showing me how to make folded newspapers into a sleeping bag that wouldn't come apart, though I must admit I never mastered it myself. A few years later, when I lived in South America working as an English teacher, I spent time with the 'street people' and with street children, and when I returned to England I started working, initially as a volunteer, with homeless young people and then homeless people more generally.

I have now worked in homelessness for over 20 years, including ten years as the operational director with lead responsibility for health and recovery at St Mungo's, Britain's largest voluntary-sector homelessness agency. For the last 15 years I have also been a psychoanalytic psychotherapist, and in this time I have worked as a clinician with rough sleepers and homeless people (amongst others) in both NHS and voluntary-sector settings.

Ill health, both mental and physical, are endemic among rough sleepers and homeless people, and they have very high morbidity and mortality rates and poor treatment experiences and outcomes. Being homeless or a rough sleeper is in itself a contributory factor in poor physical and mental health. Research suggests that homeless people are more vulnerable to ill health and early death. For example, Brodie, Carter and Perera (2013) describe 'the average age of death of a homeless person as between 40–42 years of age with the life expectancy for "rough sleepers" 40.5 years compared to the UK national average of 74 for men and 79 for women' (p.9). Furthermore, research by Brighter Futures (2011, p.13) indicates that:

> homeless people attend A & E six times as often as the housed population, are admitted four times as often and stay three times as long. A homeless drug user admitted to hospital is seven times more likely to die over the next five years than a housed drug user admitted with the same medical problem.

Older people are also more vulnerable to ill health, both physical and mental, than younger people, and the burden of ill health increases with age (Howse 2006). It therefore follows that older rough sleepers and homeless people will face particularly severe problems. In our society, where we sometimes pride ourselves on the 'universal safety net' provided by our 'welfare state' and health and social care systems (Walsh 2013), the existence and number of homeless people present a particular challenge. Those numbers are increasing, with the official count of people sleeping rough in England rising by 55 per cent between 2010 and 2015 (Homeless Link 2015). It has been argued that homeless people and rough sleepers are treated 'less well than people or groups with conventionally valued characteristics' (Payne 2005, p.272), and they often appear to be the victims of discriminatory practice.

Rough sleeping and homelessness are, I think, among the most acute examples of social exclusion. One client, who slept rough at the back of some shops on Victoria Street in the centre of London less than half a mile from the Houses of Parliament, said to me: 'I sit beside the black bin liners on the pavement and nobody notices me; the only difference between me and the bin liners is that somebody comes to collect them each day' (personal communication). This client felt so socially excluded that it was as if he were invisible, an experience similar to that described by many other homeless people. The opposite of social exclusion is, of course, social inclusion. Social exclusion can be seen as the passive or active failure of social inclusion. Inclusive practice would ensure that people do not fall into rough sleeping, homelessness and the social invisibility that this client was describing. This is not to deny agency in homeless people; rather, I am suggesting that some people (often among the most vulnerable) for various reasons (age, shame, learning difficulties, mental health problems, dependencies) do not have, or are often not able to activate, support networks or systems, and it is this vulnerability that can lead them to becoming further excluded.

Before looking at discrimination itself, I would just like to think a bit about this idea of 'failure to include' as a failure of the safety-net provision of health and social care. Safeguarding legislation has clearly established that neglect or a failure to act where there is a known or suspected (*note* 'suspected') vulnerability are forms of abuse. Under section 42 of the UK's Care Act 2014 'the local authority has a duty to "make enquiries" where there is "reasonable cause" to suspect either that an adult with care and support needs is being abused or neglected or is at risk of being abused or neglected' (Age UK 2016, p.11). When these enquiries have been made, the local authority has a duty to 'assess the needs of the adult for protection, support and redress and how they might be met' (Age UK 2016, p.12). 'Failure to include' could be viewed as a failure to meet this requirement of the Care Act 2014, and might even be viewed as abusive within the terms of the Act. People who are falling towards rough sleeping but are, for whatever reasons, unable to stop this process are vulnerable and currently largely neglected in terms of this 'failure to include'; they therefore fall within the remit of this Act. Again, this is not to deny the agency of rough sleepers, who may choose for a variety of reasons not to interact with services. However, I have experience of homeless outreach services using the safeguarding clauses of the Care Act 2014 to persuade local authority social services to care for some rough sleepers who would otherwise probably have died on the streets.

Now, let us turn our attention to discrimination. Payne (2005, p.272) has defined discrimination as treating identified 'individuals and groups with certain characteristics…less well than people or groups with conventionally valued characteristics'. If a 'failure to include' those whose vulnerability means they cannot activate support networks or systems leads to the social exclusion that both precipitates and maintains homelessness and rough sleeping, then this 'failure to include' could be seen as discriminatory practice. In effect, this is to classify being 'hard to reach' or 'hard to engage' (as such clients are so often called) as a vulnerability. The evidence of the disproportionately high number of 'hard to reach' and 'hard to engage' individuals among the rough sleeping population suggests this is true. The failure to proactively 'include' treats 'individuals and groups with certain characteristics' (people who cannot activate support networks or systems) 'less well than people or groups with conventionally valued characteristics' (those who maintain support networks) because it excludes them from support and it leads to the poor health outcomes associated with homelessness and rough sleeping. Within this logic, proactive inclusion can be seen as anti-discriminatory practice in that it seeks out those unable to seek or make use of help themselves (probably from the majority of rough sleepers, and perhaps particularly older rough sleepers, as noted below).

Discrimination is defined as an activity with an oppressive outcome (Thompson 2002). Prejudice means holding preconceived negative values about certain groups or individuals, but discrimination in its usual sense means *doing* something damaging to them – as Payne puts it, treating those individuals 'less well'. Prejudice may be behind discrimination, as may be ignorance, fear, culture, belief systems and many other social constructs, but discrimination is evidenced by an action. Discrimination can be overt or covert (College of Social Work 2014). Discrimination can also be an individual act (done by one person or a small group of people) or the act of an institution (done by an organisation or system); of course, institutions and systems act through the individuals that they are made up of.

Social exclusion, I would argue, is a case of institutional discrimination and the result of a systemic failure of inclusive practice: those who are unable to seek or are ineffective in using help, or are not compliant with the conditions of the help-givers, are excluded. It seems to me it arises from various cultural roots – for example, the value given in our society to 'standing on your own two feet' and being 'independent' and related concepts such as 'heaven helps those that help themselves'. There appears to be a strong cultural push (not least from the British government) that health and social services 'help those that help themselves' (see Health Foundation 2011). There is a residual culture of perceiving that the help-givers are benevolent and kind and that the recipients should therefore be grateful and compliant.

There continues to be a relatively strong (and indeed perhaps sometimes justified) belief that the helper or caregiver knows what is best and can therefore 'do to', rather than include, the client; it is the client's 'fault' if he or she disengages. Finally, there is a culture of restriction and intentional discrimination in most social care services (though not so much in health care) – the 'deserving poor' of the past, those who met moral criteria, are now replaced with 'target groups', those who meet (ever more restrictive) social policy criteria (Coulton and Rosenberg 2014; Heng 2007). Though there may be merit in all these positions in some situations and from some perspectives, to apply any of them across the board is to deny the reality that some people are not able to help themselves, or even to seek help effectively; they are then excluded from the 'universal' safety net of the welfare state. Older homeless people largely fall into this category.

Following on from this I argue that both the social exclusion of homelessness itself, and the poor health and outcomes associated with it, could be at least mitigated and potentially ended through anti-discriminatory, proactively inclusive practice. This would also enable local authorities to fulfil their safeguarding duties under the Care Act 2014. It is then up to health and social care professionals (you), as the guardians of the 'safety net', to be decisively and deliberately inclusive – especially where communities have failed to be – and to step in and prevent what could be termed 'social neglect'. We will look at some ideas about how this (and greater community inclusion) might be done in the conclusion of this chapter.

In summary, in this chapter I am going to focus particularly on older people who are rough sleeping or homeless, on the processes into and (to a lesser extent) out of homelessness and rough sleeping, and on the roles of health, social care and the welfare state in the prevention or otherwise of older people becoming homeless or sleeping rough. I shall argue first that homelessness and rough sleeping are instances of significant and extreme social exclusion, and second that social exclusion is a discriminatory social act. I argue that it is a 'failure to include' that leads to the high numbers of older homeless and rough sleepers. I am not intending to go as far as to say that inclusive practice, or lack thereof, is the only factor: I would always say that there are multiple interacting psychological and social factors involved in any one person becoming socially excluded. However, I am arguing that proactive inclusive practice would significantly reduce social exclusion, and particularly the extreme social exclusion of homelessness. Further, I argue that inclusive practice is a cornerstone of anti-discriminatory practice precisely because it *is* inclusive, and that there is an obligation under the Care Act 2014 to meet the needs of those who are 'hard to reach' and 'hard to engage' because they are known to be vulnerable. Not to do so is neglect and abuse under safeguarding legislation, as well as a disregard of moral obligation.

Thompson (2002, p.53) says that anti-discriminatory practice 'is any form of action that tries to prevent the sequence from diversity to difference to discrimination and on to oppression'. In the case of older homelessness, the 'difference' is social isolation and the vulnerability of not having, or not being able to summon or use, the support networks which the great majority of people have or can summon or use. We can term it (social isolation) 'vulnerability' because it exposes the person to significant negative health and social risks. For too many older people, the impact of non-inclusive practice is that this difference then leads to the social exclusion and 'oppressive' outcomes of homelessness, rough sleeping and exacerbated poor health. This is discriminatory. So inclusive practice can be viewed as anti-discriminatory. Ultimately, whether a service is discriminatory or not in any other way is irrelevant to the person who has not been included in the first place.

Although I am arguing that rough sleeping or homelessness is an extreme form of social exclusion and a specialised area of work, I also contend that the lessons about practice drawn from this work apply more widely. Inclusive practice underpins the fairest and most anti-discriminatory practice in any field; the 'failure to include' is the first discrimination. First, though, as this argument is derived from a specialised area of work, I will provide a certain amount of background on some of the concepts and categories I will be using.

Recovery

'Recovery' is a term widely used within mental health and substance dependency, and it is increasingly used in other fields of health and social care, such as homelessness. It is used internationally, and it has been given many different meanings (Davidson 2013). The Oxford Dictionary defines recovery as 'A return to a normal state of health, mind, or strength' or 'The action or process of regaining possession or control of something stolen or lost' (Oxford Dictionary 2014a).

These two definitions are essentially divisible into 'recovery of' – for example, of some control over your life, or of the ability to form or re-form sustainable relationships – and 'recovery from' – for example, from ill health or from social exclusion. The former describes a gain or increase, the latter an alleviation or diminution. The meanings I want to focus on here derive from these original definitions; they are those most common in substance dependency and those adopted by most homelessness agencies. Recovery is about gaining or regaining some control over your own life, and of your ability to achieve some kind of self-fulfilment.

Recovery in homelessness is therefore generally used to mean both 'recovery of' and 'recovery from', because most homeless people and rough sleepers need to do at least a bit of both to move on in their lives. 'Recovery of' is moving into or returning to the mainstream of life – in other words, having somewhere to live, having something purposeful to do and having regular meaningful relationships with some people. This can be a hard and long journey for many homeless people, taking many years, and this is partly a measure of how far from the mainstream of our society many homeless people have become. 'Recovery of' includes developing or regaining self-esteem, confidence, skills for positive social interaction (including perhaps work), and a sense of being able to contribute valuably to life. 'Recovery from', on the other hand, is broadly about having, or regaining, sufficiently good health and positive mental well-being to be able to do these things – having a place you can call home, worthwhile and non-destructive relationships, meaningful activity – and to enjoy them. It includes overcoming substance dependencies, working through trauma, and getting treatment for any untreated physical or mental health problems. It also means recovery from social exclusion.

Social exclusion

Social exclusion is defined by the Oxford Dictionary as 'Exclusion from the prevailing social system and its rights and privileges, typically as a result of poverty or the fact of belonging to a minority social group' (Oxford Dictionary 2014b). A report on social exclusion in Britain, commissioned by the Social Exclusion Unit of the Cabinet Office, summarised definitions of social exclusion as follows:

Social exclusion is a complex and multi-dimensional process. It involves the lack or denial of resources, rights, goods and services, and the inability to participate in the normal relationships and activities, available to the majority of people in a society, whether in economic, social, cultural or political arenas. It affects both the quality of life of individuals and the equity and cohesion of society as a whole.

This definition does not address the structural issues of inequality, polarisation, social mobility and social closure noted above... [S]tructural characteristics are best seen as drivers of social exclusion, rather than constitutive of it. (Levitas *et al.* 2007, p.25)

In the same study, Levitas *et al.* quote David Miliband, then the UK government's minister responsible for tackling social exclusion, as saying that social exclusion 'is embedded in power relations that constrain and define the capabilities and choices of individuals' (2007, p.26).

Homelessness is a powerful indicator of social exclusion because it involves the lack of a very fundamental resource in our society, a home; and that lack or loss leads to other losses, such as warmth, shelter and stability, and it makes accessing many other important resources, from social status through to health care, education or work, very difficult. Rough sleeping is an even more pronounced version of this; in fact, David Miliband talked of it in terms of 'deep exclusion' (Levitas *et al.* 2007, p.26).

Recovery from social exclusion for homeless people, then, is about recovering from years of conscious and unconscious, or intentional and unintentional, discrimination, stigma and rejection or neglect. Social exclusion is something that doesn't just happen; as Miliband suggests above, it is done by and to people through 'power relations that constrain and define the capabilities and choices of individuals' (Levitas *et al.* 2007, p.26). If it is done consistently and/or for long enough, it becomes internalised, and the person begins to exclude him- or herself. If homelessness in general, and rough sleeping in particular, are about active social exclusion – that is, people being excluded by society – then tackling homelessness comes to be not just about providing housing, support or health services (though these are of course essential) but directly about developing and fostering truly inclusive, and anti-discriminatory, practice. I will go into this in more detail below, but first let us take a brief look at who homeless people are, and specifically at who the older homeless are.

Who are homeless people?

Homeless people are, of course, not homogenous; there are as many different histories of becoming homeless as there are homeless people. However, I have suggested elsewhere (Cockersell 2011) that there are also two broad categories of homeless people:

1. Those who are *chronically and repeatedly homeless*, and who may have experienced episodes of homelessness throughout their lives.

2. Those who are homeless as a result of a discrete set of events, whom I call the *transient homeless* as they usually pass through the homelessness system into permanent resettlement relatively speedily.

Chronically and repeatedly homeless

Case study: Gareth

This is an example of a man I worked with who was chronically homeless and was rough sleeping into his seventies. His material is used with his permission, and some details have been changed to obscure his identity.

Gareth was put into temporary care by his parents when he was four, and they never took him back again; his father was in the forces and his mother said 'she couldn't manage alone'. He lived in a succession of care and foster homes (where his mother visited him sometimes) before joining the army for a couple of years as soon as he was old enough. His father died in an accident abroad while he was in foster care. After leaving the army, Gareth did casual work and stayed with his mother at first, but 'she got Parkinson's and she couldn't cope'. Gareth lived in lodgings, or hostels, depending on whether he could get casual work, though he 'worked most of [his] life'. When Gareth was 22, he was told by the Salvation Army that his mother had died. He has visited her grave once and was 'saving up to go again', perhaps on her birthday. He had lost touch with other family members by then. He lived in various cities before ending up in London, where he stayed sometimes in lodgings and sometimes in homelessness hostels or shelters. He was often moved on (many shelters are temporary) or sometimes left because he didn't like the noise or the drugs. On and off he slept on the streets because, as he put it, 'sometimes it's better on the street'.

In the 1980s he got married, having met his future wife in a day centre, and he lived with her for 17 years in her flat. She developed breast cancer. One morning he woke up, tried to talk to her, and found she was dead in the bed beside him. He had 'a nervous breakdown' and was hospitalised; the council subsequently repossessed the flat, for reasons unknown. When he left hospital, he went back to living between hostels, shelters and the streets for another ten years. He's in a small hostel now, which is run more like a hotel than a social care institution, and he feels settled because 'this place makes you feel up'. 'The neighbours are friendly', and the GP and other staff are 'very good'; it's important 'knowing you're safe'.

Transient homeless

Case study: Lily

As I mentioned at the beginning of the chapter, as a teenager I sometimes used to sleep rough in central London (never more than a couple of nights in a row). One night, when I was looking for somewhere to sleep, I met an old lady who was getting ready to bed down in a shop doorway in Oxford Street. I was 15 then, and I will never forget her. I sat down with her and we began chatting. Lily (not her real name) was 76, and she had never lived on the streets before. Lily had been married for many years but had never had children. She had lived with her husband in a council flat in another part of London. A few years previously, her husband had died, leaving her living alone.

After so many years of marriage and partnership with her husband, and (my impression was) with little outside social life, she'd felt lonely and she had got a dog for company. The dog was with her now, and I was fussing it as we talked. She said she had started finding it a bit hard to cope in her house alone; she couldn't look after it properly and got into a bit of trouble with her bills and rent payments. After a while, social services decided she needed to move into a care home. The problem was that the care homes they offered her did not allow people to have pets, so they told her she would have to rehome her dog. Lily couldn't face losing her companion again, so she abandoned her house and went to live on the streets, for the first time in her life. It still makes me want to cry. I only met her that once, and I have no idea what happened to her afterwards; when I left her to go and sleep down near Embankment tube (where in those days there used to be 24-hour public toilets and other people sleeping out, and it felt safe), she was bedding down in the shop doorway, with some blankets and her dog.

Case study: Alf

Another person who became homeless in older age was Alf (not his real name). Again, he gave permission for his story to be told. Alf spoke of a stable life, relationships and an ordinary childhood, living at home, going to the local school, and having local friends. He lived with his parents until he got a good steady job with a big company. He then worked, married, had two children and remained living locally. He was close to his family, and especially to his father and daughters. He liked a 'social drink' with mates in the pub or while watching football, but he never 'caused any trouble'.

He was a 'social drinker' all through his adult life, and this was not a problem, he said. However, his wife ended their relationship after 19 years. He would not talk about why his wife wanted to separate. Whatever led up to it, moving out of his family home and leaving his wife and children was a huge interruption in the apparently stable progress of his life. It was such a jolt that he left his locality, left his job and career, left the city altogether, went to live in the countryside (which he didn't like), and found a new relationship.

Then his father, who he'd been 'very close' to, died. Alf went to live with his mother. She wouldn't talk about his father's death – 'she would turn the telly on if I ever talked about anything' – and kept herself 'busy with just activity' while 'filling the void' left by the death of her husband. Alf was drinking more, drinking in the day in the house and drinking to the extent that he had a 'seizure' one day, but he still regarded himself as a 'social drinker'. For the first time, he was unemployed. His mother asked him to leave, and he 'didn't really believe it'; she had to insist, asking several times over a brief period, before he left.

Alf then briefly went back to his ex-wife's. She too asked him to leave again, then had to insist. Alf became homeless for the first time; he was in his late fifties, unemployed, confused and alcohol dependent. His daughter helped find him a place in a homelessness hostel, which had a lot of people with alcohol dependency problems. As he put it, this 'wasn't the best scenario drink-wise', and Alf became an even heavier drinker, although still claiming it was 'social'. He developed alcohol-related health problems and had alcohol-related falls.

Most of those who are transiently homeless have histories of relative or indeed significant stability, which are then shattered by an event or series of events that – and this is the key point, this is the vulnerability – they were not able to resolve or deal with effectively themselves, and they did not have, or were unable to mobilise effectively, supportive social networks. A significant number of older homeless people fall within this category (see the case studies of Lily and Alf) and are experiencing homelessness for the first time later in life as the result of a sequence of events they have not been able to manage or find/utilise support with. Social isolation is a known vulnerability (Campaign to End Loneliness 2013; Friedli 2009), and a failure to find ways to include these individuals led to their homelessness and its consequences. This appears to be discriminatory (the socially isolated are a social group, but a social group whose members have no connection to each other) and neglectful within the provision of the Care Act 2014.

Complex trauma

Most people who are chronically homeless have long histories of social exclusion and of complex trauma. Complex trauma is the term used by mental health clinicians to describe the experience of people who have been exposed to multiple adverse events such as violence or abuse, and/or the loss of close figures through (for example) abandonments, care proceedings or bereavements. There is a strong association between experience of complex trauma and homelessness (Maguire *et al.* 2009; National Mental Health Development Unit (NMHDU) 2010).

There is strong evidence for the association of complex trauma, adverse childhood events and damaged attachment processes with a range of poor life outcomes and the development of poor mental health (Kolk *et al.* 2009), including personality disorders (Bateman and Fonagy 2006; Schore 1994). National and international studies have shown that experience of mental health problems is very high among homeless people, with up to 30 per cent experiencing psychosis (more than 20 times the national average), over 60 per cent meeting the criteria for personality disorder (which is between 5 and 15 times the national average, depending on the criteria used), and over 40 per cent having attempted suicide (30 times the European average) (Cockersell 2011; Fazel *et al.* 2008; NMHDU 2010; St Mungo's 2009). There is also some evidence for a link between adverse childhood events and homelessness (Roos *et al.* 2013), and between complex trauma, attachment damage and long-term homelessness (Cockersell 2012).

Mental health, social inclusion, adversity and homelessness

In the brief look above at who homeless people are, I proposed that there were two identifiable groups: the chronic homeless and those who become homeless as a result of a particular set of circumstances and who probably transitioned relatively quickly through their homelessness status (transient homeless). While a history of complex trauma often characterises the long-term homeless person, this is not so true with the shorter-term cohort, whose backgrounds could be said to be more typical of the general population. They have still become homeless, however, and this implies that they have de facto moved a long way down the path of social exclusion (see above), and this in turn implies that they have lost some or many of the resources of the socially included. Relationships, as I have argued elsewhere (Cockersell 2012), are of crucial importance both in recovery from homelessness and in the process of becoming homeless. If we have the protection of a strong network of loyal and resourceful social relationships, we are unlikely to become homeless in the first place and almost certain not to become rough sleepers. Our friends and/or relatives will put us up until we 'find our feet'.

World Health Organization studies from Britain and other countries suggest that the factors 'that enable people both to cope with adversity and to reach their full potential and humanity' are things such as 'resilience, health assets, capabilities and positive adaptation' (Friedli 2009, p.45). Resilience is the quality that enables people to bounce back from adversity, and it is associated with good early care and strong social relations (Masten 2001). In a very real way, our 'health assets' depend on our social integration; there is widespread evidence that social isolation is a greater indicator of increased morbidity and early mortality than smoking, obesity or alcohol consumption (Holt-Lundstad, Smith and Layton 2010). Our capabilities are also socially produced: there are very few things that we actually do on our own, as they nearly always require engagement with and the involvement of others. Paying the rent, claiming benefits, sorting out probate when your lifetime partner has died, doing the shopping or keeping your accommodation in a habitable condition all require negotiation and relations with other people, sometimes through quite complex processes and under quite anxiety-provoking situations. Asking for help is something that many vulnerable and older people find hard to do, either through cultural values of self-reliance and pride (or denial) originating in long histories of past capability and competence, or simply because they do not know who to ask (Warnes and Crane 2006). 'Positive adaptation' requires flexibility, imagination and high levels of resilience (Masten 2001), which again is associated with positive social integration and inclusion. The capacity for positive adaptation, that is, adaptability itself, is also related to good early care (Schore 1994) and to the ability to form open and flexible relationships (Zagier Roberts 1994).

The ability to cope successfully with adversity is quite significantly dependent in all ways – from the practical to the emotional to the psychological – on our inclusion within a network of supportive and positive social relationships. Homelessness can perhaps be seen as a symptom of unsuccessful coping, but it is also undoubtedly a signifier of social isolation, and both are identifiers of vulnerability.

It seems logical, given the above, that increasing social isolation is (at least in many cases) the beginning element of the process of social exclusion, perhaps exacerbated by and exacerbating poor mental health, which is itself an isolating factor because of the long-standing stigma around mental health (Goffman 1990; YoungMinds 2015). It is the failure to recognise social isolation as rendering people vulnerable within the safeguarding sense, and therefore the importance of tackling it – in other words the 'failure to include' – that leads to the deepening of social exclusion and ultimately to homelessness.

Older age is associated with increasing social isolation anyway (Wenger *et al.* 1996; Windle, Francis and Coomber 2014). If social isolation is a vulnerability, and there is an association between social isolation and the process of social exclusion and homelessness, we might expect to see high levels of first-time homelessness in older people that would otherwise be surprising.

Homelessness among older people

A study led by Warnes and Crane (2006) found that 65 per cent of older (defined as over 55 years of age) homeless people became homeless for the first time in older age. They had seen the stability of their lives shattered and had been ill-equipped or unable to deal with it themselves, yet no services had been accessed, no one stepped in to help, and the end result was homelessness. The other side of this statistic is that around 35 per cent of older homeless people are chronically homeless – people for whom homelessness has been an ongoing or repeated experience throughout their lives, with any help that has been offered either declined or insufficient to prevent future homelessness.

There are many immediate events precipitating finding yourself without a home. In Warnes and Crane's study of older homeless people, the causes they cite include repossession or eviction (58.7%); breakdown of a marital or cohabiting relationship (22%); the death of a partner (9.9%); money problems or debts (35%), with rent arrears the most commonly cited (26.7%); work ending or retirement (19.1%); heavy drinking (25%); mental illness (22.1%); and physical illness (18.3%). Many other causes are cited, from criminal charges to problems with neighbours, and people frequently gave more than one reason for their becoming homeless (Warnes and Crane 2006).

However, many people face adverse events such as those listed in Warnes and Crane's study but do not become homeless. In light of the discussion on social exclusion, we can assert that becoming homeless for these people was a result of their vulnerability because of their social isolation, in addition to the specific negative life events that they cited. Therefore, the figures that Warnes and Crane give say something quite disturbing. We are proud in the UK that we have a safety net to protect us – and especially the vulnerable among us – from the worst levels of poverty and distress. Yet despite this safety net, these older people are homeless; some have been socially excluded all their lives, while some were included but became socially excluded later in life. How could this be? What happened to the safety net?

I have argued elsewhere and above that social exclusion is a process, something that is done to people (who then react in a way that colludes or exacerbates the process); we are not born socially excluded, though the processes of exclusion may start very early (Cockersell 2015). However, the evidence from studies of older homeless people suggests that the processes of social exclusion may become acute at any time, even well into people's old age. In Warnes and Crane's sample population, 18 per cent were aged 65 or over and just under 5 per cent were aged 70 or over when they became homeless (Warnes and Crane 2006). Their evidence is corroborated by evidence from the US (Center for Supportive Housing (CSH) and Hearth 2011). However, in the US there is no safety net in the way that there is in European countries, and poverty, whatever its cause, can much more easily lead to homelessness. The strange thing, then, is that in Britain our safety net still allows this to happen: 12 per cent of St Mungo's clients are 55 or over (and of these over-55s, 67% have identified mental health problems, 50% alcohol issues, and 39% both; St Mungo's 2014a).

Therefore, if we look at the processes of becoming homeless from another perspective, what we in fact have evidence of again is a failure of social inclusion. The safety net is supposed to operate when the normal social mechanisms of support, adaptability and survival are either failing or not present. The safety net comprises statutory and voluntary sector services designed to mitigate or relieve suffering, prevent homelessness, treat illness and tackle social exclusion: these are their objectives (e.g. Health and Social Care Act 2013). Both the chronically homeless and the transiently homeless have, in the great majority of cases, been in contact with some form of statutory or voluntary-sector services (St Mungo's 2009, 2014b; Warnes and Crane 2006); many have been in contact with multiple services over a period of time, sometimes many years (especially in the case of the chronically homeless) (Making Every Adult Matter (MEAM) 2010). This fact – that people have sought help but they have not been able to find the help they need, or in a form they can engage with – is sometimes used to suggest that homeless people are somehow being difficult or are in some way wilfully obstructive and making a 'lifestyle choice'. The other possibility is that this is evidence of a significant and widespread failure of inclusive practice; it is discrimination against the socially isolated, often those whose vulnerability is that they find social interaction and seeking or accepting help difficult.

This is not to deny homeless people any agency, as the very behaviours that mainstream services often find very challenging to work with can be understood as responses to the processes of exclusion themselves (Brown 2015). Homeless people, like the rest of us, have responses adapted to their experience of life. Many agencies and services behave as if the only change required is in their client: the experience of life has to change as well to enable the socially excluded person to make sustained change. I am suggesting here that the change that agencies and services need to make is to become proactively inclusive, and that this would be one of the life-experience-changing acts that would facilitate a reduction in social exclusion.

Applying this line of thinking to the case studies

It may be useful to look at this in the light of the case studies given earlier. Gareth was taken into care at four years old, so social services were involved at this point and possibly earlier (usually children are not taken into care until there has been quite a long history of social services and possibly voluntary-sector intervention). He was in and out of foster care, the army and then hostels. He had a period of stability for 17 years when he was married, but when his wife died it appeared that he could not cope alone. He acquired a psychiatric diagnosis, was hospitalised and had follow-up outpatient treatments, but returned to a life on the streets and in hostels. Although I never discussed this with him, much of this happened without an apparent resulting reduction in Gareth's social exclusion. It appears that the services he met with, who worked with him, did not manage to tackle his lack of social inclusion. For whatever reason, they did what they did, but that did not involve helping him to develop the social networks and sense of connectedness or attachment that might have enabled him to regain stability and end his homelessness. They were actually neglecting what could be considered his core vulnerability and his core need.

Leicester City Council's anti-discriminatory guidance suggests that 'there is a tendency to overlook social identity as one of the causes of a problem. The problem is redefined as a personality conflict or an individual's fault' (Leicester City Council 2014, p.13). It goes on to say the following:

Institutional discrimination has three key features:

- It is triggered by social identity

- It is systemic – it is built in

- so it keeps happening, which results in patterns

These features distinguish institutional discrimination from other random and individual forms of bad treatment. (Leicester City Council 2014, p.13)

Gareth, I think, was treated as a series of largely impoverished social identities, and his human needs for deep, sustaining and lasting social relationships were never prioritised, except perhaps by the woman he met in the homelessness day centre and within the life he lived with her for 17 years.

Anti-discriminatory practice would suggest that more could and should have been done by those involved with him at every stage of his life. Anti-discriminatory practice would suggest asking 'What does this infant/child/youth/person need to make his/her life better?', not 'What does this service do? Does he/she meet the organisational criteria for us to offer services to him/her?' We live in an imperfect world and resources are limited, so we need to remain open to alternatives that enhance anti-discriminatory practice. If social exclusion is discriminatory, then anti-discriminatory practice must be inclusive, and that means working with people whatever their social identity to increase their social inclusion. Anti-discriminatory practice has to *challenge* institutional discrimination, not merely acknowledge it.

The cases of Lily and Alf are of people who were for a long time socially included but became socially excluded in older age. In the case of Lily, the local authority acted within defined criteria, which was also applied by social services or the relevant voluntary agency, resulting in Lily becoming homeless for the first time in her life in her mid-seventies. She chose to remain with her dog – her only social and emotional connection – and be homeless, as the care home was unable to accept pets. These rigid criteria seem morally and pragmatically wrong and indeed self-defeating: the purpose of social services is to provide a social safety net. I would say it was abusive. There was nobody asking the questions 'What does this person want and need?' or 'What really matters to this person?' and then creating a flexible response that enabled Lily to remain housed, let alone anyone trying to support her in redeveloping a social network. Instead, she ended up homeless and even more isolated and vulnerable.

In the case of Alf, it is perhaps less obvious where the intervention points were up until he became homeless, because he was within relationships and he was working. However, there seems to be a history and pattern of people not talking about what really mattered in his family/families: his wife 'suddenly' asked him to leave after 19 years, and his mother wouldn't talk about his father's death. This might be considered a private affair, but it becomes public because it becomes a cost for public spending. Because there was no chance of resolution within the families, Alf ended up living in a homelessness hostel for 18 months and damaged his health through unrecognised or at least unacknowledged alcohol dependency. It becomes a public health issue when people bottle up their feelings and try to drown them or make them disappear rather than process them or deal with them. This kind of social isolation – being with people but having nobody to talk to about what really matters – can lead to ill health just as much as the social isolation of having nobody at all. It is the quality of relationships that makes them good for health and well-being, not just the quantity (Holt-Lunstad, Smith and Layton 2010). Had Alf or members of his family known about or believed that there was help available, they might have sought it earlier. Support and treatment need to be proactively inclusive. This matters for a country with a welfare system – especially in times of austerity – as prevention and early intervention are both associated with more positive outcomes and lower longitudinal cost.

It could be argued that it is institutional discrimination for services to wait within their institutions for people's lives to unravel and then only to see them if they meet the required level of acuteness in their distress. Inclusive, anti-discriminatory service provision would advertise its existence and strive to ensure that it is available to help with whatever distress the client brings, and within a short time frame. The prevalent argument put forward by the government and main political parties in Britain is that the country cannot afford comprehensive support services. I argue here that this is dangerous for many vulnerable people because they do not, or cannot, effectively access rationed services (which tend to be rationed by excluding criteria). It is also cost-ineffective as many vulnerable people go on to cost a lot more in health and social care than they would have done if they had been picked up earlier. Inclusive services are the bedrock of prevention and early intervention.

I want to challenge here the idea that we cannot afford these services. This is a political position and decision, not a clinical or even an economic one: there are choices, and they are being made. Currently, welfare resources are rationed by becoming increasingly focused on responding only to acuity and criticality; earlier intervention is arguably more equitable, likely to reach more people and likely to be cheaper in the long term (Friedli 2009; Public Health England (PHE) 2015). This is certainly clinically true for health care, including mental health care. The economic necessity is also a political judgement and not unchallengeable. The post-war British government introduced a free and universal healthcare system and free education for all to tertiary level, and it launched a huge social house-building programme at a time when the country's debt to GDP ratio was far worse than it is now. Arguably, that led to the prosperity of Britain in the 1960s, with the Conservative Prime Minister Harold Macmillan famously telling the public in 1957 that they had 'never had it so good' (Macmillan 1957). Despite the commitment to massive new government spending in creating the welfare state, the debt ratio actually fell in the ensuing 20 years. The decision that we could afford a welfare state was a political decision. The current decision to cut and/or redirect social care and welfare resources continues to be political.

Homelessness and inclusive practice

I have argued that transient homelessness is related to adverse life events, and that chronic or long-term homelessness is often related to complex or compound trauma. I have also argued here that in both these cases it is a failure in the processes of social inclusion – a 'failure to include' – that actually delivers the individual concerned into homelessness. This, I suggest, is discriminatory and also falls foul of statutory safeguarding duties in the Care Act 2014. It discriminates against those who are vulnerable because of their social isolation and inability to activate social networks or systems of care. While Gareth's case study describes a history of compound and multiple broken attachments, Lily's and Alf's do not. In both situations and in all three cases we have seen how social isolation can turn into social exclusion through failures in active inclusion, or failures in (or in the existence of) inclusive practice.

From an individual psychological perspective, social exclusion might be understood in terms of broken attachments and their associated processes. From a social rather than an individual perspective, both situations and all three cases suggest a pattern of vulnerability through social isolation not being recognised and not being responded to, and thereby becoming social exclusion. For social services in the broad sense – that is, health services, social care, local authority services, and many voluntary-sector and community services – tackling social isolation is often seen as a relatively low priority. By November 2013, out of 152 Health and Wellbeing Board Strategies across the country, only 10 had plans with measurable actions to tackle loneliness and isolation, with a further 33 acknowledging that there was a problem but saying that they needed to learn more, and around half not mentioning loneliness and isolation as a factor at all (Campaign to End Loneliness 2013). This is perhaps understandable given the competing demands on an ever-shrinking public purse and the ignorance around the importance of social inclusion, but it is also a costly mistake given the evidenced correlation between social isolation and increased morbidity and mortality (VicHealth 2005), as well as the link that I am suggesting here between social isolation and homelessness, and particularly older homelessness. Ignorance may be understandable, but it often underpins discriminatory action. The ignorance of the importance and impact of social isolation underpins the common institutional discrimination against the proactively inclusive practice that would enable the inclusion of those whose vulnerability is that, for whatever reasons, they do not have or cannot effectively utilise support systems or networks.

Social inclusion and anti-discriminatory practice

Social exclusion is a dynamic process arising from the interplay between a series of actions and inactions by society (family, institutions, agencies, etc.) and by an individual; it is this duality of agency that distinguishes social exclusion from social isolation. Individuals can become isolated on their own by gradually interacting less and less with others. Isolation is the result of a process of withdrawal. Social exclusion, on the other hand, is the result of a process of closure of opportunity; the opportunity to engage with and be part of society reduces or is reduced. Levitas *et al.*'s (2007, p.25) definition of social exclusion was offered earlier: 'Social exclusion is a complex and multi-dimensional process. It involves the lack or denial of resources, rights, goods and services, and the inability to participate in the normal relationships and activities, available to the majority of people in a society.'

In our society, the creation of social exclusion is not usually intended (though it may be, for example with certain groups of immigrants or some offenders). However, there are still many different ways in which social exclusion is practised. It is often the result of systemic barriers (such as referral criteria, restricted opening times, narrowly defined care pathways or difficult locations) where the design of services has the intended or unintended consequence of making them inaccessible for certain people or groups of people. This may stem from unconscious and unspoken prejudices – for example, against people who take drugs or drink too much, or people experiencing mental health problems – which makes accessing some services a negative experience for many homeless people. It may also be the result of direct exclusion through rules and regulations or cultural norms which proscribe certain behaviours or appearances. It can also be through inaction as well as action; for example, not tackling social isolation is a form of social exclusion. We know that social interaction and social activities are good for people's physical and mental health (e.g. the 'five ways to well-being' – Connect, Be Active, Take Notice, Keep Learning and Give; Aked *et al.* 2014), and that social isolation often increases morbidity and premature mortality. Therefore, not proactively intervening to reduce social isolation is an act of social exclusion, discrimination, neglect and abuse under safeguarding legislation. If isolation is an act of individual withdrawal, then not intervening is a response of social uncaringness. It says, loudly: 'We don't care if you are lonely and isolated.' Psychologically, attachment is at the core of our human social behaviours, and yet health and social care often pay little or no attention to people's attachment situation.

In addition to the more gradual process of social isolation through attachment attenuation, most homeless people, as noted earlier, have also experienced single or multiple traumatic events. One of the reasons that many older people do not have the capacity to cope with this trauma is that their social relations have already become limited, often to just one or two individuals. The implication of this is that social exclusion and homelessness could be preventable to a large degree if we systematically tackled social isolation by proactive social inclusion. At the least, social isolation should be seen as a vulnerability and should therefore trigger safeguarding actions when adverse events or neglect are (as the legislation says) suspected. As discussed, in the case of older homelessness it is not inevitably the catastrophic event per se that leads to homelessness (many people experience catastrophes and do not become homeless), but the context of social isolation within which it occurs means the person does not have the resources to prevent the outcome of homelessness. If homelessness is the result of not recognising the vulnerability associated with social isolation, then it is institutional discrimination not to promote social inclusion and inclusive services. It is also the role of anti-discriminatory practice to challenge the processes of exclusion.

This is particularly important for older people if we are to prevent shocking statistics, such as that 65 per cent of our older homeless people are in their first episode of homelessness. Social isolation is more prevalent among older compared to younger people in our society (Wenger *et al.* 1996). Tackling social isolation by actively promoting social inclusion and championing anti-discriminatory services could be the cornerstone for a policy to eliminate social exclusion and homelessness among older people. This need not be expensive, because it is not necessary (or probably even desirable) to have professional support services for everything and everywhere. Many southern or eastern European and Scandinavian countries, as well as the US, have much more developed cultures of volunteering and charitable activity. In Britain, there are many older people who have been made redundant or been retired as firms downsize as well as large numbers of unemployed or underemployed youth. With organisation and the safeguard of links into formal services, these people hold the potential to form a safety net of proactive and inclusive community support networks to tackle social isolation. A political and cultural shift is required to facilitate this social resource, but the implications for protecting those who are vulnerable due to social isolation, and of generally becoming a more inclusive and cohesive society, are compelling.

Anti-discriminatory practice

Despite rhetoric about the need for and value of prevention or early intervention, in practice it is often suggested that we cannot actually implement such measures because of austerity and the tightness of funding for social care and support. Putting aside the arguments about prioritisation of spending (and that there seems to be unlimited funding to support business and banks), it seems to me that we are actually missing the point here. Tackling social isolation requires human relationships and multi-personal and ongoing contact. It often requires the involvement of people with time, rather than just money. In the great majority of cases, I would argue it is the lack of this sort of activity to tackle social isolation that means that expensive professional interventions are needed later down the line. Some people do need professional interventions, that is undoubted; but in many cases social inclusion is simply that – a social act that includes someone within a social network in a meaningful way. In these cases, it is not large amounts of financial resources that are required but a different application of existing resources and a change of priorities and values. In the medium term, I suggest this would become cheaper than the system we have now because there would be less demand for emergency and acute responses (PHE 2015).

Here are a few of the things you can do to put this into practice:

- Social exclusion is a process performed by systems and institutions; you can embrace anti-discriminatory practice by challenging excluding practice and promoting inclusivity and inclusive services. Clearly, it is a complex process to change the criteria of a service. However, one simple way of making a service more inclusive is to have an up-to-date and as comprehensive as possible list of local resources. That way, if your service cannot meet someone's needs, you can at least offer them some suggestions as to where they might be able to find what they need. Many services can also benefit from creative thinking about how to widen access by making more people who do meet the criteria aware of the service and working with other agencies to ensure they refer people who could benefit from this service. Gently challenge the idea of 'demand management': services are actually there to meet need, not to avoid it. (What percentage of the people who come to your service do you actually offer *something* helpful to? Why can't it be 100%, even if that something helpful is to refer them to a different service?)

- Social isolation may be turned into social exclusion and homelessness by the institutional response. Tackling social isolation is anti-discriminatory practice; expecting the socially isolated to access services and use them according to service criteria could be viewed as institutional discrimination. How can you help reach the socially isolated? One way is through proactive outreach. If your service cannot do that, is there some allied (perhaps voluntary) service that can do it for you? Also, it is important to establish which aspects of your criteria are *really* critical. It may be useful to form a focus group with service users to explore this.

- Enabling social inclusion requires system change, and system change means doing things differently to how they have been done in the past. Change is a funny thing: there is a tendency to want everyone else to do the changing. You can do things differently by asking open questions about how people are and what troubles them, rather than what brings them to your service and how they meet the criteria (which you may have to do in addition, but it does not have to be the first question). Whatever you do, kindness and positive regard will make the experience more positive for the service user. Greater institutional change requires participation by more people, often from different agencies: try taking a problem-solving approach to cases, rather than an approach based on what each agency can do. Establishing shared values – such as a principle of inclusion – could be part of establishing local communities of practice, where people working in related areas try to find joint solutions to the problems their clients face.

- Focusing joint energy on resolving the clients' problems, rather than on discussing what the agencies can (or cannot) offer, is often illuminating for the agencies and helpful for the client. There are many places where multi-agency responses to seemingly intractable problems in delivering effective services to 'challenging' groups have resulted in successful joint working and successful interventions. These include the development of the Multi-Agency Risk Assessment Conference (MARAC) approach in domestic abuse (Robinson 2004; Robinson and Tregidga 2005), the Multi-Agency Public Protection Arrangements (MAPPA) approach to managing sex offenders (Scottish Government 2014), and, more specific to homeless people, the current Big Lottery-funded Fulfilling Lives programme that works with homeless people with complex needs (Fulfilling Lives 2016). All of these involve statutory agencies, including health, social care and criminal justice, working with third-sector and community agencies and are successful examples of what have been termed 'communities of practice' (Cornes *et al.* 2014).

- The system change needed is to one that recognises the importance of social connectedness and social interaction as the basis of well-being. You can promote these values by recognising the importance of relationships, the fact that you are in a relationship (however brief or limited) with your clients, and whether or not they are in other relationships. This will impact on the effectiveness or otherwise of your intervention as well as the experience of the service user. Social connectedness and social interaction for your clients can be significantly enhanced by forming groups within your own and related services that meet regularly to try to enable the most effective responses to client need. Solution-focused service meetings will also help your clients to connect.

- 'One of the things I learned…was that until I changed myself, I could not change others' (Mandela 2014). You need to be prepared to change and prepared to change your service; it is simply ineffective (as well as morally wrong) to expect the socially excluded to be the ones who make all the changes.

- The biggest change you can make in your practice is to think of the person in front of you as a person, not as a 'service user' defined by the service's criteria. Ask them how you can help them, then work with them on finding a response that really matters for them. Most recovering homeless clients say that there was someone really important for them, usually a worker, in enabling them to move themselves out of homelessness (Groundswell 2014). You can be one of the most important people in somebody else's life.

- Think how you can include people – colleagues, commissioners and service users themselves – who are involved in the service or could collaborate with the service. Inclusive practice begins by including people around you.

Conclusion

We *can* change the dynamic that leads older people from social isolation to social exclusion and homelessness. It 'just' requires proactively working to increase the inclusiveness of our services. System change, like culture change, happens because a determined number of people want to make that change, and they persist – so be patient. Smaller changes in inclusivity can be easier to make, and multiple small changes in practice underpin system and culture change.

Promoting social inclusion is a social act. Doing this by organising a community of practice between professionals and the communities they work within, perhaps using or developing links with volunteers and charitable activity as I suggested above, is likely to be beneficial for everyone. It would activate the 'five ways to well-being' – Connect, Be Active, Take Notice, Keep Learning and Give (Aked *et al.* 2014) – for all the participants. Social and health care in a neighbourhood could be jointly designed and jointly delivered by multiple participants including the local community; there have been several experiments in community commissioning as well (Turning Point 2015). This could have effects on public health, mental health, crime and disorder, antisocial behaviours and the whole panoply of social and health issues. Moreover, it would almost certainly turn out to be cheaper than what we are doing now.

Fortunately, we also already have the main resources to do it: ourselves; existing services in health, social care and the voluntary sector and the professionals within them; and the people around us (PHE 2015). Of all initiatives, ending social isolation and proactively working towards social inclusiveness lends itself very much to 'localism' because it is in each of our own localities that the socially isolated are living, right now. This will require strong leadership – leadership at all levels – and you can be part of that leadership. Professionals working in health and social care are in a prime position to provide such leadership.

Perhaps we need to decide what sort of society we want to live in: socially exclusive or socially inclusive? The well-being of all of us may depend on it, and our professional lives give us a platform from which to work towards the changes we want to see. So lastly, I'd like to leave you with a question to think about: when people in your community need help, do you and your service tell them 'This is what we offer'? How much difference would it make to them, and to you, if instead you could ask them 'What is it that you want and need?', and then (as part of a local network of inclusive services) offer them help to find it? Wouldn't you and they both feel better at the end of the day?

References

Age UK (2016) *Factsheet 78: Safeguarding Older People from Abuse and Neglect.* London: Age UK. Available at www.ageuk.org.uk/Documents/EN-GB/Factsheets/FS78_Safeguarding_older_people_from_abuse_fcs.pdf?epslanguage=en-GB?dtrk=true, accessed on 6 November 2016.

Aked, J., Marks, N., Cordon, C. and Thompson, S. (2014) *Five Ways to Wellbeing.* London: New Economics Foundation. Available at http://b.3cdn.net/nefoundation/8984c5089d5c2285ee_t4m6bhqq5.pdf, accessed on 6 November 2016.

Bateman, A. and Fonagy, P. (2006) *Mentalization-based Treatment for Borderline Personality Disorder.* Oxford: Oxford University Press.

Brighter Futures (2011) *Rough Treatment for Rough Sleepers.* Available at www.brighter-futures.org.uk/images/uploads/Rough_Treatment,_Rough_Sleepers.pdf, accessed on 25 September 2016.

Brodie, C., Carter, S. and Perera, G. (2013) *Rough Sleepers: Health and Healthcare.* London: NHS Central London CCG, NHS Hammersmith & Fulham CCG and NHS West London CCG.

Brown, R. (ed.) (2015) 'Special issue: Homelessness – the extreme of social exclusion.' *Clinical Psychology Forum 265,* 1–48.

Campaign to End Loneliness (2013) 'Just over half of England's health and wellbeing boards now acknowledge loneliness and isolation.' Available at www.campaigntoendloneliness.org/blog/just-over-half-of-englands-health-and-wellbeing-boards-now-acknowledge-loneliness-and-isolation, accessed on 25 September 2016.

Cockersell, P. (2011) 'Homelessness and mental health: Adding clinical mental health interventions to existing social ones can greatly enhance positive outcomes.' *Journal of Public Mental Health 10,* 2, 88–98.

Cockersell, P. (2012) 'Homelessness, Complex Trauma and Recovery.' In R. Johnson and R. Haigh (eds) *Complex Trauma and Its Effects.* Hove: Pavilion Publishing.

Cockersell, P. (2015) 'The processes of social exclusion.' *Clinical Psychology Forum 265,* 13–18.

College of Social Work (2014) *Module 5: Equality and Diversity.* Available at http://cdn.basw.co.uk/upload/basw_25529-2.pdf, accessed on 6 November 2016.

Cornes, M., Manthorpe, J., Hennessy, C., Anderson, S., Clark, M. and Scanlon, C. (2014) 'Not just a talking shop: Practitioner perspectives on how communities of practice work to improve outcomes for people experiencing multiple exclusion homelessness.' *Journal of Interprofessional Care 28,* 6, 541–546.

Coulton, C.J. and Rosenberg, M. (2014) 'Social justice and rationing social services.' *Journal of Sociology and Social Welfare 8,* 2, Article 14. Available at http://scholarworks.wmich.edu/jssw/vol8/iss2/14, accessed on 25 September 2016.

CSH and Hearth (2011) *Ending Homelessness Among Older Adults and Elders through Permanent Supportive Housing.* New York: Center for Supportive Housing.

Davidson, L. (2013) *Recovery: Challenging the Paradigm.* Available at http://old.recoverydevon.co.uk/resource?task=document.viewdoc&id=11127, accessed on 6 November 2016.

Fazel, S., Khozla, V., Doll, H. and Geddes, J. (2008) 'The prevalence of mental disorders among the homeless in Western countries: Systematic review and meta-regression analysis.' *PLoS Medicine 5,* 12, e225, doi:10.1371/journal.pmed0050225.

Friedli, L. (2009) *Mental Health, Resilience and Inequalities.* Copenhagen: World Health Organization.

Fulfilling Lives (2016) *Fulfilling Lives: Supporting People With Multiple Needs.* Available at www.biglotteryfund.org.uk/prog_complex_needs, accessed on 25 September 2016.

Goffman, E. (1990) *Stigma.* London: Penguin.

Groundswell (2010) *The Escape Plan.* Available at http://groundswell.org.uk/the-escape-plan, accessed on 25 September 2016.

Health Foundation (2011) *Evidence: Helping People Help Themselves.* London: The Health Foundation. Available at http://personcentredcare.health.org.uk/sites/default/files/resources/helping_people_help_themselves_0.pdf, accessed on 25 September 2016.

Heng, S. (2007) 'Social workers rationing services: The unhappy gatekeepers.' *Community Care,* 7 November. Available at www.communitycare.co.uk/2007/11/07/social-workers-rationing-services-the-unhappy-gatekeepers-by-simon-heng, accessed on 25 September 2016.

Holt-Lunstad, J., Smith, T.B. and Layton, J.B. (2010) 'Social relationships and mortality risk: A meta-analytic review.' *PLoS Med 7,* 7, e1000316, doi:10.1371/journal.pmed.1000316.

Homeless Link (2015) *Rough sleeping in England up 55% in Five Years*. Available at www.homeless.org. uk/connect/news/2015/feb/26/rough-sleeping-in-england-up-55-in-five-years, accessed on 25 September 2016.

Howse, K. (2006) *Increasing Life Expectancy and the Compression of Morbidity*. Working Paper No. 206. Oxford: Oxford Institute of Ageing. Available at www.ageing.ox.ac.uk/files/workingpaper_206. pdf, accessed on 25 September 2016.

Kolk, B.A. van der, Pynoos, R.S., Cicchetti, D., Cloitre, M. *et al.* (2009) *Proposal to Include a Developmental Trauma Disorder Diagnosis for Children and Adolescents in DSM-V*. Available at www. traumacenter.org/announcements/DTD_NCTSN_official_submission_to_DSM_V_Final_ Version.pdf, accessed on 6 November 2016.

Leicester City Council (2014) *Anti-discriminatory Practice*. Leicester: Leicester City Council.

Levitas, R., Pantazis, C., Fahmy, E., Gordon, D., Lloyd, E. and Patsios, D. (2007) *The Multi-dimensional Analysis of Social Exclusion*. Bristol: University of Bristol. Available at http://dera.ioe. ac.uk/6853/1/multidimensional.pdf, accessed on 25 September 2016.

Macmillan, H. (1957) '1957: Britons "have never had it so good".' *BBC News*. Available at http:// news.bbc.co.uk/onthisday/hi/dates/stories/july/20/newsid_3728000/3728225.stm, accessed on 25 September 2016.

Maguire, N.J., Johnson, R., Vostanis, P., Keats, H. and Remington, R.E. (2009) *Homelessness and Complex Trauma: A Review of the Literature*. Southampton: e-prints.soton.ac.uk.

Mandela, N. (2014) 'Quotes about negotiating change.' *goodreads*. Available at www.goodreads.com/ quotes/tag/negotiating-change, accessed on 25 September 2016.

Masten, A. (2001) 'Ordinary magic: Resilience processes in development.' *American Psychologist 56*, 3, 227–238.

MEAM (2010) *Multiple Needs and Exclusions*. Available at www.meam.org.uk/multiple-needs-and-exclusions, accessed on 25 September 2016.

NMHDU (2010) *Meeting the Psychological and Emotional Needs of People Who Are Homeless*. Available at http://eprints.soton.ac.uk/187695/1/meeting-the-psychological-and-emotional-needs-of-people-who-are-homeless.pdf, accessed on 6 November 2016.

Oxford Dictionary (2014a) 'Recovery.' *Oxford English Dictionary*. Available at www.oxforddictionaries. com/definition/english/recovery, accessed on 25 September 2016.

Oxford Dictionary (2014b) 'Social exclusion.' *Oxford English Dictionary*. Available at www. oxforddictionaries.com/definition/english/social-exclusion?q=social+exclusion, accessed on 25 September 2016.

Payne, M. (2005) *Modern Social Work Theory*. Basingstoke: Palgrave Macmillan.

PHE (2015) *Local Action on Health Inequalities: Reducing Social Isolation Across the Lifecourse*. London: Public Health England.

Robinson, A.L. (2004) *Domestic Violence MARACs (Multi-Agency Risk Assessment Conferences) for Very High-Risk Victims in Cardiff, Wales: A Process and Outcome Evaluation*. Cardiff: Cardiff University.

Robinson A.L. and Tregidga, J. (2005) *Domestic Violence MARACs (Multi-Agency Risk Assessment Conferences) for Very High-Risk Victims in Cardiff, Wales: Views from the Victims*. Cardiff: Cardiff University.

Roos, L.E., Mota, N., Afifi, T.O., Katz, L.Y., Distasio, J. and Sareen, J. (2013) 'Relationship between adverse childhood experiences and homelessness and the impact of axis I and II disorders.' *American Journal of Public Health 103*, Suppl. 2, s275–s281, doi:10.2105/AJPH.2013.301323.

Schore, A. (1994) *Affect Regulation and the Origin of the Self: The Neurobiology of Emotional Development*. Hillsdale, NJ: Lawrence Erlbaum.

Scottish Government (2014) *Multi-Agency Public Protection Arrangements (MAPPA) in Scotland: National Overview Report*. Available at www.gov.scot/Resource/0046/00462072.pdf, accessed on 25 September 2016.

St Mungo's (2009) *Happiness Matters: Homeless People's Views about Breaking the Link between Homelessness and Mental Ill Health*. London: St Mungo's. Available at www.mungos.org/documents/1043/1043. pdf, accessed on 25 September 2016.

St Mungo's (2014a) *Annual Client Survey* (internal report). London: St Mungo's Broadway.

St Mungo's (2014b) *Homeless Health Matters: The Case for Change*. London: St Mungo's Broadway. Available at www.mungosbroadway.org.uk/documents/5390/5390.pdf, accessed on 25 September 2016.

Thompson, N. (2002) 'Developing Anti-discriminatory Practice.' In D.R. Tomlinson and W. Trew (eds) *Equalising Opportunites, Minimising Oppression*. London: Routledge.

Turning Point (2015) *Explaining Connected Care*. London: Turning Point. Available at www.turning-point.co.uk/media/23688/connectedcarebrochure.pdf, accessed on 25 September 2016.

VicHealth (2005) *Social Inclusion as a Determinant of Mental Health and Wellbeing*. Carlton, Australia: VicHealth. Available at www.vichealth.vic.gov.au/search/social-inclusion-as-a-determinant-of-mental-health-and-wellbeing, accessed on 25 September 2016.

Walsh, K. (2013) *Homelessness, Ageing and Dying*. Cork: Simon Community.

Warnes, A. and Crane, M. (2006) 'The causes of homelessness among older people in Britain.' *Housing Studies 21*, 3, 401–421.

Wenger, G.C., Davies, R., Shahtahmasebi, S. and Scott, A. (1996) 'Social isolation and loneliness in old age: Review and model refinement.' *Ageing and Society 16*, 333–358.

Windle, K., Francis, J. and Coomber, C. (2014) *Preventing Loneliness and Social Isolation: Interventions and Outcomes*. Research Briefing 39. Available at www.scie.org.uk/publications/briefings/files/briefing39.pdf, accessed on 25 September 2016.

YoungMinds (2015) *Stigma – A Review of the Evidence*. London: YoungMinds. Available at www.youngminds.org.uk/assets/0000/1324/stigma-review.pdf, accessed on 25 September 2016.

Zagier Roberts, V. (1994) 'The Organisation of Work.' In A. Obholzer and V. Zagier Roberts (eds) *The Unconscious at Work*. London: Routledge.

PART III

Additional Information and Practical Guidance to Support Positive Practice

The Rough Guide to Working with Interpreters in Mental Health

Rachel Tribe and Pauline Lane

A ten-minute training film on working with interpreters in mental health services was developed by Pauline Lane and Rachel Tribe for the Department of Health, and it can be located on YouTube at www.youtube.com/watch?v=k0wzhakyjck.

While some of the other chapters in this volume have used the terms 'service user', 'client' or 'patient', this chapter will use the term 'expert by experience' in order to denote and emphasise the importance of acknowledging the expertise, knowledge and insights about their own histories and mental distress held by the people who use health and social care services.

Introduction

Some experts by experience will not be fluent in the official language of the country where the consultation is taking place and will require the services of an interpreter to enable them to access services and for effective communication to take place. For instance, it is not uncommon for professionals to speak unthinkingly when working with older adults and to address carers or younger family members rather than the older adult. This practice often happens even when a shared language is spoken by both the expert by experience and the practitioner, so it can become even more complex and important to note when there is not. Working in partnership with an interpreter is a skill which all health and social care practitioners should acquire through training so as to ensure that anti-discriminatory practice is promoted and upheld and that services are accessible to all.

Working effectively with interpreters is imperative for equitable service delivery. Moreover, the provision of interpreters in public-sector services needs to be informed by and observe the relevant equalities legislation. Many countries have a range of legislation that relates to promoting equality and anti-discrimination; in the UK, for example, this includes the Human Rights Act 1998, the Race Relations (Amendment) Act 2000, the Disability Discrimination Act 2005 and the Equality Act 2010. Relevant legislation will cover the use of interpreters to support and enable access to public services for all members of the community, regardless of their fluency in English or another relevant language. Although legislation may not always mention directly the use of interpreters, it may contain a number of concepts which relate to this. For example, concepts such as preventing indirect discrimination, statements about it being unlawful to discriminate on racial grounds, the right to freedom of expression or a legal duty to eliminate unlawful discrimination and advance equality of opportunity between different groups will be present in legislation in many countries. All of these legal requirements broadly encompass a right to access public services through an interpreter for an expert by experience who is not fluent in English or the language of the country in which he or she is living. If you need to find out the language spoken by an expert by experience, this can be checked at the following web site, which provides a guide to languages by country: www.ethnologue.com/country_index.asp.

Some older adults may never have learned to speak English fluently due to migration issues, living and working within one language community, a lack of opportunity to do so or for other reasons (Tribe 2011). On occasion, older adults who have been fluent in English as a second language when they were younger may lose their fluency when suffering from disorders such as dementia, and therefore it is often good practice to offer the option of using an interpreter to ensure that their needs are properly understood and addressed. This needs to be discussed with the expert by experience and approached with sensitivity and diplomacy. Shah has written about the potential tensions and associated good practice relating to working with interpreters, specifically relating to the issue of mental capacity (see Chapter 5, this volume).

Being dependent on another person to convey one's words and meanings, as in the context of using an interpreter, can lead to anxiety and feelings of discomfort as it requires placing one's complete trust in another person to represent one's words, private thoughts and feelings accurately. It is important that practitioners are sensitive to this and the changed dynamics that can occur, and that they take this into account in their work. Additionally, accessing health and social care services per se may be viewed with anxiety or suspicion by some experts by experience, and this can be exacerbated when someone is not fluent in the English language or belongs to a community which has experienced discrimination and social exclusion in the past. Likewise, it may be that if an older adult has not accessed services previously, he or she may feel unsure about what to ask for or be unclear on what service providers can offer and what his or her health and social care entitlements might be. It is important that practitioners do not underestimate these kinds of life-embedded nuances and that they remain mindful of the personal and relational dynamics that can unfold.

The role of carers

The option of using an interpreter may need to be discussed with a carer for an older adult in order to ascertain and engage with the wants, needs and concerns the older adult may have. It is possible that a carer may also require an interpreter if he or she is not fluent in English. In this context, issues of trust and confidentiality may require particular attention from the practitioner working with older adults and from their family members or carers. Good practice stipulates that a practitioner should use an interpreter even if other family members or a carer speaks English. This is to ensure that the expert by experience is enabled to understand everything that is being discussed in the meeting (perhaps between the carer and the practitioner) and does not become or feel unnecessarily excluded. The carer has a particular role, and family members may bring their own interpretation or views of the issue in question, and these may differ from those of the older adult who is the expert by experience. It ensures that the voice of the older adult is not filtered through the experiences or wishes of a family member or carer. In an initial meeting, when an older adult may have some anxieties, or when the purpose is only information exchange (e.g. a change of appointment time or a change in a medication regime), it may be appropriate for a family member to be used. Nonetheless, the older adult should be consulted, and if he or she confirms to the health or social care professional that it is an appropriate way forward, this direct exchange can allow immediate issues to be dealt with promptly. Also, if there is anxiety or suspicion about health and social care services on the part of the expert by experience, the use of a family member or carer in an initial meeting can on occasion enable trust to be developed between the worker and older adult before a professional interpreter is introduced. Such a negotiation requires skill on the part of the worker to ensure that boundaries and issues of confidentiality are adequately managed (Resera, Tribe and Lane 2015; Tribe and Thompson 2016).

The process of working with an interpreter

We will now identify the different phases of working with an interpreter. We have inserted references throughout the text which the interested reader may wish to consult.

Preparation
Booking an interpreter

This may be done through an interpreting agency or, if available, your organisation's own panel of interpreters. If an interpreting agency is to be used, it is important to check that it is registered with a reputable national organisation[17] and that the interpreter is qualified to National Vocational Qualification Level 3 or holds the Diploma in Public Service Interpreting. The issue of qualifications for interpreters is still developing, and there are a range of different qualifications currently available, although national standards are being produced. It is good practice to avoid using family members as interpreters, apart from initial meetings when practicalities (e.g. booking a time) are being addressed, as detailed earlier, and *never* use children. When working with older adults in the family setting, it may be tempting to use family members, but some older adults want to discuss personal issues (or may even be vulnerable to abuse), and therefore it is important to employ a professional interpreter.

Before making a booking

It might appear obvious, but it is important to find out what is the expert by experience's first language and try to find an interpreter for this language. It is always preferable to use an interpreter who is proficient in the expert by experience's mother tongue, or preferred language (even though, for example, some Asian experts by experience may speak multiple languages). Ensure that the correct dialect is spoken, as otherwise communication may be negatively affected (Tribe 2009). This is particularly important within mental health services where the expert by experience's exact meaning and purpose may be extremely important. Language usually embodies something of the culture it represents (Anderson and Goolishian 1992), so if a third language is used, particular nuances and subtleties may be lost or compromised.

If you have not had an opportunity to undertake training in working with interpreters, you may find it useful to prepare yourself by arranging to spend time talking with an experienced interpreter in advance of your meeting. Many professional organisations and health trusts run training sessions on working with interpreters. A possible training curriculum for working with interpreters can be located in Tribe with Sanders (2003). Research shows that the more experienced interpreters are, the more likely they are to regard training as beneficial both in terms of their own skill development and for the person they are interpreting for (Granger and Baker 2003). It has also been found that training health professionals in working with interpreters helps increase their readiness to work alongside interpreters (Stolk *et al.* 1998).

It is bad practice to invite interpreters to wait without you prior to the meeting with the older adult, carers or the family, as they may be put under pressure to take on tasks beyond their remit. Razban (2003) has written on the pressures she experienced from individuals and families when working as an interpreter. These included being invited to partake of meals and being asked to intercede on behalf of the individual and family. The former may be something that is culturally appropriate but could feel like it blurs the professional's boundaries for both parties. It may be different if the interpreter is specifically employed as a health advocate or link worker by your organisation and is expected to advocate on behalf of the expert by experience or community, as this will be part of his or her role.

Schedule extra time for the meeting or consultation

Since all conversation needs to be interpreted, practitioners may need to give themselves more time than they would schedule for a normal meeting. This will enable those involved not to feel rushed, and it is more likely to lead to better outcomes and the expert by experience feeling he or she has been treated with respect, properly listened to and understood (Kline *et al.* 1980).

Employ the right interpreter

It is helpful, in selecting an interpreter, to employ someone who is familiar with working in mental health settings and has undertaken some training in this field. If the interpreter is used for an assessment under the Mental Health Act 1983, it is important to familiarise yourself with the relevant guidance (Department of Health 2015). It is also important to rule out any interpreters who feel uncomfortable or anxious about working within mental health as well as those who may have a special sensitivity to the subject matter. For instance, it might be inappropriate to expect someone who has negative views about mental health or who holds ageist views to interpret for an older adult with mental health issues. Anti-discriminatory practice requires that older adults are given a choice about the interpreter selected, as it is important that they feel comfortable and able to discuss issues openly.

Gender, age, nationality and religion

It is usually helpful to match the gender of the interpreter to that of the expert by experience, particularly when this may have a bearing on the mental health issue under discussion (Shah and Heginbotham 2008). For example, when discussing sexual health or a sexual assault, an expert by experience may be more likely to feel comfortable with an interpreter of the same gender. However, this may not always be the case; for example, if an older man had been raped, he may not feel that he would want to discuss this in front of a male interpreter.

Another dynamic in interpreting involves religious beliefs. These may form an important part of an individual's world, and they may also be a valuable source of support and assist in promoting resiliance and compassion. In addition, people from different cultural backgrounds may account for their mental health in terms of spiritual beliefs, for example believing that a Jinn or the devil is talking to them. Therefore, matching the older person and the interpreter by religion may be significant. It may come to be a useful resource, or it may not be significant – either way, exploring the matter as part of the selection process will be extremely beneficial. In addition, age can be positioned differently across cultures, and this may require consideration in ensuring that an older adult gets the best interpreter to meet their needs, as some older people may not be comfortable sharing private feelings with a younger interpreter. Therefore, it is important to take the personal characteristics of the interpreter into account to support and promote anti-discriminatory practice.

Booking the same interpreter

It is good practice to use the same interpreter for a series of consultations or meetings. You may need to emphasise this when you make the original booking with the interpreter and, if possible, make a series of bookings. This will enable trust to be built up in the therapeutic setting and is likely to lead to the expert by experience feeling more comfortable, respected and contained. It is also good practice to create an atmosphere in which the interpreter feels able to ask for clarification of a word or sentence and to say when something is not clear to them. Most health and social care professionals use a range of jargon or abbreviations without even realising that they are doing so, and therefore it is useful to check that the interpreter follows what you are saying. Indeed, it may be helpful to explain some specific terminology in the pre-meeting with the interpreter.

The importance of a pre-meeting

Once you have selected an interpreter, having gone through the points above, it is useful to arrange to meet the interpreter for 10 or 15 minutes before meeting the expert by experience to decide how you will work together, explain the objectives of the meeting and to share any relevant background information. This is likely to be time well invested. It will provide an opportunity to clarify any technical concepts and vocabulary which may be used, as well as to check whether there are any cultural issues likely to have relevance to the meeting. Interpreters are not only proficient in two languages but also likely to be an invaluable source of relevant cultural information if you allow them to be.

If a carer is to be present for the meeting or consultation, the health and social care professional should decide whether or not it is appropriate for the carer also to attend the pre-meeting without the older adult. In general, this is not recommended, as it can lead to the older adult feeling excluded and disempowered and is not in line with anti-discriminatory practice.

Depending on the nature of the meeting and its objectives, you may need to speak with the interpreter in the pre-meeting to choose a method of interpreting that best suits the consultation. For example, in a psychotherapeutic encounter you may be most concerned with understanding the intended meanings, feelings and emotions which are being expressed, while if you are writing a medico-legal report you may be more concerned with a word-for-word interpretation (Raval 2003; Tribe 1999). While a meeting about medication or the provision of aids may be more factual and outcome-focused, interpreters may move between interpreting for psychiatric assessments, outpatient medication monitoring sessions and a range of therapies, all of which make different demands of the interpreter. It is helpful to discuss this with the interpreter in advance of the session so that you are both clear about how you will work together. This is likely to lead to better outcomes for the expert by experience. Remember that having an interpreter as a conduit or intermediary makes you and the expert by experience dependent on another person, and this may alter the dynamics of all the interactions during the meeting (Resera, Tribe and Lane 2015).

The physical layout of the room

Before you start the meeting, consider how you will physically manage a three-way consultation or, if a carer is present, a four-way consultation. You may wish to move the furniture around before the expert by experience arrives, and there are several schools of thought on the best arrangement. We recommend a triangular-shaped arrangement (with the carer, if there is one, sitting close to the expert by experience), allowing everyone to see everyone else. However, some practitioners believe that the interpreter should sit behind the expert by experience and act merely as the expert by experience's voice, with all speech delivered in the first-person singular. The use of the first person is usually viewed as being more respectful and as better able to convey immediacy, vocal expression and emotion. This is therefore the best option, regardless of the selected layout of the chairs (Tribe and Thompson 2016). If the older adult is frail, has restricted mobility or is in bed, it is important to think about where you and the interpreter will sit, so that the expert by experience feels respected and can see and hear everybody.

Ground rules

It is important that you create an environment in which the interpreter feels able to ask for clarification if the issues are not understood. You are working in partnership with the interpreter, and without his or her contribution your meeting could not take place. It may be helpful to reflect upon this in advance and during the session. Interpreters bring a range of skills and they are not just technicians; they can offer useful cultural and contextual information too, though any information should always be checked out with the expert by experience. Languages are not interchangeable, and one word in one language may need several sentences in another (Mudakiri 2003). Grammatical structures vary wildly, so do not feel uncomfortable if a long exchange appears to be taking place as the result of one sentence from you. Working in a triad as opposed to a dyad can lead to feelings of exclusion for one party, and it may be helpful to be mindful of this. This may be further exacerbated if a carer can speak both languages, and therefore this may require acknowledgement and open discussion. It is good practice to state that everything that is said in the session will be translated, so that no one feels excluded.

Remember that interpreting is often exhausting. The interpreter is constantly either listening, interpreting or talking, so schedule time accordingly. The older adult may also find a long session tiring, so both of these factors need consideration.

Trust

The health and social care practitioner and the interpreter need to gain the trust of the expert by experience if they are to be able to work together effectively. The health or social care practitioner needs to work at ensuring that a comfortable and professional atmosphere is created in the room to assist with this process. Issues of trust may have particular meaning and significance for people from communities who have experienced discrimination, disempowerment or disenfranchisement. Older adults may not be used to talking about their feelings and needs to people outside of their family, and therefore it is very important to establish a good therapeutic alliance and clear communication. The latter can be made more complex when working through an interpreter and with a carer present, who may want to speak on behalf of the older adult, especially if the older adult has diminished mental capacity. However, it is always important to make time to listen and to remember that the expert by experience is the one who has come to see you. Pivotal to building trust is openness of rapport, and non-verbal communication holds a particular place within this. Remember to look at and address when appropriate the person who has come to seek your services rather than the interpreter. You will find that a natural rhythm is established with different people looking at each other at different times.

The session
During the consultation
Allow some time for the interpreter and the expert by experience to introduce themselves. Should an expert by experience bring a carer with them to a meeting, it is important not to have conversations with the carer which the older adult cannot understand as this may lead to them feeling excluded.

In spite of all preparations, you may find that the expert by experience is initially uneasy with the presence of an interpreter. You may find it useful in these circumstances to reintroduce the interpreter in your own words and, with the help of the interpreter, confirm that the interpreter is a professional doing his or her job. Reiterate and stress that the interpreter is independent and is present to facilitate communication between you and the expert by experience. Clarify that he or she is not there to make any evaluations, has no decision-making powers and is bound by the agency's confidentiality policy. Health and social care practitioners may also feel uncomfortable working with an interpreter, but usually they find that they gain confidence with experience (Raval 1996).

Plain English
Try to avoid using specialist terminology unless it is essential, and try to explain any technical terms that you are using. By using straightforward language, you can reduce the possibility of misunderstandings and misinterpretations. For example, if you refer to OCD (obsessive-compulsive disorder), PTSD (post-traumatic stress disorder), dementia

with Lewy bodies (DLB) or Pick's disease, this may not have any meaning to an interpreter if they are not trained in mental health terminology in both languages. Also avoid using proverbs and sayings. Many proverbs do not translate into other languages easily, and any attempt to translate them can result in misunderstandings. A good rule to follow is that whatever does not make literal sense will not translate well into another language.

While in the presence of the expert by experience, avoid discussing issues with the interpreter that do not require interpretation (e.g. discussing external issues such as the time of the next client's appointment). Such discussion can lead to the expert by experience feeling excluded and disenfranchised. Keep external matters for after the meeting.

Pace of the session

You may need to slow down the pace of your delivery, as the interpreter has to remember what you have said, translate it and then convey it to the expert by experience. If you speak for too long, the interpreter may be hard pressed to remember the first part of what you said and may inadvertently summarise it. Conversely, if you speak in segments that are too short, you may find that your speech becomes fragmented and that you and the interpreter lose the thread of what is being said. You will find that, with open communication and trust, a natural rhythm becomes established which everyone feels comfortable with. Some older adults may have experienced hearing loss, and everyone may benefit from openly discussing and thinking through the best ways of managing this.

Idioms of distress

Different cultures present their distress in different ways, so it is important that the practitioner is receptive to other explanatory health beliefs and idioms of distress. (An idiom of distress is the way that distress is presented, and it may be culturally located and defined.) Exploring this meaning-making process through an interpreter when working with someone who has a different mother tongue and culture can be a fascinating process, and it may lead to a new understanding of the mental health issue in question. On occasion, however, interpreters may find themselves interpreting between different world views. You need to be receptive to this if you are to fully understand what the expert by experience is trying to describe, and you should also be mindful of the interpreter's role in explaining this.

After the consultation
Debriefing your interpreter

Remember that you and your organisation have a duty of care to your interpreter. They may have heard very difficult and traumatic material being discussed, and they are as susceptible to vicarious or secondary traumatisation as anyone else. It is important to remember that they may not have anywhere else to discuss their feelings since many interpreting agencies do not offer support or supervision to their interpreters, and most interpreters will not have had comprehensive health or social care training (unlike a practitioner). Therefore, each organisation should consider how they will support their interpreters. Spending 10 to 15 minutes with the interpreter after each meeting should always form part of your practice. Make the interpreter comfortable enough to give his or her impression of the meeting. You will often find that interpreters, relieved from the pressure of the meeting, produce useful observations and information. You can also use the time to ask the interpreter to clarify any relevant issues that arose from the meeting. Welcome criticism of yourself, as this may help you to improve your practice when working with interpreters in the future.

Discuss your own observations of the interpreter's performance. If you have any serious doubts about the interpreter's conduct, make sure you provide this feedback to the interpreter's agency after having first discussed it with him or her. This is crucial in the development and improvement of the quality of the service provided to experts by experience by your organisation.

Conclusion

In summary, interpreters provide a valuable and highly skilled service to experts by experience who are not fluent in English, and without them it would not be possible to provide services to non-English-speaking experts by experience. Their invaluable and skilled contribution is frequently not recognised.

Acknowledgements

We would like to acknowledge the Department of Health for its assistance in producing an earlier version of these guidelines.

References

Anderson, H. and Goolishian, H. (1992) 'Client as Expert.' In S. McNamee and K. Gergen (eds) *Therapy as a Social Construction*. London: Sage.

Department of Health (2015) *Mental Health Act 1983: Code of Practice*. Published August 1993 pursuant to Section 118 of the Act. London: The Stationery Office. Available at www.gov.uk/government/uploads/system/uploads/attachment_data/file/435512/MHA_Code_of_Practice.PDF, accessed on 26 September 2016.

Granger, E. and Baker, M. (2003) 'The Role and Experience of Interpreters.' In R. Tribe and H. Raval (eds) *Working with Interpreters in Mental Health*. London: Brunner-Routledge.

Kline, F., Acosta, F., Austin, W. and Johnson, R.G. (1980) 'The misunderstood Spanish-speaking patient.' *American Journal of Psychiatry 137*, 1530–1533.

Mudakiri, M.M. (2003) 'Working with Interpreters in Adult Mental Health.' In R. Tribe and H. Raval (eds) *Working with Interpreters in Mental Health*. London: Brunner-Routledge.

Raval, H. (1996) 'A systemic perspective on working with interpreters.' *Clinical Child Psychology & Psychiatry 1*, 1, 29–43.

Raval, H. (2003) An Overview of the Issues in the Work with Interpreters.' In R. Tribe and H. Raval (eds) *Working with Interpreters in Mental Health*. London: Brunner-Routledge.

Razban, M. (2003) 'An Interpreter's Perspective.' In R. Tribe and H. Raval (eds) *Working with Interpreters in Mental Health*. London: Brunner-Routledge.

Resera, E., Tribe, R. and Lane, P. (2015) 'An introductory study into the experiences of interpreters and counsellors working with refugees and asylum seekers.' *International Journal of Culture & Mental Health 8*, 2, 192–206.

Shah, A.K. and Heginbotham, C. (2008) 'The Mental Capacity Act 2005: Some implications for black and minority ethnic elders.' *Age and Ageing 37*, 242–243.

Stolk, Y., Ziguras, S., Saunders, T., Garlick, R., Stuart, G. and Coffey, G. (1998) 'Lowering the language barrier in an acute psychiatric setting.' *Australian and New Zealand Journal of Psychiatry 32*, 434–440.

Tribe, R. (2011) 'Migrants and Mental Health: Working Across Culture and Language.' In D. Bhugra and S. Gupta (eds) *Migration and Mental Health*. Cambridge: Cambridge University Press.

Tribe, R. (2009) 'Working with interpreters in mental health.' *International Journal of Culture & Mental Health 2*, 2, 92–101.Tribe, R. and Thompson, K. (2016) *British Psychological Society's Guidelines on Working with Interpreters in Health Settings*. Leicester: British Psychological Society.

Tribe, R. with Sanders, M. (2003) 'Training Issues for Interpreters.' In R. Tribe and H. Raval (eds) *Working with Interpreters in Mental Health*. London: Brunner-Routledge.

Tribe, R. (1999) 'Bridging the gap or damming the flow? Using interpreters/bicultural workers when working with refugee clients, many of whom have been tortured.' *British Journal of Medical Psychology 72*, 567–576.

Further reading

Abdallah-Steinkopff, B. (1999) 'Psychotherapy of PTSD in co-operation with interpreters.' *Verrhalensterapie 9*, 211–220.

Bansal, A., Moore, D. and Singh, D. (2015) 'Consulting through interpreters.' *InnovAiT: Education and Inspiration for General Practice 8*, 5, 306–311.

Barrington, A.J. and Shakespeare-Finch, J. (2014) 'Giving voice to service providers who work with survivors of torture and trauma.' *Qualitative Health Research 24*, 12, 1686–1699.

Barron, D.S., Holterman, C., Shipster, P., Batson, S. and Alam, M. (2010) 'Seen but not heard – ethnic minorities' views of primary health care interpreting provision: A focus group study.' *Primary Health Care Research & Development 11*, 2, 132–141.

Bischoff, A., Bovier, P.A., Isah, R., Francoise, G., Ariel, E. and Louis, L. (2003) 'Language barriers between nurses and asylum seekers: Their impact on symptom reporting and referral.' *Social Science & Medicine 57*, 503–512.

Brisset, C., Leanza, Y. and Laforest, K. (2003) 'Working with interpreters in health care: A systematic review and meta-ethnography of qualitative studies.' *Patient Education and Counselling 91*, 131–140.

Drennan, G. and Swartz, L. (1999) 'A concept overburdened: Institutional roles for psychiatric interpreters in post-apartheid South Africa.' *Interpreting 4*, 2, 169–198.

Edelson, M. (1975) *Language and Interpretation in Psychoanalysis.* New Haven, NJ: Yale University Press.

Farooq, S. and Fear, C. (2003) 'Working through interpreters.' *Advances in Psychiatric Treatment 9*, 104–108.

Gerrish, K. (2001) 'The nature and effect of communication difficulties arising from interactions between district nurses and South Asian patients and their carers.' *Journal of Advanced Nursing 33*, 566–574.

Green, H., Sperlinger, D. and Carswell, K. (2012) 'Too close to home? Experiences of Kurdish refugee interpreters working in UK mental health services.' *Journal of Mental Health 21*, 3, 227–235.

Greenhalgh, T., Robb, N. and Scambler, G. (2006) 'Communicative and strategic action in interpreters' consultation in primary health care: A Habermasian perspective.' *Social Science & Medicine 63*, 170–187.

Hoffman, L. (1989) *Lost in Translation.* London: William Heinemann.

Hsieh, E. and Nicodemus, B. (2015) 'Conceptualizing emotion in healthcare interpreting: A normative approach to interpreters' emotion work.' *Patient Education and Counseling*, S0738-39915 (epub).

Karliner, L.S., Jacobs, E.A., Chen, A.H. and Mutha, S. (2007) 'Do professional interpreters improve clinical care for patients with limited English proficiency? A systematic review of the literature.' *Health Service Research 42*, 726–754.

Kuay, J., Chopra, P., Kaplan, I. and Szwarc, J. (2015) 'Conducting psychotherapy with an nterpreter.' *Australasian Psychiatry 23*, 3, 282–286.

Leanza, Y., Boivin, I., Moro, M.R., Rousseau, C. *et al.* (2014) 'Integration of nterpreters in mental health interventions with children and adolescents: The need for a framework.' *Transcultural Psychiatry 52*, 3, 353–375.

Leanza, Y., Miklavcic, A., Boivin, I. and Rosenberg, E. (2014) 'Working with Interpreters.' In L. Kirmayer, J. Guzder and C. Rousseau (eds) *Cultural Consultation.* New York: Springer.

National Register of Public Service Interpreters (2011) *Code of Professional Conduct.* Available at www.nrpsi.org.uk/for-clients-of-interpreters/code-of-professional-conduct.html, accessed on 26 September 2016.

Papadopoulos, R. (2003) 'Narratives of Translating-interpreting with Refugees: The Subjugation of Individual Discourses.' In R. Tribe and H. Raval (eds) *Working with Interpreters in Mental Health.* London: Brunner-Routledge.

Patel, N. (2003) 'Speaking with the Silent: Addressing Issues of Disempowerment when Working with Refugee People.' In R. Tribe and H. Raval (eds) *Working with Interpreters in Mental Health.* London: Brunner-Routledge.

Pavlenko, A. (2012) 'Affective processing in bilingual speakers: Disembodied cognition.' *International Journal of Psychology 47*, 6, 405–428.

Searight, H.R. and Armock, J.A. (2013) 'Foreign language interpreters in mental health: A literature review and research agenda.' *North American Journal of Psychology 15*, 1, 17–38.

Splevins, K., Cohen, K., Bowley, J. and Joseph, S. (2010) 'Vicarious posttraumatic growth amongst interpreters.' *Qualitative Health Research 20*, 12, 1705–1715.

Steinberg, A.G., Sullivan, V.J. and Loew, R.C. (1998) 'Cultural and linguistic barriers to mental health service access: The deaf consumer's perspective.' *American Journal of Psychiatry 155*, 7, 982–984.

Travesse, M. (2008) *An Interpreter in the Therapy Room. G6 Information Sheet.* Lutterworth: The British Association for Counselling and Psychotherapy.

Tribe, R. (2005) 'Working with Interpreters in Legal and Forensic Settings.' In K. Barrett and B. George (eds) *Race, Culture, Psychology and the Law.* New York: Sage.

Tribe, R. and Raval, H. (eds) (2003) *Working with Interpreters in Mental Health.* London: Brunner-Routledge.

CHAPTER 13

Ageing, Food and Malnutrition

Pauline Lane and Rachel Tribe

This final chapter offers the reader a quick overview of some of the key issues concerning ageing and food. Good food is essential for our physical and mental well-being, but our individual approach to food and eating is influenced by a wide number of factors. These can be understood at three interdependent levels – namely:

1. *Micro level (personal characteristics)*: While we all need money to buy good food (or grow food), there are other things that influence our food choices, such as our dietary or health needs, religion and culture, childhood or family food traditions, and our experience of food education. In addition, people's household income, location and mobility all influence their access to good food.

2. *Meso level (structural characteristics)*: This relates to the organisational structure of the food industries (incorporating, for example, supermarkets, agro-industry, factory farming, etc.) and the impact these have on food. All of these issues have an impact on older people, as their diets are influenced by the availability of local food, access to shops and transportation, and the cost of food in the shops.

3. *Macro level (national and global economy)*: All of our food consumption is influenced by governmental policies and global food markets (with transnational companies controlling most of the food markets in the world). The macro politics of food has an impact on not only the kinds of foods available to us

but also the cost of those foods and the impact of agricultural and trading policies on local people and the environment.

While these three levels of food politics are interlinked, this chapter will look only at the impact of food on older people at the micro level (i.e. the personal level), as that is the level where most professionals are able to bring about any impact or change. However, it may be useful to understand some of the broader political and structural boundaries that influence our access to food, and so a very short reading list is also provided at the end of the chapter.

Barriers to healthy eating for older people

People approach their food choices, preparation and consumption in very different ways.

How we obtain food, share it and receive it are all part of our daily social practices. These practices tell us a lot about what a society values. While many older people retain responsibility for their own food shopping and cooking, others will have their food provided by families or commercial companies, and thousands of others will have their food provided for them in hospitals and care homes.

There is very limited research on older people living with long- or short-term mental health problems and their access to good nutrition. However, there are a few studies that identify the apparent complexity of the relationship between older people, food and mental health. Because eating well is vital for both physical and mental health, how older people eat at home represents an important part of their physical and mental health management (Berman, Kendall and Bhattacharyya 1994). However, many older people find it difficult to sustain good nutrition, and this may be the result of a number of issues:

- Poor appetite, cognitive impairment, and physical and sensory disabilities can all impact on an older person's eating and drinking patterns. Some older people may be unable to recognise that they are hungry or thirsty. Specific forms of cognitive impairment, such as dementia (Chen *et al.* 2010).

- Other mental health problems and physical disabilities may also impair communication so that the older person is unable to express his or her needs. Eating by oneself may be a risk factor for mental illness among older men, but this may also be influenced by cohabitation status (Tani *et al.* 2015).

- Eating disorders are usually seen as affecting young people, but a recent study suggests that there has been a gradual increase in eating disorders among middle-aged and older women related to their concerns about body image (Mangweth-Matzek, Hoek and Pope 2014). These findings are echoed in an earlier study with men in the USA, which found that older men can also suffer from a syndrome similar to anorexia nervosa (Miller *et al.* 1991).

- A study by Haw and Stubbs (2010) looked at the practice of mixing medication in food (covert drug administration) for older inpatients with severe mental illness. The researchers suggest that while this may be common practice, the process raises important medical and legal issues. (Although it was beyond the scope of the study, it would have been useful to know if this process had an effect on the level of food consumption.)

At a more general level, research has shown that there are a number of barriers to healthy eating for older people.

Poverty

Poverty has a significant impact on the quality of older people's lives, and, unsurprisingly, research has shown that poverty is a major barrier to healthy eating (Jones *et al.* 2009). In some cases, the cost of fuel and other bills means that older people cut back on food. Some older people who arrived in the UK in the 1950s and 1960s had little or no opportunity to build pensions and consequently are living in extreme poverty in their old age (Joseph Rowntree Foundation 2014; Lane, Tribe and Hui 2010).

Ethnicity

Black, Asian and Minority Ethnic (BAME) older people are more likely to face a greater level of poverty, live in poorer quality housing and have less access to benefits than White older people. Research suggests that many BAME older people feel that the majority of public-sector services do not meet their cultural and personal needs (Joseph Rowntree Foundation 2004). Access to the majority of public-sector services for BAME older people remains problematic due to language barriers, a lack of knowledge as to what is available, and the attitudes and practices of service providers (Joseph Rowntree Foundation 2004). Many BAME older people may need support and advice on food if they need to make changes to their diet later in their life. Some traditional and religious foods (such as samosas, pakoras, gatya and kachoris) may contain high levels of saturated fat, salt and sugar. BAME elders often have limited information on healthy eating (Age UK 2007), but family members and professionals can help by offering information and advice on healthier alternatives.

Homelessness

Homeless people (old and young) have little or no food security, and they often do not know where their next meal will come from. Many homeless people are also living with drug and alcohol dependency, which can affect their nutrition and general health (Shaw and MacDonald 2007).

Bereavement

Bereavement often has a significant impact on older people's eating patterns; this is particularly the case when it is a life partner who has died, as most couples will have had a lifetime of sharing meals. People who are newly bereaved can often find it difficult to adjust to cooking for one. For people living alone, being able to buy small amounts of food is very important for their health, but a recent project noted that small quantities of food (such as tinned food and meat) are often much more expensive than larger quantities, and the UK food industry does not really cater for people living alone (Pilmeny Development Project 2011). Research suggests that older men who live alone often have less variety in their diets and a lower intake of fruit and vegetables than older women who live alone (Hughes, Bennett and Hetherington 2004), and this could be linked to the fact that older men often have poorer cooking skills than women (Lilley 2002).

Transport

Many older people living in rural areas do not have access to local shops, and only 52 per cent of people aged over 70 hold a full driving licence. Most older people find taxis unaffordable, and many areas have cut local bus services, while some older people physically struggle to use free public transport facilities (Age UK 2011). This means that many rural older people are travelling long distances to source their food.

Technology

Although some older people are able to use online shopping, many are not able to use the internet or do not have a computer. Most supermarkets also have a minimum spend limit for delivery and sometimes a delivery charge. In addition, a report by Age UK (2012a) suggests that online shopping does not facilitate the social interaction that some older people value, especially if they live alone.

Modern diets

When thinking about food and nutrition, it is important to recognise that many people will adapt and change their food preferences and practices over time. For example, in the past, Gypsies would often cook traditional food, such as rabbit stew, to keep their families fed while they were on the road. Nowadays, many Gypsy and Traveller families eat fast and convenience foods, and due to government policy many Gypsies and Travellers are forced to live on permanent sites, and diabetes and cardiovascular disease are now on the rise in many Gypsy and Traveller communities (Greenfields 2014; Vozarova de Courten *et al.* 2003). Therefore, practitioners may want to work with older people in these communities to encourage them to consider traditional cultural foods that may be healthier than some of the modern fast-food alternatives.

Local authority budgets

Due to central funding cuts, one-third of all UK local authorities have abandoned 'meals on wheels' provision to their older and vulnerable residents, though some older people are using their social care budgets to source their meals from elsewhere (Butler 2014).

Malnutrition in older people

As a consequence of the barriers identified above, many older people in the UK suffer from malnutrition. BAPEN (a charitable association that raises awareness of malnutrition) states that it affects more than one in ten older people (BAPEN 2006). Malnutrition is largely both preventable and treatable, and it is not a natural consequence of older age (Malnutrition Task Force 2013). Malnutrition is an important risk factor for older people becoming vulnerable to illness and their independence becoming compromised, and malnourished older people will often experience an increased risk of infection and greater antibiotic use, longer recovery time from illness as well as an increased risk of mortality (Wilson 2013). In 2015, the total public expenditure on tackling malnutrition in health and social care services was estimated to be £19.6 billion, with older adults accounting for 52 per cent of the total amount (BAPEN 2015). So better nutritional care for individuals at risk from malnutrition could result in better outcomes for the individual, as well as substantial cost savings to the NHS (Elia *et al.* 2005).

Research suggests that 1.3 million people over 65 suffer from malnutrition, and the vast majority (93%) live in the community (BAPEN 2014). The risk of malnutrition increases significantly with age, often due to many of the barriers identified above together with the fact that people often have increased frailty and physical dependence as they age. Of those at risk from malnutrition in the UK, 93 per cent live at home and have little or no link with health services (Age UK 2014). Those who live on their own are almost twice as likely to be undernourished compared to those who live with someone else (Age UK 2014). One-third of all older people admitted to hospital are at risk of malnutrition (Age UK 2014). However, 36 per cent of patients in hospital who said they needed help to eat their meals did not always get it (Care Quality Commission 2013).

Research suggests that in the winter there is an increase in hospital admissions of people with malnutrition, especially among people aged over 80 years (Age UK 2014). Malnourishment has a considerable impact on health: malnourished patients stay in hospital longer, are three times as likely to develop complications during surgery, and have a higher mortality rate than people who are well nourished (Age Concern 2006).

In 2012, the Care Quality Commission released a report that identified that one-fifth of 1362 nursing homes and 15 per cent of 258 NHS hospitals were not helping older patients to access the food and drink they required. While the national minimum standards for care homes require that 'service users receive a wholesome appealing balanced diet in pleasing surroundings at a time convenient to them' (Department of Health 2003), nearly 2000 care homes in England did not meet this standard in 2006 (Commission for Social Care Inspection 2006).

However, in recent years there has been a culture change in health and social care, and BAPEN (2015) have reported that:

> substantial changes in clinical practice have occurred since 2007, with more nutritional screening taking place in hospitals, and more attention being given to inspections in both hospitals and care homes. For example, the Care Quality Commission undertook both general and specific inspections on dignity and nutrition/hydration to evaluate quality of care against their standards. The Francis Inquiry into the failing of the mid-Staffordshire Health Authority also highlighted various types of problems due to poor nutrition and hydration. It concluded that there was a need to produce a culture change in order to improve clinical standards of care, with potentially important economic consequences. (BAPEN 2015, p.6)

Promoting good nutrition for older people eating in their own homes

Research by Vesnaver *et al.* (2012) looked at how older people who are healthy and active manage to eat well despite the dietary obstacles of old age. The researchers noted that most of the older people who were successful in maintaining their health and activity developed 'dietary resilience' that involved the following:

- prioritising eating well

- personal food resources such as food and nutrition knowledge, cooking skills, good physical health and financial adequacy

- Independent transport facilitated the development of adaptive strategies among participants to overcome their nutritional vulnerabilities.

The importance of relying on oneself was mentioned frequently. Participants became aware of services through their social network. For example, they knew about calling meals on wheels and were aware of who else they could call on if they needed support. How such lunch and social clubs are advertised can be critical for engagement. For example, research by Dwyer and Hardill (2011) suggests that many older men regard lunch clubs as being for women only.

Another long-term study (by EPIC) of health and ageing based in Norfolk also looked at the positive and negative eating habits of older people. EPIC-Norfolk is part of a Europe-wide project that is the largest study of diet and health ever undertaken. It involves over half a million people in ten countries. They recruited 25,000 people aged 40 to 80 to take part in a 20-year Europe-wide study of health. Previous research had demonstrated that people who consume extra vegetables each week have a 13 per cent lower risk of developing Type 2 diabetes. However, the researchers in the Norfolk study found that many people who were widowed had poorer diets than those who lived in partnerships and ate considerably fewer vegetables. But the good news is that the same research shows that improving older people's social ties has a positive impact, not only on people's social lives but also on their eating and overall health (Myint *et al.* 2007).

In traditional gender roles, the purchasing and preparation of food tends to be seen as the role of women, especially in households where people are older. However, when traditional gender roles are challenged by ill health (such as a stroke or dementia), some men see this as a new opportunity to cook and show their caring skills (Mattsson Sydner and Fjellström 2007).

From the research studies outlined above, it is clear that there are a number of social factors that can both mitigate against good nutrition and also promote good nutrition and the well-being of older people. As practitioners, we are rarely in a position to be able to influence national and global food policies, but we can make a difference at the individual level by supporting people to build their 'dietary resilience' and to ensure that the services we work with facilitate access to all and support the improved nutrition.

Food festivals and religious observances

For many older people, eating is associated with memories and food from their past (Lyman 1989). Although many European countries are increasingly secularised, a lot of older (and younger) people continue to follow religious observances where food rituals and food taboos form part of their wider belief system, and these may also set a boundary between believers and non-believers (Grumett 2013). While specific foods are sometimes deemed sacred, other food may be blessed or have spiritual qualities bestowed upon it (Mintz and Du Bois 2002). Because people's religious practices are so diverse, it is not possible here to cover all religions' food obligations and taboos. However, many websites offer information about religion and food, and those listed below are just a small sample of those that are available:

- BBC guide to world religions: www.bbc.co.uk/religion/religions

- BBC guide to religious festivals: www.bbc.co.uk/religion

- FAQs.org Religion and Dietary Practices: www.faqs.org/nutrition/Pre-Sma/Religion-and-Dietary-Practices.html.

Ideas and resources for promoting anti-discriminatory practice and healthy eating

For older people who cook and eat at home

Ideas

- Improving the diets of older adults might include offering cooking classes, especially those focusing on cooking for older men and for people living on a restricted budget.

- The introduction of direct payments and personal budgets can give older people more choice and control over their food and can promote mental well-being. For example, an older Chinese man may wish to use his budget to pay a local Chinese restaurant to provide a hot meal on a daily basis.

- Information needs to be provided in appropriate languages and formats to enable BAME older people who are not fluent in English to access the whole range of services offered by personalisation.

- Older people can often be a useful resource for local communities and schools for heritage teaching. Bringing young and older people together to make food can support and encourage intergenerational understanding as well as pride in cultural foods.

- Volunteers run local lunch clubs in many areas, but it can be difficult for some people to find out about them, especially if they don't speak English, or to access them if they have a disability. Information needs to be available in a number of formats and languages, and the lunch clubs need to be accessible.

- It is important for older people to be encouraged to enjoy their traditional foods, but it is also necessary to help people to focus on dishes that are low in fat and salt and rich in fruit and vegetables.

- For many older people, eating several (5–6) small, non-fatty meals each day can be helpful. This pattern is associated with greater food variety and lower body fat, blood glucose and lipid levels, especially if meals are eaten early in the day.

- Encouraging older people to be more physically active on a regular basis, including exercises that strengthen muscles, improves balance and should help to prevent falls. This might include joining a walking group, attending dancing or swimming classes, or gardening.

- Religious and cultural issues often heavily influence the diets of people including older adults.

- Maintaining nutrition during fasting periods can be difficult for some older people, and some religions allow exemptions from strict adherence. (For example, Muslims who are ill or frail would be exempt from fasting during Ramadan.) Where necessary, seek advice from religious leaders.

Resources

- The Scottish Older People Services Development Project has developed a useful downloadable leaflet titled *Healthy Diet and Lifestyle for Ethnic Minority Older People: Providing Information, Raising Awareness* (2015): www.communityfoodandhealth.org. uk/wp-content/uploads/2015/11/Healthy-Living-Final-English.pdf. (The guide is available in Arabic, Chinese, Urdu, Punjabi and Hindi, and other languages on request.)

- Age UK's report *Fit as a Fiddle: Engaging Faith and BME Communities in Activities for Well-being* contains many positive practice examples: www.ageuk.org.uk/Documents/EN-GB/ FaithGood%20Practice%20GuideWEB.pdf?dtrk=true

- Third-sector organisations have always been involved in providing food for people who are marginalised in our communities, and many charities and faith communities are involved in running soup kitchens, food banks and lunch clubs. For example:

  » the Trussell Trust provides food banks across the UK: www.trusselltrust.org/map

  » the Royal Voluntary Service provides lunch clubs to bring older people together to enjoy a hot, nutritious meal and socialise with friends at the same time (they host 450 community and lunch clubs across England, Scotland and Wales): www.royalvoluntaryservice.org.uk/get-help/ social-activities/lunch-clubs

For older people who are eating in a hospital or care home
Ideas

- Offering people choice and control over their food is important, not only because it helps people to enjoy their food more, but also because food is often part of people's social and cultural identity.

- Eating together, cooking tasty food and offering small, frequent meals can encourage older people to eat better.

- The environment really matters; people need an appropriate space to eat and time to do so.

- Older adults may need help and encouragement to eat, and this can also help to tackle malnutrition.

- In a day centre, home or hospital, it is useful to have a copy of religious festivals and observances close at hand so that staff can provide the appropriate food and understand if someone is fasting.

- If your service offers food, offering culturally appropriate food can make a real difference to people's well-being, so it is helpful to develop menus in consultation with the people who are going to eat the food.

- Older people may sometimes like to share traditional recipes and be involved in food preparation. Food-related reminiscence may also help to engage older people in discussions about their cultural heritage. In addition, this could be used as an opportunity to discuss the adaptation of traditional foods to meet the dietary needs for specific conditions (e.g. diabetes).

- Some older people may like to say prayers before or after meals; always allow time and space for this.

Resources

- The National Patient Safety Agency (NPSA) has produced a series of nutrition factsheets to support the delivery of the ten key characteristics of good nutritional care: www.nrls.npsa. nhs.uk/resources/?entryid45=59865. Their website also contains links to other nutrition factsheets.

- The Royal College of Nursing (RCN) have developed guidance (titled *Enhancing Nutritional Care*) on how to raise standards of nutrition and hydration in hospitals and in the community: www2.rcn.org.uk/__data/assets/pdf_file/0006/187989/003284.pdf

- The Care Quality Commission has introduced basic enforceable nutritional and hydration standards for service providers:

www.cqc.org.uk/content/regulation-14-meeting-nutritional-and-hydration-needs.

- BAPEN's Malnutrition Universal Screening Tool ('MUST'), a standardised and validated tool, is freely available to all care workers for screening adults for malnutrition in the community. 'MUST' is a five-step screening tool to identify adults who are malnourished, at risk of malnutrition (undernutrition), or obese: www.bapen.org.uk/screening-and-must/must-calculator.

References

Age UK (2007) *Fit as a Fiddle: Engaging Faith and BME Communities in Activities for Well-being*. London: Age UK.

Age UK (2011) *Agenda for Later Life*. London: Age UK.

Age UK (2012a) *Food Shopping in Later life: Barriers and Service Solutions*. London: Age UK.

Age UK (2012) *Factsheet: Later Life in the United Kingdom*. London: Age UK.

Age UK (2013) *Later Life in the United Kingdom*. London: Age UK.

Age UK (2014) *Age UK Inquiry Submission: APPG on Hunger and Food Poverty Inquiry, June 2014*. London: Age UK.

BAPEN (2014) *Introduction to Malnutrition*. Available at www.bapen.org.uk/about-malnutrition/introduction-to-malnutrition?showall=&start=4, accessed on 26 September 2016.

BAPEN (2015) *The Cost of Malnutrition in England and Potential Cost Savings from Nutritional Interventions*. Southampton: Malnutrition Action Group of BAPEN and the National Institute for Health Research Southampton Biomedical Research Centre. Available at www.bapen.org.uk/pdfs/economic-report-full.pdf, accessed on 26 September 2016.

Berman, P., Kendall, C. and Bhattacharyya, K. (1994) 'The household production of health: Integrating social science perspectives on micro-level health determinants.' *Social Science and Medicine 38*, 2, 205–215.

Butler, P. (2014) 'A third of councils cut "meals on wheels" elderly care lifeline.' *Guardian*, 11 November. Available at www.theguardian.com/society/patrick-butler-cuts-blog/2014/nov/11/third-councils-cut-meals-on-wheels-social-care, accessed on 26 September 2016.

Care Quality Commission (2014) *National Findings from the 2013 Inpatients Survey*. Available at www.cqc.org.uk/sites/default/files/inpatient_survey_national_summary.pdf, accessed November 2015.

Chen, Y., Chen, T., Yip, P., Hu, C., Chu, Y. and Chen, J. (2010) 'Body mass index (BMI) at an early age and the risk of dementia.' *Archives of Gerontology and Geriatrics 50*, Suppl. 1, S48–S52.

Davis, M.A., Randall, E., Forthofer, R.N., Lee, E.S. and Margen, S. (1985) 'Living arrangements and dietary patterns of older adults in the United States.' *Journal of Gerontology 40*, 434–442.

Department of Health (2003) *Care Homes for Older People: National Minimum Standards*. London: HMSO.

Dwyer, P. and Hardill, I. (2011) 'Promoting social inclusion? The impact of village services on the lives of older people living in rural England.' *Ageing and Society 31*, 243–264.

Elia, M. and Russell, C. (eds) (2009) *Combating Malnutrition: Recommendations for Action. A Report from the Advisory Group on Malnutrition, Led by BAPEN*. Redditch: BAPEN.

Elia, M., Stratton, R., Russell, C., Green, C. and Pang, F. (2005) 'The cost of disease-related malnutrition in the UK and economic considerations for the use of oral nutritional supplements (ONS) in adults.' *Health Economic Report on Malnutrition in the UK*. Redditch: BAPEN.

Greenfields, M. (2014) 'It's a sweet life travelling: Meeting the healthcare needs of Travellers with diabetes.' *Journal of Diabetes Nursing 18*, 193–198.

Grumett, D. (2013) 'Food and Theology.' In K. Albala (ed.) *Routledge International Handbook of Food Studies*. Abingdon: Routledge.

Hill, K., Sutton, L. and Hirsch, D. (2011) *Living on a Low Income in Later Life*. London: Age UK.

Hughes, G., Bennett, K. and Hetherington, M. (2004) 'Old and alone: Barriers to healthy eating in older men living on their own.' *Appetite 43*, 269–276.

Jones, J., Duffy, M., Coull, Y. and Wilkinson, H. (2009) *Older People Living in the Community – Nutritional Needs, Barriers and Interventions: A Literature Review*. Edinburgh: Centre for the Older Person's Agenda, Queen Margaret University.

Joseph Rowntree Foundation (2004) *Black and Minority Ethnic Older People's Views on Research Findings*. Written by Jabeer Butt and Alex O'Neil. York: Joseph Rowntree Foundation. Available at www.jrf.org.uk/report/black-and-minority-ethnic-older-peoples-views-research-findings, accessed on 26 September 2016.

Lane, P., Tribe, R. and Hui, R. (2010) 'Intersectionality and the mental health of elderly Chinese women living in the UK.' *International Journal of Migration, Health and Social Care 6*, 4, 34–41.

Lilley, J.M. (2002) *Food Choice in Later Life*. London: Food Standards Agency.

Lyman, B. (1989) *A Psychology of Food: More than a Matter of Taste*. New York: Van Nostrand Reinhold Co.

Malnutrition Task Force (2013) *A Review and Summary of the Impact of Malnutrition in Older People and the Reported Costs and Benefits of Interventions*. London: International Longevity Centre – UK.

Mangweth-Matzek, B., Hoek, H. and Pope, H. (2014) 'Pathological eating and body dissatisfaction in middle-aged and older women.' *Journal of Foodservice 18*, 119–129.

Mattsson Sydner, Y. and Fjellström, C. (2007) 'Illuminating the (non-)meaning of food: Organization, power and responsibilities in public elderly care – a Swedish perspective.' *Journal of Foodservice 18*, 119–129.

Millen, B. (1999) 'Preventive Nutrition Services for Aging Populations.' In W.O. Seiler and H.B. Strahelin (eds) *Malnutrition in the Elderly*. New York: Springer.

Miller, D.K., Morley, J.E., Rubenstein, L.Z. and Pietruszka, F.M. (1991) 'Abnormal eating attitudes and body image in older undernourished individuals.' *Journal of the American Geriatrics Society 39*, 462–466.

Mintz, S.W. and Du Bois, C.M. (2002) 'The anthropology of food and eating.' *Annual Review of Anthropology 31*, 99–119.

Myint, P.M., Welch, A.A., Bingham, S.A., Surtees, P.G. *et al.* (2007) 'Fruit and vegetable consumption and self-reported functional health in men and women in the European Prospective Investigation into Cancer-Norfolk (EPIC-Norfolk): A population-based cross-sectional study.' *Public Health Nutrition 10*, 1, 34–41.

Pilmeny Development Project and Edinburgh Food and Health Training Hub (2011) *Case Study into the Quality, Scope and Nature of Food Services for Older People in North East Edinburgh*. Available at http://pilmeny.wdfiles.com/local--files/reports/Food%20Services%20for%20Older%20People%20Case%20Study%20Final.pdf, accessed on 26 September 2016.

Tani, Y., Sasaki, Y., Haseda, M., Kondo, K. and Kondo, N. (2015) 'Eating alone and depression in older men and women by cohabitation status: The JAGES longitudinal survey.' *Age and Ageing 44*, 6, 1019–1026.

Vesnaver, E., Keller, H., Payette, H. and Shatenstein, B. (2012) 'Dietary resilience as described by older community-dwelling adults from the NuAge study "If there is a will – there is a way!".' *Appetite 58*, 730–738.

Vozarova de Courten, B., De Courten, M., Hanson, R., Zahorakova, A. *et al.* (2003) 'Higher prevalence of type 2 diabetes, metabolic syndrome and cardiovascular diseases in Gypsies than in non-Gypsies in Slovakia.' *Diabetes Research and Clinical Practice 62*, 2, 95–103.

Wilson, L. (2013) *A Review and Summary of the Impact of Malnutrition in Older People and the Reported Costs and Benefits of Interventions*. London: International Longevity Centre and Malnutrition Task Force.

Further reading on national and global food politics

Lang, T. and Heasman, M. (2004) *Food Wars: The Global Battle for Mouths, Minds and Markets.* London: Earthscan.

Lang, T., Barling, D. and Caraher, M. (2009) *Food Policy Integrating Health, Environment and Society.* Oxford: Oxford University Press.

McMahon, P. (2014) *Feeding Frenzy: Land Grabs, Price Spikes, and the World Food Crisis.* Vancouver: Greystone Books.

Milestine, E. (2008) *The Atlas of Food: Who Eats What, Where and Why?* California: University of California Press.

Pretty, J.N., Lang, T., Morison, J. and Ball, A.S. (2005) 'Farm costs and food miles: An assessment of the full cost of the UK weekly food basket.' *Food Policy 30*, 1, 1–20.

Contributors

Editors

Pauline Lane is a Reader in Mental Health at Anglia Ruskin University. Originally trained as a nurse and later as a sociologist, Pauline has worked on numerous national and international projects concerning social inclusion and minority communities and she has authored/co-authored a large number of governmental reports. She has expertise in ethnographic research methods and is an experienced filmmaker.

Rachel Tribe is Professor of Applied Psychological Practice at the School of Psychology, University of East London. In 2014 she was awarded the British Psychological Society Award for Challenging Social Inequalities in Psychology. She is a Fellow of the British Psychological Society. She has experience obtained over 30 years of developing clinical services and conducting research. She is active in national and international consultancy and training work. She has experience of working in the private, public, charity and academic sectors. She has worked clinically with a range of diverse communities.

Contributors

Matt Broadway-Horner is an experienced consultant in psychological and behavioural health, treating anxiety, depression and trauma using many approaches like CBT, mindfulness and ACT, to name a few. He consults in the NHS, private and charitable sector in the restructuring of services and brand development. Currently he is studying for his PhD at Kings College London on intimate partner violence.

Maria Castro Romero has been Senior Lecturer and Academic Tutor on the Professional Doctorate in Clinical Psychology at the University of East London for the past seven years. Her teaching, research and writing focus on problems faced by elders (including dementia diagnoses), narrative therapy, community and liberation psychology. Before this, Maria was a Highly Specialist Clinical Psychologist in Mental Health Care for Older People. Since then, she has worked collaboratively alongside older adults, women, minorities and other largely marginalised groups, to co-construct with the people who seek help, and their families and communities, a humanising mental health care.

Peter Cockersell is a UKCP-registered Psychoanalytic Psychotherapist with over 20 years' experience of working in homelessness. He has worked in health, mental health, homelessness and social exclusion as a psychotherapist and as a Director of Health and Recovery of a third-sector homelessness agency. Peter currently lectures, consults in Britain and Europe on Psychologically Informed Environments and psychosocial interventions with homeless and socially excluded people, and acts as a clinical supervisor. He also has a small private psychotherapy practice. Peter has published various works on mental health and social exclusion.

Dr Afreen Huq is a Consultant Clinical Psychologist and Neuropsychologist who is retired from the NHS after over 27 years. Dr Huq is a passionate advocate for older adults, working with diversity, maintaining their personhood and addressing social inequalities. Afreen is committed to championing the rights of others by mentoring, supporting and empowering people.

Rena Kydd-Williams commenced her career in 1993 by training as a nurse for people with a learning disability. After qualifying, she held a number of roles before completing her BSc (Hons) in Community Practice. Later she became a school nurse for children with special needs and also conducted research. As her career developed, she took up the post of senior lecturer at Anglia Ruskin University where she worked for over nine years. Rena is currently a PhD student researching the lived experiences of carers of people with learning disabilities on a Caribbean island.

Dr Maureen McIntosh is the current chair of the Division of Counselling Psychology. She has worked in the National Health Service for 14 years with older adults. Maureen belongs to numerous committees, including the North Thames Faculty for the Psychology of Older People and the British Psychological Society Presidential Taskforce on the future of Applied Psychology training. She is facilitator of the NHS Psychology Network which is open to all Applied Psychologists. She has co-authored a book chapter about Professional and Ethical Issues in working with older adults, and her Doctorate research about Older Adults' Experience of Psychological Therapy has been published.

Musthafar Oladosu has worked extensively in services for people with learning disabilities and mental health problems in England. He has worked in both long-stay hospitals and community-based residential facilities, as well as in specialist community multidisciplinary teams in London. Musthafar is currently the Service Manager of the Hackney Integrated Learning Disability Service where he is directly responsible for the specialist health team – a post he has held for several years. He belongs to various leadership forums in London and nationally. His interests include promoting an integrated agenda, health inequality and safeguarding adults.

Ajit Shah is an old age psychiatrist and honorary Professor of Ageing, Ethnicity and Mental Health at the University of Central Lancashire. He has spent the bulk of his clinical and academic career addressing mental health and mental capacity issues in older ethnic minority individuals.

Romany Gypsy **Siobhan Spencer** is studying for a PhD at Anglia Ruskin University. She works in a national capacity on Gypsy planning and health community issues. In 2005 she set up the National Federation of Gypsy Liaison Groups (NFGLG), which provides a network group that encourages and enables members of the Gypsy and Traveller community to participate more effectively with Government and agencies. Between 2007 and 2009 she represented Gypsy Communities on the Government Task Group on Accommodation and Enforcement Issues. She received an MBE for community relations in 2009. In 2012 she she received a Law Degree from Derby University. In 2015 she was appointed to the Government Commission for the Holocaust.

Endnotes

1   Freud used the word 'seele', meaning soul, in his original German writings.
2   From a British and masculine point of view.
3   That is, the processes through which subjectivities are degraded.
4   I use the term structure broadly to include physical/environmental, logistical, discursive (policy), relational and hierarchical elements.
5   Those that are evidence-based, with a reductionist view of evidence presented: 'We can only improve what we can actually measure' (Department of Health 2008, p.49).
6   Taking into account inflation, national investment in mental health services for elders increased by 8.2 per cent from 2008/09 but decreased by −3.1 per cent in 2011/12 (Mental Health Strategies 2012).
7   Former Chief Executive of NHS England Sir David Nicholson earned £211,249 versus £14,294 for Band 1, Point 1. Non-medical consultants on the highest level – Band 9, Point 54 – get paid £98,453.
8   The most basic junior trainee starting salary is £22,636, with consultants and GPs earning £101,451.
9   In plural form, to acknowledge the multiplicity of 'knowledges' that people have, rather than a body of knowledge.
10 Hence it is best expressed as a verb in the gerund form.
11 Curiously, the adjective for someone acting in/with solidarity is not commonly used in English as it is in other languages (e.g. Spanish).
12 It is worth noting that some women from some BME groups may be reluctant to be admitted into hospital or placed in a nursing home out of fear that they might not be able to continue to wear culturally and religiously appropriate clothing. This could trigger an assessment of decision-making capacity, particularly if there are communication barriers if the person lacks fluency in English.
13 Phase 2 of the Carers Act 2014, which was meant to be implemented in 2015, has now been delayed until 2020. Most notably this has delayed the 'cap on care costs' for individuals – it was hoped that this would set a limit on how much money an individual would have to use for care costs.
14 Healthwatch is a statutory watchdog in England that ensures that health and social care services listen to people's views and experiences and act on them.
15 These are a set of checks that aim to make sure that any restrictions on a person's liberty are both appropriate and in their best interests.
16 Note: LGBTi will be used to refer to all people that can be incorporated under the LGBTi banner, and throughout this chapter it will refer to not only lesbian, gay, bisexual, transgender and intersex people, but also queer/questioning, pansexual, asexual, genderqueer non-binary people and all other people who consider themselves to be represented by the banner.
17 The Institute of Translating and Interpreting, the Chartered Institute of Linguists, and Signature (formerly known as CACDP, for sign language interpreters) can all provide further information. There is a National Register of Public Services Interpreters which can be accessed online.

Subject Index

About Dementia (British Institute of Learning
  Disabilities) 201
active ageing theory
  description of 33–4
Adults with Incapacity (Scotland) Act (2000)
  122
advance care planning
  for end of life 190–2
age discrimination
  and intersectionality 22–4
  older people's experience of 7, 22–4
  overview of 38–9
anti-discriminatory practice
  for carers 166–9
  end of life 193–5
  for gypsies and travellers 274–8
  for healthy eating 337–41
  for homeless people 302–7
  for learning disabled people 225–6
  for LGBTi 245–50
  in mental health services 102–4
  for practitioners 42–4, 118–19
  resources for 118–19
anxiety
  and gypsies and travellers 264
  statistics on 80–1, 103
associative discrimination 160

BAME people
  access to mental health services 82–5, 93–5
  as carers 152–5, 162–3, 165
  case studies 71, 73, 77, 141–2
  cultural construction of ageing in 71–3
  culture and identity 69–71
  demographics of 69
  diagnosis of mental illness 86–7
  and discrimination 73–7, 88
  and distress 87, 88–90
  and end of life 178, 185–6, 200
  health beliefs 88–90
  and healthy eating 331–2

improving access to mental health services
  93–5
and intersectionality 22–4, 85
indirect discrimination in mental health
  77–8
and LGBTi people 233–4
marginalisation among 73–7
and Mental Capacity Act (2005) 127–8,
  129–43
mental health service provision for 90–2,
  93–5
parity of esteem in mental health services
  83–5
social exclusion among 73–7
statistics on mental health 81–2
and stigma 88
bereavement
  and healthy eating 332

capabilities
  description of 30–1
  and mental health 27, 28–32
Care Act (2014) 174
  and health of carers 159
  and homeless people 284, 286, 287, 293,
    301
  non-family carers in 157
  and role of carers 148
  support for carers 162
carers
  age of 150–1
  anti-discriminatory practice for 166–9
  attitudes towards 148
  BAME 152–5, 162–3, 165
  cost of 147, 161–2
  definition of 147
  discrimination against 160
  gender of 149–50
  gypsies and travellers 269–74
  health issues 157–9
  hours of 150

impact on 151–2
  and interpreters 317–18
  isolation of 159–60
  learning disabilities 155–6, 224–5
  legislation for 174
  LGBTi 152–3, 156–7, 162–3
  local carers groups 173
  partnership working with 165–6
  and personal budgets 163–5
  and personalisation 163–5
  resources for 172–3
  role of 148–9
  social exclusion of 159–60
  social factors in 149
  support for 162–3
Carers and Disabled Children Act (2000) 174
Carers (Equal Opportunities) Act (2004) 174
Carers (Recognition and Services) Act (1995) 174
case studies
  BAME people 71, 73, 77, 141–2
  dementia 110
  diagnostic systems 110
  end of life 191
  gender 136
  gypsies and travellers 37, 267, 271–4
  homeless people 290–2, 298–301
  humanisation 53–4, 56–7, 62–3
  intersectionality 23–4
  learning disabled people 219, 222, 225
  LGBTi people 250–2
  Mental Capacity Act (2005) 123, 124, 126, 136, 141–2
  mental health 79, 111–123
  older people and mental health 79
  vulnerabilities 28–9
citizenship
  for older people 64–5
communication
  in Mental Capacity Act (2005) 128–34
Community Catalysts 92
Confidential Inquiry into Premature Deaths of People with Learning Disabilities (CIPOLD) 222
countertransference
  and therapists 114–15
Court of Protection 127
Cultural Formulation Interview (CFI) 86
culture
  in caring role 154–5
  construction of ageing 71–3
  and identity 69–71
  and interpreter use 325
  and Mental Capacity Act (2005) 134–5, 136–43
  and mental health service provision 90–2, 94–5

death *see* end of life
Death by Indifference (Mencap) 187, 222
delirium
  statistics on 81, 103
Delivering Race Equality in Mental Health Care (Department of Health) 143
dementia
  and BAME people 81
  case studies 110
  description of 109–10
  diagnosis of 109–11
  and learning disabled people 210, 212, 214
  statistics on 25, 80, 81, 103
demographics
  of older people 7, 20–1, 102, 103
depression
  and BAME people 81
  and carers 152
  and gypsies and travellers 264
  statistics on 80, 81, 103
Diagnostic and Statistical Manual of Mental Disorders (DSM-V) 86, 89, 106
  and diagnosis of mental health 106
  and LGBTi people 236
diagnostic systems
  case studies 110
  for dementia 109–11
  and medical expertise 109
  for mental health services 106–9
Disability Discrimination Act (2005) 316
discrimination
  associative 160
  and BAME people 73–7, 88
  and carers 160
  and Equality Act (2010) 40–1
  forms of 36–8, 40–1
  gypsies and travellers 262–3
  and homeless people 284–5
  and LGBTi people 232–6
  structural 52–4
disengagement theory
  description of 33
distress
  and BAME people 87, 88–90
  as emotional defect 107–8
  and interpreter use 325
  and mental health 107
dying *see* end of life

Employment Rights Act (1996) 174
end of life
  advance care planning for 190–2, 200
  anti-discriminatory practice for 193–5
  for BAME people 178, 185–6, 200
  barriers to good palliative care 189–90
  case studies 191

end of life *cont.*
　death rates 176–8
　definition of 189
　and gypsies and travellers 178, 192
　and homeless people 177, 188, 200
　idea of 'good death' 178–9
　and learning disabled people 177, 187–8,
　　200
　and LGBTi people 186, 200
　and Mental Capacity Act (2005) 181, 188,
　　190, 195, 196, 201
　and mental health services 177, 181–3
　and palliative care 179–81, 189–90
　and religion 183–4
　resources for 200–1
　responsibility for 190
　social context for 176–9
　staff training for 189–90
Equal Treatment Bench Book (Judicial College)
　143
Equality Act (2010)
　and carers 152, 160, 167–8, 174
　and end of life 175
　and gypsies and travellers 275, 276
　and interpreter use 316
　and mental health service provision 90
　overview of 39–41
　practitioner awareness of 42–3
　protected characteristics in 152, 160, 167–8
　and public sector Equality Duty 41–2, 275
equality in humanisation 59–60
Equality Impact Assessments 127–8
ethnic minorities *see* BAME people

food
　anti-discriminatory practice for 337–41
　barriers to healthy eating 330–3
　interdependent levels of 229–30
　malnutrition in older people 334–5
　promoting healthy eating 335–6
　and religion 337
Gay British Crime Survey (Stonewall) 242
gender
　and ageing 20
　in caring role 149–50
　case studies 136
　and end of life 176–7
　and health inequalities 26
　and interpreter use 320
　and Mental Capacity Act (2005) 135–6
Global AgeWatch Index (HelpAge International)
　22
gypsies and travellers
　accommodation for 266–8, 274
　anti-discriminatory practice for 274–8
　carers for 269–74

case studies 37, 267, 271–4
　and end of life 178, 192
　government policy towards 259–61
　and healthy eating 333
　intergenerational reciprocity 269–74
　mental health needs of 264–6
　and Mochadi 266
　population of 259
　resilience of 268–9
　social determinants of health 261–4
　terminology for 258–9

health beliefs
　and BAME people 88–90
health inequalities
　overview of 24–6
Health and Social Care Act (2012) 84, 106,
　206, 297
Healthcare for All (Michael) 222
High Quality Care for All (Department of Health)
　51
homeless people
　anti-discriminatory practice for 302–7
　and Care Act (2014) 284, 286, 287, 293,
　　301
　case studies 290–2, 298–301
　categories of 290–3
　complex trauma 293
　discrimination against 284–5
　and end of life 177, 188, 200
　and healthy eating 332
　among older people 295–7
　recovery in 287–8
　resilience among 294–5
　social exclusion 282–4, 285–7, 288–9,
　　295–6, 301–2
Human Rights Act (1998) 175, 316
humanisation
　as active process 57–8
　case studies 53–4, 56–7, 62–3
　and citizenship 64–5
　dehumanising practices 55–7
　equality in 59–60
　ethical commitment to 58–61
　integrality in 59
　lack of in institutions 50–2
　new horizons for 61–2
　overview of 48–50
　participation in 60–1
　reciprocity in 61
　research on 65–6
　as social task 65
　solidarity in 59
　structural discrimination 52–4
Improving Access to Psychological Therapies
　(IAPT) 28, 75, 84, 105

Independent Mental Capacity Advocate 135, 137, 143
inequality
    health 24–6, 94–5
    and intersectionality 22–4
integrality in humanisation 59
    structural 54–5
intergenerational caring 8
    and gypsies and travellers 269–74
intergenerational conflict theory
    description of 35–6
International Classification of Diseases (ICD) 86, 106, 236–7
International Classification of Functioning, Disability and Health (ICF) 208
interpreter use
    after sessions with 326
    and carers 317–18
    legislation on 132–3, 316
    preparation for working with 318–24
    sessions with 324–5
intersectionality 22–4, 85
isolation
    among carers 159–60
    among learning disabled people 222–3

Joint Commissioning Panel for Mental Health 92–3

lasting power of attorney 126
learning disabled people
    anti-discriminatory practice for 225–6
    access to mental health services 206–7, 216–23
    care provision for 206–7
    as carers 155–6
    carers for 224–5
    case studies 219, 222, 225
    definitions of 208–9
    diagnosis of mental health issues 217–20
    and early-onset ageing conditions 210, 212
    and end of life 177, 187–8, 201
    frequency of falls 223–4
    isolation of 222–3
    and Mental Capacity Act (2005) 211
    and mental health issues 212–16
    and POhWER advocacy group 205–6
    premature ageing of 211
    prevalence of 209–10
    social exclusion of 222–3

LGBTi people
    anti-discriminatory practice for 245–50
    and BAME people 233–4
    as carers 152–3, 156–7, 162–3
    case studies 250–2

discrimination against 232–6
    and end of life 186, 200
    history of 233–4, 252–4
    mental health challenges of 240–2
    mental health needs of 239–40
    and mental health services 236–9
    and queer theory 243–5
    resilience of 242–3
    as service users 243
Liberating the NHS: No Decision About Me Without Me (Department of Health) 51
Living and Dying with Dignity: The Best Practice Guide to End-of-life Care for People with a Learning Disability (Mencap) 201

marginalisation
    among BAME people 73–7
Marriage Act (2013) 248, 254
Mental Capacity Act (2005) 42
    advance decisions in 127
    assessment of decision-making capacity 123–4
    and BAME people 127–8, 129–43
    'best interests' assessment 125–6
    and carers 174
    case studies 123, 124, 126, 136, 141–2
    Code of Practice 125, 126, 128, 130, 131, 133, 134, 135, 138
    communication in 128–34
    Court of Protection 127, 133, 137
    and cultural background 134–5, 136–43
    and end of life 181, 188, 190, 195, 196, 201
    and Equality Impact Assessments 127–8, 133, 135, 137, 143
    and gender 135–6
    interpreter use 132–3
    lack of decision-making capacity in 125
    lasting power of attorney 126, 140
    and learning disabled people 211
    overview of 122–3
    and parity of esteem 84
    personal appearance 136–7
    principles of 123
    and religious beliefs 134–5, 136–43
    and second languages 129–34
mental health
    and capabilities 27, 28–32
    case studies 79, 111–13
    diagnostic systems for 106–9
    and end of life 177, 181–3
    and learning disabled people 212–16
    needs of gypsies and travellers 264–6
    needs of older adults 111–12
    overview of 27–8
    and physical health 112–13

mental health *cont.*
referral pathway 105
seeking help for 104–5
statistics on BAME older people 81–2
statistics on older people 78–81
and vulnerabilities 27, 28–32
Mental Health Act (1983)
and use of interpreters 320
Mental Health Act (2003)
and BAME people 84
Mental Health Act (2007)
and end of life 183
practitioner awareness of 42–3
mental health services
anti-discriminatory practice in 102–4
BAME access to 82–5, 93–5
BAME provision for 90–2, 93–5
diagnostic systems in 106–9
and end of life 177, 181–3
learning disabled people access to 206–7, 216–23
and LGBTi people 236–9
and medical expertise 109
partnetship with carers 165–6
referral pathway 105
seeking help for 104–5

National Health Service (NHS)
humanisation in 50–2
National Health Service and Community Care Act (1990) 215
National Service Framework for Older People (Department of Health) 210
Northern Ireland Act (1998)39

older people
age discrimination 7, 22–4
celebration of 8
citizenship for 64–5
and commissioners of older people's mental health services 92–3
demographics of 7, 20–1, 102, 103
global well-being 22–3
health inequalities 24–6
mental health needs of 110–12
multiple health problems 111–13
poverty 22
statistics on mental health 78–81
and therapeutic alliance 113–17

Older People – Positive Practice Guide (IAPT) 79
On Death and Dying (Kübler-Ross) 179

palliative care 179–81, 189–90
participation in humanisation 60–1
personal appearance

and Mental Capacity Act (2005) 136–7
personal budgets
for carers 163–5
personalisation
for carers 163–5
POhWER advocacy group 205–6
poverty
and healthy eating 331
among older people 22
public sector Equality Duty
overview of 41–2

Race Relations (Amendment) Act (2000) 316
reciprocity in humanisation 61
referral pathway
for mental health services 105
religion
and end of life 183–4
and healthy eating 337
and interpreter use 320–1
and Mental Capacity Act (2005) 134–5, 136–43

Sexual Offences Act (1967) 235–6, 252, 243
social care
decline in funding 26
social exclusion
among BAME people 73–7
among carers 159–60
definition of 288–9
among gypsies and travellers 262–3
among homeless people 282–4, 285–7, 288–9, 295–6, 301–2
among learning disabled people 222–3
solidarity in humanisation 59
structural discrimination 52–4
structural inequality 54–5

therapeutic alliance
and older people 113–17
Think Local Act Personal partnership 92

Valuing People (Department of Health) 208, 211, 217
Valuing People Now (Department of Health) 211
vulnerabilities
and mental health 27, 28–32

women
and ageing 20
in caring role 149–50
and end of life 176–7
and health inequalities 26
and Mental Capacity Act (2005) 140
World Health Organisation Disability Assessment Schedule 2.0 (WHODAS 2.0) 208

Author Index

Abel, J. 192
Abrams, D. 33, 38
Academy of Medical Royal Colleges 104, 181
Academy of Medical Sciences 77
Adams, J. 180
Adamson, J. 154
Afuape, T. 49, 59
Age Concern 74, 90, 103, 334
Age Platform Europe 34
Age UK 35, 41, 72, 151, 161, 223, 284, 332, 333, 334, 339
Age UK Buckinghamshire 74
Ahmed, I. 75
Ahmed, Z. 212
Aked, J. 303, 308
Alborz, A. 187
Almack, K. 157
Alzeheimer's Association 110
Alzheimer's Society 80, 81, 109, 110, 176, 214
American Psychiatric Association (APA) 86, 89
Amory, D.P. 233
Anderson, D. 73, 77, 80, 88
Anderson, E. 62
Anderson, H. 319
Andrew, M.K. 112
Antonicci, T.C. 74
Artazcoz, L. 24
Atchley, R.C. 184
Atkins, D. 114, 115, 116
Atterbury, J. 266
Audit Commission 158
Ayme, C. 42

Backes, D.S. 58, 59, 60, 64, 65
Bailey, L. 238, 241
Baker, M. 319
Bakker, T.J.E.M. 149
Ball, S.L. 224
Banerjee, S.D. 87
BAPEN 334, 335

Barbui, C. 88
Barker, J. 130
Barker, P. 106
Barrett, H.A. 244
Barros, M.E.B. 49
Bateman, A. 293
Bayer, R. 236
Beaumont, J. 80, 103
Beecham, J. 73
Beilby, J.J. 62
Bell, D. 138, 210
Bellamy, G. 157
Benbow, S.M. 220, 221, 223
Bender, M. 110, 111
Bennett, K. 332
Bennett, T. 39
Bentall, R. 78, 106, 107
Berger, M. 106
Berkman, B.J. 75
Berkman, L. 269
Bermajo, J.C. 49, 65
Bermajo Higuera, J.C. 52, 53, 58, 65, 66
Berman, P. 330
Bernard, C. 214
Berry, J.W. 74
Bhalia, A. 129
Bhattacharyya, K. 330
Bhugra, D. 70, 81, 91, 130
Bhui, K. 70, 84, 85, 89, 91, 130
Bick, J. 107
Biggs, S. 34, 109, 116
Bjertness, E. 159
Blakemore, K. 129
Blauner, R. 176
Blaxland, M. 148
Boen, H. 159
Boland, S.M. 38
Bolliger, M. 183
Borowsky, S.J. 82
Borthwick-Duffy, S.A. 214
Boseley, S. 213

Bot, K. 83
Bouras, N. 221
Bowes, A. 74, 90
Bowling, A. 34
Boyer, J.M. 240
Boyle, M. 62, 78, 106
BPS 105, 106
Bracken, P. 86, 106
Bradford, J. 239, 243
Brake, M. 33
Bretschneider, J.G. 245
Brewer, M.B. 38
Bright, C. 187
Brighter Futures 283
Bristol Mind 265
British Institute of Learning Disabilities 211, 222
British Psychological Society 213, 218
Brodie, C. 283
Brodolini, F. 150
Brooks, J. 164
Brotman, S. 243
Brown, C. 88
Brown, P. 259
Brown, R. 297
Brown, S. 177
Bruton, L. 266
Burnett, A. 92
Burns, A. 75, 182
Busby, N. 152
Butler, P. 333
Butler, R.N. 38, 113

Cahill, S. 240
Cairns, R. 128
Calanzani, N. 185
Campaign to End Loneliness 293, 302
Cappeliez, P. 77
Care Quality Commission 81, 334
Care Services Improvement Partnership 77
Carers Trust 147, 151, 161
Carers UK 150, 153, 158, 159, 161
Carers Week 158
Caring for Carers 160, 165
Carr, S. 74, 90, 152, 153
Carter, S. 283
Carvalho, R. 49, 59
Cass, B. 148
Castro Romero, M. 48, 49, 52, 54, 57, 59, 60, 62, 64
Ceccim, R.B. 60
Cemlyn, S. 260, 270
Center for Supportive Housing 296
Centre for Ethnicity and Health 132
Centre for Local Economic Strategies 22
Centre for Policy on Ageing 76

Chakraborty, A. 74, 82
Challis, D. 190
Chan, M.Y. 55
Chauncey, G. 234
Chavira, V. 269
Chellingsworth, M. 105
Chen, Y. 330
Chidgey-Clark, J. 186
Chowdhury, N.A. 87
Cinnirella, K. 88, 91
CIPOLD 222
Clark, C. 269
CNA 223
Cochran, S.D. 37
Cochrane, R. 81
Cockersell, P. 290, 293, 294, 296
Cohen, C. 75
Cohen, S. 159
Cole, P. 138
College of Social Work 285
Combs, G. 59
Commission on Improving Dignity in Care 48
Commission for Racial Equality 259, 260, 261
Commission for Social Care Inspection 335
Condeluci, A. 109
Conner, K.O. 88
Conrad, P. 106
Conway, S. 49, 64
Cook, M. 233
Coomber, C. 295
Cooper, S. 213, 214, 218, 219
Copeland, V. 88
Coppel, D.B. 152
Coppock, V. 106
Cormier, R. 243
Cornes, M. 306
Cornwell, E.Y. 74
Corrigan, P. 36, 85, 88
Cortina, K.S. 74
Costa, S.C. 55
Coulton, C.J. 286
Council of Europe 263
Coupland, C. 79
Craig, R. 74
Crane, M. 188
Crane, M. 295, 296, 297
Crawshaw, P. 64
Crenshaw, K. 23
Cromby, J. 106
CSH and Hearth 296
CSIP 83
Cullen, S. 267
Cumming, E. 33
Curfs, L. 188
Cutler, D. 176

Dahlin-Ivanoff, S. 151
Davidson, L. 287
Davies, E. 189
Dawson, R. 263, 266
DCP 107
Deacon, S. 245
Deaton, A. 176
Deb, S. 187
Delor, F. 29
Demo, D.H. 269
Denson, L.A. 62
Department of Communities and Local
    Government 35
Department for Constitutional Affairs 125,
    128, 130, 131, 133, 143
Department of Health 51, 52, 55, 81, 95, 103,
    105, 117, 132, 143, 181, 187, 208, 210,
    211, 217, 225, 320, 335
Department for Work and Pensions 210
Derbyshire Gypsy Liaison Group 265, 267,
    268, 277
Devine, M. 213
Dickenson, D. 128, 129
Diener, E. 55
Dighe-Deo, D. 75
Division of Clinical Psychology (DCP) 106
Dixon, J. 176
Donovan, J. 154
Dorfman, R. 244
Drennan, G. 91
Driskell, J. 239
Druss, B.G. 177
D'Augelli, A. 242
Du Bois, C.M. 337
Duivenvoorden, H.J. 149
Dull, V. 38
Duncan, R.L. 114
Dwyer, P. 336

Eccles, F.J.R. 103
Ekdawi, I. 108
Elia, M. 334
Elliott, R. 116
Ellis, H. 233, 238, 239
Emerson, E. 155, 187, 209, 210
Emery, T. 35
Epiphaniou, E. 186
Equal Ground 234
Equality and Human Rights Commission 178,
    260, 261, 263, 264, 271, 274
Erdmann, A.L. 58
EuroHealthNet 177
European Commission 259, 263
European Court of Human Rights 263
Evison, F. 85

Falco, K.L. 237
Farquhar, C. 241
Fassil, Y. 92
Fazel, S. 293
Featherstone, M. 245
Fernandez, J.-L. 80
Fernando, S. 70, 74, 82, 83, 84, 86, 87, 154
Ferraro, K.F. 38
Figeiredo, M.R.B. 55
Fillit, H. 113
Finch, J. 150
Fiori, K.L. 74
Fish, J. 156
Fisk, J.D. 112
Fjellström, C. 336
Flynn, A. 220
Fonagy, P. 293
Forbes, L.J. 75
Forder, J. 73, 80
Fortin, M. 77
Foster, J. 89
Foucault, M. 60
Foundation for People with Learning
    Disabilities 207
Fountain, J. 264
Francis, J. 295
Francis R. 117
Fredriksen-Goldsen, K.I. 237, 238
Fredman, G. 62
Fredman, S. 38
Freedman, J. 59
Friedli, L. 293, 294, 300
Friere, P. 65
Froggatt, K. 190
Fulfilling Lives 306
Fuller, A. 263

Gabbay, S. 242
Gaines, J. 39
Gallian, D.M.C. 62
Galvin, K.T. 49
Ganguli, M. 140
Garstka, T.A. 38
Gawande, A. 72
Gibson, G. 87
Gill, P. 262, 277
Gilleard, C. 34, 35
Gilmour, S. 44
Glendinning, C. 164, 187
Glover, G. 85
Goffman, E. 295
Goldsmith, M. 184
Gomes, R.S. 49
Gonçalves Brito, N.T. 49, 59
Gooding, P.A. 76
Goolishian, H. 319

Gosman-Hedström, G. 151
Gott, M. 189, 190
Goudie, F. 75, 88
Government Office for Science 7
Goward, P. 264, 265
Grace, J.A. 186
Granger, E. 319
Gravestock, S. 220
Green, J. 233
Green, M. 24, 26
Greenfields, M. 260, 261, 263, 269, 270, 333
Gregory, C. 153
Griffiths, A. 189
Griffiths, F. 269
Grohmann, S. 186
Grossman, A. 242
Groundswell 307
Groves, D. 150
Grumett, D. 337
Gruskin, E.P. 241
Gupta, S. 70

Hall, V. 263
Hansen, E. 108
Hardill, I. 336
Harding, R. 186
Harold, R.D. 240
Harper, D. 78, 106
Hart, B. 179
Hassiotis, A. 210
Hatton, C. 155
Hauser, J. 180
Hayes, P. 267
Health Careers 55
Health Foundation 285
Health and Social Care Information Centre 85
Health Survey for England 74
Heaphy, B. 157, 240
Hearsum, S. 91, 153
Hegde, R. 138, 143
Heginbotham, C. 129, 130, 132, 135, 136, 138, 140, 144, 320
Helgeson, G. 183
Helman, C. 90, 91
Help the Aged Housing Trust 90
HelpAge International 19, 22
Hemmings, C. 221
Henderson, M. 182
Heng, S. 286
Henry, W. 33
Herek, G.M. 237
Herzog, D. 234
Heslop, P. 177, 207, 210, 222
Hetherington, M. 332
Hettiaratchy, P. 130
Hickling, F.W. 81-2

Higginson, I. 185
Higgs, P. 34, 35
Hillman, J. 246, 247, 250
Hinrichsen, G.A. 246, 247, 250
Hinton, D.E. 89
Hodges, N. 260
Hoek, H. 331
Hoggs, J. 188
Holewa, H. 181
Holland, A. 215, 217, 218
Holloway, I. 49
Holloway, M. 194
Holmes, J.D. 81, 103
Holt Barrett, K. 78
Holt-Lundstad, J. 294, 300
Home, R. 270
Homeless Link 283
Hopton, J. 106
Horowitz, A. 152
House, A.O. 81, 103
House of Commons Health Committee 189, 191, 192
Howse, K. 283
Hoxey, K. 130
Hubert, M. 29
Hughes, A.K. 240
Hughes, G. 332
Hughes, L. 267, 269
Hughes, M. 242
Hughes, T. 52
Hui, R. 24, 331
Hummert, M.L. 36, 38
Hutt, P. 44
Hyer, L. 112, 113

IAPT 76, 79
Improving Access to Psychological Therapies (IAPT) 75, 91
Inouye, S.K. 81
Institute for Fiscal Studies 22
Institute for Research and Innovation in Social Service 149
International Longevity Centre 20
Irish Traveller Movement in Britain 259

Jacob, K.S. 91
James, E. 116
James, N. 225
Jenkins, R. 187
Jennings, R. 232, 233
Jesper, E. 269
Johnson, V.E. 245
Johnstone, L. 106
Joint Commissioning Panel for Mental Health 92, 104, 162, 216
Jones, A. 260, 262, 264, 274

Jones, D.W. 242, 250
Jones, J. 331
Joseph Rowntree Foundation 148, 331, 332
Joung, H. 34
Judicial College 143

Kahn, R. 245
Kannabiran, M. 207
Kaplan, D.W. 75
Karlsen, S. 82
Karlsson, M. 149
Kaskett, E. 116
Kawachi, L. 269
Kelber, M.S. 149
Kellehear, A. 178
Kendall, C. 330
Kennedy, C. 106
Kessler, R.C. 159
Kidd, W. 210
Kim, J. 89
Kimmel, D. 232, 235
King, M. 241
Kinsey, A.C. 245
Kirkwood, T. 7, 8
Kishita, N. 105
Kitwood, T. 110
Kleinman, A. 89
Kline, F. 132, 320
Knight, B.G. 105, 107, 109, 114, 116
Knight, T. 36
Knocker, S. 234, 235, 236, 237, 240, 247
Koerich, M.S. 58
Koffman, J. 185
Kolk, B.A. 293
Kübler-Ross, E. 179
Kumar, A. 190

Laidlaw, K. 105
Lane, P. 24, 91, 94, 153, 260, 261, 262, 263,
    265, 268, 269, 270, 318, 322, 3331
Latoo, J. 151
Lau, A. 265
Lawrie, L. 104
Layton, J.B. 294, 300
Leadership Alliance for the Care of Dying
    People 181
Lee, M. 25
Leeds GATE 278
Leicester City Council 298
Leonard, R. 37
Levine, M.P. 37
Levitas, R. 289, 302
Lewis-Fernandez, R. 89
Licata, S. 233, 249
Lilley, J.M. 332
Lindberg, E. 52

Lindesay, J. 130, 132, 133
Linn, L. 182
Litwin, H. 74
Livingston, G. 70, 90
Lleras-Muney, A. 176
Lloyd-Williams, M. 184
Loewenthal, K.M. 88, 91
Loft, H. 80, 103
Lokae, V. 87
London Gypsy and Traveller Unit 263
Lowenthal, D. 114, 115, 116
Lui, L.L. 38
Lyman, B. 337

MacInnes, T. 22
MacKenzie, S. 86, 129, 130
MacKinlay, E. 183
MacLachlan, M. 82, 89
Macmillan, H. 301
Maguen, S. 241
Maguire, N.J. 293
Making Every Adult Matter 297
Malutrition Task Force 334
Mandela, N. 307
Mangweth-Matzek, B. 331
Manning, L.K. 184
Manthorpe, J. 130
Marcos, L.R. 132
Marianti, R. 30, 31
Marin, M.J.S. 53
Markowitz, F. 36
Marmot, M. 177
Martin, J. 192
Martin, C.E. 5
Martin, P. 259
Martinsen, E.H. 8
Martinsen, K. 8
Marwaha, S. 88, 91
Masini, B.E. 244
Masten, A. 294, 295
Masters, W.H. 245
Matín-Baró, I. 60
Mattos, R.A. 49, 59
Mattson Sydner, Y. 336
Mayengo, N. 72
Mays, V.M. 37
McCabe, M. 218
McCallum, J. 83, 90
McCann, E. 241
McCoy, N.L. 245
McCready, M. 260
McFarquhar, T. 34
McGee, R.E. 177
McGillivray, J. 218
McGrath, P. 181
McIntosh, M. 103, 111, 114

McKenzie, K. 74, 82
McKeown, E. 241
McLornian, P. 213
McNally, R. 187
McNeil, J. 238
Meier, D.E. 190
Meikle, J. 238
Mencap 187, 201, 207, 222
Mendes, V.L.F. 57
Mental Health Foundation 54, 74, 85, 111, 155
Merhy, E.E. 60
Merom, D. 226
Meyer, I.H. 37
Mezzich, J.E. 86
Mhaol'ain, A.M. 105
Michael, J. 187, 222
Midlands Psychology group 107, 108
Miller, D.K. 331
Miller, N. 34
Milne, E. 153
Mind 27, 78, 83, 84, 161
Mindell, J. 74
Ministry of Justice 133, 134, 137, 143
Minority Ethnic Carers of Older People Project in Scotland 270
Mintz, S.W. 337
Mir, G. 154
Mitchell, S.L. 182
Mitchell, W. 164
Mkandawire, T. 26
Mohebati, L. 82
Moncrieff, J. 106, 107
Moore, P. 35
Moravcik, M.Y. 53
Moreno-Leguizamon, C. 186
Moriarty, J. 27
Morrison, R.S. 190
Mortimer, J. 24, 26
Mota, C.S. 62
Moulaert, T. 34
Mudakiri, M.M. 323
Mukherjee, S. 128, 129, 130
Mullick, A. 192
Muran, C.J. 113
Murtagh, F. 190
Myint, P.M. 336

Nare, L. 74
National Black Carers and Carers Workers Network 154
National Council on Aging 85
National Institute for Health and Care Excellence (NICE) 53, 103, 105, 181, 184, 187
National Mental Health Development Unit (NMHDU) 293

National Patient Safety Agency 224
Naylor, C. 177
Nazroo, J. 81, 82
Nelson, T. 38
New Pathways 215
Newton, N.A. 113
Ng, C.H. 88, 91
NHS Choices 223, 224
NHS England 27, 84
NHS Information Centre 80, 148
Nichter, M. 89
Nnatu, I. 129
Nystrom, N.M. 242

Odell, S.M. 82
OECD 22
Office for National Statistics 21, 69, 81, 103, 148, 150, 158, 176, 177, 210, 259, 270
Oishi, A. 190
Okitikpi, T. 42
Orel, N.A. 242, 243
O'Shea, E. 153
Otis, M.D. 242
Ott, C. 149
Oxford Dictionary 287

Page, B. 266
Palmore, E.B. 39
Parkman, S. 130, 132
Parry, G. 178, 262, 264, 265, 267
Pasche, D.F. 49, 58, 61, 65
Patel, N. 70, 75, 78, 87, 90, 95
Payne, M. 283
Peinado–Gorlat, P. 192
People First 207
Perera, G. 283
Petersen, R.P. 233, 249
PHE 305, 308
Phelan, M. 130, 132
Phillips, L.H. 104
Phinney, J.S. 269
Pickard, L. 149
Pickett, K.E. 59
Pilmeny Development Project 332
Pincus, F.L. 36, 37
Política Nacional de Humanização 49
Pomeroy, W.B. 245
Pope, H. 331
Poverty Site 75
PRIAE 69
Price, R.H. 159
Prince, M. 103
Public Health England 300
Puchalski, C. 184
Putnam, R.D. 269

Quayhagen, M. 151
Quayhagen, M.P. 151

Rabow, M. 180
Rait, G. 75, 78, 89
Raval, H. 94, 132, 322, 324
Razban, M. 319
Royal College of Psychiatry (RCP) 81, 82, 88, 103, 104, 105
Read, J. 107
Reginato, V. 62
Reid, A.H. 215
Resera, E. 318, 322
Restakis, J. 60
ReThink Mental Illness 36
Rhondda Cynon Taff People First 215
Rhue, S. 37
Ricciardelli, L. 36
Richards, M. 182
Ridge, M. 265
Roberts, G. 32
Roberts, J. 62, 224
Robertson, A.E. 241
Robinson, A.L. 306
Rocha, A.A.R.M. 49, 51, 55
Rockwood, K. 112
Rodgers-Johnson, P. 81–2
Roos, L.E. 293
Rosenberg, M. S286
Rothblum, E.D. 243
Rowe, J. 245
Royal College of Psychiatrists 216
Rueda, S. 24
Ryan, C. 243
Ryder, A. 261, 270
Ryder, S. 180, 189, 190

Sadouni, M. 263
Safran, J.D. 113
Sainsbury, P. 179
St Mungo's 293, 297
Sallnow, L. 192
Sampson, E.L. 182
Samstag, L.W. 113
Sandberg, L. 244
Sanders, M. 319
Sanders, S. 149
Santos Filho, S.B. 49, 57
Saraceno, B. 88
Sashidharan, S.P. 70, 263
Schaurich, D. 55
Schmidt, D.F. 38
Schope, R.D. 240
Schore, A. 293, 295
Schröder-Butterfill, E. 30, 31
Scottish Government 306

Scottish Parliament 260
Scullion, L. 259
Seabrooke, V. 153
Sembhi, S. 70, 90
Sen, A. 30
Sexton, H.C. 113
Seymour, J. 157, 189, 190
Shah, A.K. 75, 76, 83, 86, 89, 91, 94, 128, 129, 130, 132, 135, 136, 138, 140, 144, 151, 161, 320
Sharpley, M.S. 82
Shelter 263
Shenk, D. 110
Shepherd, G. 266
Shindleman, L.W. 152
Shipherd, J. 241
Shipman, B. 157
Short, S. 179
Siddiqi, N. 81, 103
Simpson, J. 103
Sjostrand, M. 183
Skinner, W. 242
Smart, C. 157
Smiley, E. 212, 214, 216, 217
Smith, D. 186, 261, 266
Smith, T.B. 294, 300
Smyth, C. 148
Snell, J. 211
Sontag, S. 38
South London and Maudsley NHS Foundation Trust 32
South West London and St George's Mental Health NHS Trust 32
Souza, L.A.P. 57
Spencer, S. 260, 266
Spiegelhalter, D. 245, 249
Stanley, N. 144
Steffen Dalgard, O. 159
Stenner, P. 34
Stocks, T. 234, 236, 238
Stolk, Y. 319
Stonewall 234, 235, 236, 239, 240, 241, 242, 246, 247, 248, 249
Storniolo, L.V. 53
Stott, J. 62
Strydom, A. 214
Summerfield, D. 86
Sutton, D. 223
Swartz, L. 91
Sykes, C. 103
Szyf, M. 107

Taggart, L. 213
Talbott, J.A. 182
Tani, Y. 331
Taylor, B. 260

Thomas, M. 177, 187
Thomas, P. 55
Thompson, D. 157, 240
Thompson, K. 132, 318, 322
Thompson, N. 285, 287
Thorpe, L. 216
Tiwari, G. 233
Todres, L. 49, 65
Torrey, E.F. 82
Tovey, P. 154
Trad, A.A.B. 49, 51, 55
Traveller Movement 261
Travers, V. 103
Tregidga, J. 306
Treise, C. 266
Tribe, R. 24, 70, 82, 83, 86, 89, 91, 94, 132,
    153, 154, 262, 316, 318, 319, 322, 331
Truss, K. 87
Tuffrey-Wijne, I. 188
Tunariu, A. 70
Turnbull, A. 210
Turner, S. 214
Turning Point 308

UK Network of Sex Work Projects 249
United Nations 7, 20, 211
University of Glamorgan 215
University of Leeds 161
Ustun, B. 106

Valanis, B.G. 241
Van Cleemput, P. 265
Van der Lee, J. 149
Van Dyck, S. 34
Van Oorschot, W. 26
Van Wagenen, A. 239, 241
Varney, J. 233, 243
Vesnaver, E. 335
VicHealth 302
Villacieros Durbán, M. 52, 53, 58, 65, 66
VoiceAbility 207
Vozarova de Courten, B. 333

Wadoo, O. 151
Wahler, J. 242
Waite, L.J. 74
Walker, A. 155, 156
Walker, C. 155, 156

Walker, E. 177
Wallace, S.P. 239
Wallcraft, J. 165, 166
Walsh, K. 74, 153, 283
Wanless, D. 80
Ward, C. 223
Warfa, N. 81
Warner, M. 244
Warnes, A.M. 188
Warnes, A. 295, 296, 297
Warren, E. 103
Watson, A. 36, 85
Watt, L.M. 77
Weltens, B. 83
Wenger, G.C. 295, 304
Wernick, A. 245
West Sussex Local Involvement Network 270
Whitaker, H.R. 107
Whitbourne, S. 39
White, M. 62
Whittaker, D. 241
Wilkinson, H. 90
Wilkinson, J.A. 38
Wilkinson, R.G. 59
Williams, R. 209
Willis, S. 39
Willis, T.A. 159
Wilson, L. 334
Wilson, M. 158
Windle, K. 295
Winefield, H.R. 62
Windsor, J. 223
Wirral Carers Strategy 148
Wolfson, P. 32
Woolf, L.M. 242
Woolfe, R. 72
World Health Organization 28, 43, 72, 74, 76,
    79, 80, 85, 208, 223
World Psychiatric Association 166
Wortman, C.B. 159

Yeandle, S. 147, 154
Yip, K. 157, 240
YoungMinds 295

Zagier Roberts, V. 295
Zaidi, a. 262